HEALTH RESEARCH IN CYBERSPACE: METHODOLOGICAL, PRACTICAL AND PERSONAL ISSUES

HEALTH RESEARCH IN CYBERSPACE: METHODOLOGICAL, PRACTICAL AND PERSONAL ISSUES

PRANEE LIAMPUTTONG
EDITOR

Nova Science Publishers, Inc.
New York

LIBRARY OF CONGRESS CATALOGING-IN-PUBLICATION DATA
Health research in cyberspace / Pranee Liamputtong (editor).
p. ; cm.
Includes index.
ISBN 1-59454-819-6
1. Internet in medicine. 2. Internet research. 3. Medical care --Research--Methodology. I. Liamputtong, Pranee, 1955- .
[DNLM: 1. Internet. 2. Research--methods. W 20.5 H4337 2006]
R859.7.I58H42 2006
610.285--dc22 2005031859

Published by Nova Science Publishers, Inc. ✢ New York

Dedication

To my daughters
Zoe Sanipreeya Rice and Emma Inturatana Rice

CONTENTS

PREFACE

This book is a product of my effort online. Considering my cyber conversations with Janne, one of the contributors in this volume, below:

From: Pranee Liamputtong
Sent: Tue 11/2/2004 9.18 AM
To: Janne C.Haugnes Bromseth
Subject: RE: Contributing in a book!

Dear Janne,
Re: Health Research in Cyberspace: Methodological, Practical and Personal Issues.

My name is Pranee Liamputtong and I am an Associate Professor at the School of Public Health, La Trobe University in Melbourne, Australia. I came across your work in Researching ICTs in Context. I was interested in your new projects on gender and sexuality (lesbian and bisexual women and women who want to become pregnant). I hope by now you have done the research!

I would like to ask if you could write a chapter on methodological, practical and personal issues in doing this research which sits well with the title of my upcoming book (titled above). The book will be published by Nova Science in New York. I would need a chapter of about 6000 words by 31 January, but this is negotiable.

At this stage, I am inviting colleagues to contribute and will need an abstract very soon.

Would you be kind enough to write a chapter for me? I hope you can contribute in this new and exciting book, however.

Please get back to me and I will supply more information soon.

I look forward to hearing from you soon and hope that we can work together on this project.

Best Regards,
Pranee

From: Janne C.Haugnes Bromseth
Sent: Thu 11/4/2004 8:10 AM
To: Pranee Liamputtong
Subject: Re: Contributing in a book!

Dear Pranee – thank you so much for your request - it is always nice to hear that my work is actually read by someone out there ;)!

Your book sounds very interesting and important, and I would very much like to contribute. I am actually writing the last part of my dissertation these months and my schedule is quite tight to be able to finish by March 1st, so I would like to ask you how much the date could be negotiated..?

It still would be very useful for me to write it too, as my methodology chapter is not written yet. What happened after the article you have read, is that I had to give up using the pregnant women as material as the owner of the site did not want to cooperate. So I ended up with just using the discussion group for lesbian and bisexual women. Methodologically, there are many issues that could be discussed in relation to the process I went through with this group. It took very long to get my final permissions from the list owners, and that process is one part. More interestingly, I think, is the process of finding a participant position within the group as a participant researcher, trying to develop a 'voice' that reaches through in the subcultural context and creates credibility and trust- and the dilemmas of balancing the use of personal information/ being too private.

An additional ethical aspect also turned up during the time I spent in the group because four of the long term participants in the group were revealed to be written by one man, something that created chock and gradually so much distrust in the group that it dissolved at the end of my study. Since this group was based on anonymous self presentations, I had to be very careful of 'proving' my identity afterwards (as the crossdresser even had the same first name as myself).

So there are enough issues to address..! Can I think it through this week and try to come up with an abstract? If you think any of these ideas sounds interesting, comments are very welcome on a possible angle!

Thanks again for your interest - more soon!
All the best,
Janne

From: Pranee Liamputtong
Sent: Wed 11/4/2004 2.00 PM
To: Janne C.Haugnes Bromseth
Subject: RE: Contributing in a book!

Dear Janne,

Thanks heaps for getting back to me. What you said on this email is extremely interesting and important for online researchers to know. I am looking for this sort of thing in this book, as I don't want people to think that doing research online is easy.... Your one would sit neatly with that chapter too.

I don't need to submit my final manuscript to the publisher until the end of June. But I need some time to edit the chapter and it may need some addition etc. So, what about May? Would this help?

What about writing something along what you said on this email using the research on lesbians and bisexual groups as a case study?

Please find enclosed my book proposal that I submitted to Nova. Most people in the proposal have agreed to write for me, except two from whom I have had difficulties getting responses. I think I will have to forget about them in the next few weeks (if I still can't get them to commit).

When I have got all abstracts and biographies in, I will finalise it. The instructions for contributors will tell you what I am looking for in this book.

Thanks again and talk to you more soon too.
Best Regards,
Pranee

From: Janne C.Haugnes Bromseth
Sent: Fri 11/5/2004 4:37 AM
To: Pranee Liamputtong
Subject: RE: Contributing in a book!
Dear Pranee –

Thank you so much for your thorough response. And May is just perfect - couldn't be better! I will look at the attachment and get back to you soon.
Have a great day,
Janne

These conversations occurred spontaneously. They occurred over a few days due to a time lag between Australia and Sweden. This has also been my experience with other contributors in this volume. Most often when I turned on my computer in the morning, people's responses would be there for me to read and then get back to them. This is to reiterate that communication between individuals nowadays is so fast. We can connect with our families, friends and colleagues across the world in a flash of time. Social researchers are also quick with this trend and this is reflected in the work of many contributors in this volume.

Chen and colleagues (2004: 157) contend, online technologies provide "researchers with an array of alternative arenas for data collection". As we shall see in this volume, there are numerous ways for social researchers to undertake their research. In many ways, online research provides researchers with numerous attractive environments that offline research may not be able to do. But we shall see too that online researchers have come to realise that many issues that we have adopted for offline research can be problematic when we attempt to do the same for online research and this includes the methods of data collection and ethics. Online research can also be problematic and there are important issues which researchers need to think through and deal with. I have attempted to cover these issues in the chapters in this volume. Essentially, contributors discuss more or less along the methodological, practical and personal issues in doing their online research. Some chapters may lean towards a more formal type of writing and are more theoretical while others may be more subjective and practical. But this is the intention of this book, as reflected in its title.

REFERENCE

Chen, S-L.,S., Hall, G.J., and Johns, M.D., 2004, 'Research Paparazzi in Cyberspace: The Voices of the Researched', in M.D. Johns, S-L.S. Chen, and G.J. Hall (eds), Online Social Research: Methods, Issues, and Ethics, pp. 157-175. Peter Lang, New York.

ABOUT THE BOOK

This book comprises 19 chapters. In chapter one, I introduce the issue of online research. I contend that as our lives and societies are being transformed by new technology, there are new forms of data for qualitative researchers to collect and new ways for us to obtain and analyse the data. In this chapter, I point to several salient issues concerning doing qualitative health and social science research in cyberspace. I will first look at the definition of online qualitative research and then discuss some positive aspects of going online. This follows with its pitfalls. I then proceed to examine the private and pubic issues of online information, as these have implications for ethics in cyber research. The rest of the chapter discusses ethical issues in conducting cyber research.

In chapter two, I outline some of the methodological perspectives in doing research online. In this chapter, I first discuss some practical ways in conducting research in cyberspace. In particular, I will first examine some important issue in conducting research online. Second, I will suggest some practical ways to access research participants in cyber-research and third how to obtain informed consent is given. I then proceed to provide some discussions on qualitative research methods which are commonly employed in online research as well as some detailed examples from exiting literature.

In chapter 3, Antionette Cotton argues that the research universe has undergone enormous, rapid expansion with the genesis of cyberspace, which has and continues to spawn a plethora of virtual and social worlds, offering healthcare professionals unprecedented opportunities to conduct diverse, innovative modes of online health research. Whilst virtual worlds may operate substantially differently than offline worlds, it is important to note their symbiotic relationships. Further, collision between many of the different worlds involved in cyber health research, (such as offline and online, private and public, global and local, real and virtual, connected and unconnected, researcher and participant), may occur with serious consequences for either or both participants and researchers. Indeed, health research in cyberspace presents unique conceptual, theoretical, professional, ethical and methodological challenges along with opportunities to engage in new and different research settings, ways of collecting, analyzing, interpreting, presenting and disseminating data, and types of participant and researcher subjectivities and relationships.

Internet-based research, however, requires a critical examination beyond its utility as a research tool, and needs to be understood in terms of its socio-historical contexts as well as its agencies and effects. It is not politically neutral, but is structured by and through collective discourses, arguably replicating and perhaps magnifying many of the heterogeneous, hierarchical structures of health research offline in addition to creating new, unique power knowledge structures. Health care professionals researching in cyberspace need to be cognizant that technologies and methodologies are affected by socio-political contexts and institutional interests, and be reflexive about their participation in cyber research and cyber participant and cyber researcher relationships. Antionette's chapter seeks to interrogate the phenomenon of health research in cyberspace, particularly as it relates to the constitution of the discursive and non-discursive worlds of health research in cyberspace, their relation to pertinent symbiotic, merging, complementary and colliding worlds, and draw out implications for healthcare professionals conducting research in cyberspace.

In chapter 4, Radhika Gajjala and Melissa Altman propose a methodology, based in epistemologies of doing, that suggests that the researcher studying the production of race in cyberspace should engage in the production of culture and subjectivity in the specific context while interacting with others doing the same. This enables them to really talk about the meaning-making that goes on there. Thus, "race in cyberspace" can benefit from a much more complex analysis and response than what has been pursued so far by scholars studying race in cyberspace.

Virtual space cannot exist without a perceiver. Likewise, techno-mediated subjectivities cannot be understood unless the observer enters these spaces and tries living in them, working with them, doing things with and in them. Based on such a premise, they develope a methodology called "cyberethnography" and draws on ongoing debates in cultural anthropology, feminist epistemology, postcolonial theory and feminist ethnography and combines them with debates regarding the problematics of studying online spaces. The approach emphasizes the doing of technology, building of cyberspatial environments and sustained interaction and "being" online in order that the researchers may understand the everyday practices associated with the context, as well as begin to engage the specifics of such a an engagement. Living online, thus, emphasizes immersion so that there are relational links between the ethnographer and the subject(s) being studied and so that the ethnographer understands how the spatio-temporal praxis of being in such environments might shape his or her subjectivity. Thus, the researcher not only inhabits such spaces, s/he also learns to code herself into existence within such spaces by building, interacting and collaborating within them. Thus, s/he dialogically produces cyberselves.

The increasing availability and access to various synchronous and asynchronous interactive communication tools online has instigated much discussion and experimentation during this past decade or so regarding the potential for the use of these interactive tools within a variety of work and play activities. Subjectivities produced in the context of virtual/real interaction and within related techno-mediated environments cannot be understood unless the "observer" enters these spaces and tries living in them, working with them, doing things with them. In other words, academic analyses of techno-mediated subjectivities must self-reflectively engage and observe the Self (and the Other within the Self) "inside" technospaces.

Radhika and Melissa suggest that the notion that there is no race or gender in cyberspace has long been contested by critical scholars and inhabitants of online spaces. Although analyses of static texts are proliferating, fewer scholars are actually observing the processes of production of culture within such online spaces. Thus, their chapter focuses on the actual production of cultural experience and materiality of virtuality, as it is experienced by participants in online environments.

Even in these virtual environments, participants do not leave their bodies behind. Hence the virtual/real distinction sets up a false binary that cannot be substantiated when they analyze engagement with online environments. Part of what their analysis does is to try to unravel the dichotomy between the virtual and the real. Physicality of the body is expressed through everyday material practices, even when those practices involve online production of self. The practice of engaging such a technological environment produces the subject/agent. Meaning, therefore, is made through doing—doing among other things in this case, is coding, programming, typing one's self into existence through building objects and interacting socially, textually.

An interesting writing on researcher, women and lesbian is presented in chapter 5 by Janne Bromseth. Her chapter focusses upon the methodological and ethical challenges related to doing ethnographic research in mediated discussion groups. Using a study of lesbian and bisexual women in Scandinavia as a point of departure, this chapter points in particular to the process of finding a position within the group in doing situated participant observation. How is it possible to create credibility and trust in presentations of the project and the self in a text-mediated environment? What is the process of developing a 'voice' that reaches through in a subcultural context based on gender and sexual orientation as participant criteria? What are the dilemmas in trying to balance the use of personal information/being too private when communicating with the group? And what happens with the established trust when the group is suddenly shaking with distrust following the revelation of a multiple-identity cross-dresser..?

In chapter 6, Richard Hessler presents his study which was funded by the Missouri Department of Health and Senior Services, Bureau of Disabilities Prevention and Injury Control. The chapter focuses on a methodological analysis of an innovative study of adolescent risk through the use of e-mail diaries. In this study, teens eighteen years and younger were paid to keep personal diaries on line in the form of daily e-mail sent to the investigator. Richard discusses advantages and disadvantages of this approach, including enhanced rapport and trust, problems with quality control, and ethical issues surrounding threats to confidentiality.

Similarly, Brian Mustanski discusses in great length of methodology of researching sex online in chapter 7. Although his chapter is geared toward positivist approach, it sits neatly within the methodological experience of doing online research. Brian's chapter discusses methodological aspects of using the Internet as to conduct sexuality research. Benefits, such as larger samples, and risks to validity, such as lying and sabotage, are discussed in the context of an Internet-based daily diary study on the association between mood and sexual interest, behavior, and risk-taking. Brian offers some suggestions for how to maximize utility as well as combat potential risks and ethical dilemmas. Special attention is paid to the use of the Internet to collect data from groups that are traditionally underrepresented. The chapter ends with a look to the future of sex research over the Internet, especially experimental and ideographic approaches.

Anthony Lombardo and James Gillett, in chapter 8, contend that the Internet has become a vast, interactive, and even overwhelming source of information for people living with critical illness. Access to this information resource has drastically transformed the health and health care landscape in late industrial societies. But the Internet as an information resource only tells one side of a much more complicated story. People with critical illnesses have also created their own online spaces as a form of communication and self expression. This chapter examines the practical and methodological challenges of conducting research on Internet use regarding critical illness. In the first section, Anthony and James review current methodological approaches in the literature on health, illness and the Internet. They draw on two cases studies about Internet use and HIV/AIDS. The second section draws on two case studies to illustrate the application of qualitative methodologies to the study of HIV/AIDS and the Internet. First is a study of narratives posted to the "ask the expert" section of the "thebody.com", an Internet site devoted to providing online information about HIV/AIDS. The second case study examines Internet sites created by and for people living with HIV/AIDS. A critical appraisal of methodological approaches to the study of Internet use is discussed in the third section. They explore the strengths and weaknesses of taking the methodological approach used in the case studies regarding HIV/AIDS. Their conclusion explores future directions for research on Internet use among people with illnesses.

In chapter 9, Eun-Ok Im and Wonshik Chee look at Email Group Discussion Among Cancer Patients: Feminist Issues. They argue that e-mail group discussion is the oldest and most popular form of interactions on the Internet, yet issues in conducting e-mail group discussion among a specific group of people have been rarely discussed. In this chapter, from a feminist perspective, issues in using e-mail group discussion among cancer patients are explored and discussed by analyzing a study on gender and ethnic differences in pain experience among cancer patients. Eun-Ok and Wonshik discuss issues raised during the research process while considering essential components of research from a feminist perspective. The issues include: a low response rate, white male dominance, confidentiality and privacy issues, security issues, a lack of guidelines for human subject protection, relevance issues, and difficulties in using general topics. Based on the discussion, ethnic and gender specific approach, motivation strategies, consciousness raising about confidentiality and privacy in electronic communication, identification of participants' own needs, and consideration on timing issues are proposed for future studies.

In chapter 10, Bibi Holge-Hazelton, in a study of young people with diabetes, shows how the Internet became an ethnographic field comparable to other social fields. Despite the absence of concrete physical bodies in cyberspace, Bibi shows how conducting research via the Internet can establish rewarding research relationships founded in a meaningful context for young people and where issues of lived life with chronic illnesses have fruitful conditions to unfold.

Sex in cyberspace and personal experiences in doing this type of research is discussed in chapter 11 by Danielle Couch and Pranee Liamputtong. In this chapter, they discuss in details about the experience of doing this research. First, Danielle talks about her own online dating which has prompted her to carry out a minor research for her postgraduate study with Pranee. Some practical and problematic aspects that they encounter in their research are given in great details. These include recruiting potential research participants, using chat interviewing as a research tool, emoticons and acronyms used in this kind of research, the ways researchers can introduce other participants into the research cycle and so on. Danielle and Pranee cautiously conclude their chapter that chat interviews provide data that is very different to what an interviewer might gather in a face-to-face interviews, but if chat is a common method of communication to the context being researched then it can offer a useful method for exploring how people participate in that context.

Monika Merkes, in chapter 12, suggests that with a growing proportion of older people in the Australian population and increased longevity, paid work after the age of 65 years may become an option or a necessity in the future. However, there is scant research on issues of future generations' work-retirement decision and its policy implications, including implications for unpaid work such as volunteering and caring. Most research to date has focused on early retirement, on men, and on the economic implications of an ageing population. In this chapter, Monika reports on a research study with a focus on Australian women of the baby boom generation, their working futures, and the work-retirement decision. The study included computer-mediated communication and futures studies, involving an Internet website with four future scenarios for the year 2020 (Oztopia, Bladerunner, the Island Nation, Australia on a Bad Day), a set of questions, and an online discussion board. The research participants included people with a personal and/or research interest in the topic. The women and men who participated in this study valued aspects of the Oztopia and Island Nation scenarios such as spirituality, equality, strong social and environmental values, an emphasis on sustainability, and a valued role for Indigenous people. The study identified a range of broad and specific strategies that governments should embrace in their planning for an ageing population to create a future where older women - and men - have work and retirement choices and a valued role in a diverse and inclusive community. To achieve the research participants' preferred future, change has to occur in the following areas: the work-life balance, the health, education and retirement income systems, housing arrangements, support for people with caring responsibilities, attitudes towards the environment, and the reflection of Australia's diverse community across all spheres of life.

In chapter 13, Monique Solomon argues that talking about illness in our society today has reached epidemic proportions. Television, radio, newspapers, magazines, and the Internet keep our thoughts occupied with stories of illness while offering the latest health and wellness information. These stories of illness carry powerful messages about how a person *does* illness and what meanings society, in general, attributes to the idea of illness. Embedded in the personal stories that we tell about illness are larger cultural ways of talking about illness and numerous narrative resources that are drawn upon to story identity. Monique's chapter explores the way members of an online support group for chronic illness (Multiple Sclerosis) draw on available social and cultural narrative resources to communicate about their illness experiences with one another and accomplish their identities in an online context. Her chapter considers narrative resources that arise in an online group message board (such as medical talk, social meanings, personal expressions and local group narratives of storying the experience of MS) and how these narrative resources are practiced in everyday talk to accomplish identity.

Michael Hardey, in chapter 14, explores the way the Internet has opened up new spaces for people to write about their health, illness and other experiences. Web pages and blogs have proliferated as we grasp the opportunity to make connections with others and contribute to what he argues is the new genre of 'digital life-stories'. This new genre has long established roots in auto/biographical writing that in the past has reflected economic inequalities that include access to literacy, the printing press and distribution systems. Most people were, therefore, dependent on oral traditions to tell stories of their lives while others kept their accounts confined to their dairies. The Internet has changed this. As researchers, Michael argues, we have a unique opportunity to gain insights into the experience of health and illness through digital life-stories. In the course of the chapter, Michael highlights the important topic of ethics and explores how we might analyze, understand and make use of this new genre in our research.

Stephen Bradley and Bernie Carter, in chapter 15, provide an account of a research project, conducted from the UK, which sought to address the paucity of empirical research that investigates young peoples' perspectives on child and adolescent mental health (CAMH) issues and experiences. Stephen and Bernie tell the story of their qualitative inquiry project because, in seeking to access young people's accounts of mental health experiences, they investigate the Internet as a promising source of appropriate material. This led them to focus particularly on exploring the potential of Internet newsgroups as a rich resource for healthcare researchers of, largely untapped, data. They share lessons from the project so as to indicate some of the issues that researchers need to consider, the sources they found helpful in addressing these issues and some of the solutions that they arrive at. Stephen and Bernie concentrate particularly on conceptual and methodological issues, but also include some of the outcomes of the project as indication of the potential of such research. Their hope is that their chapter might encourage others to consider investigating Internet newsgroup materials in their own healthcare research.

The emphasis of chapter 16 by Yeslam Al-Saggaf and Radwan Kharabsheh is on the philosophical underpinnings of a study that took place in 2005 and on the ways in which silent observation and thematic content analysis were used in their study. The purpose of their study was to understand how healthcare-related web forums are being used by people in Saudi Arabia. After a brief discussion of the philosophical aspects of the study, Yeslam and Radwan discuss the study design highlighting the rationale for using the above mentioned techniques. They go on to discuss, in detail, the procedures carried out using these techniques in the collection and analysis of their data, including the selection and descriptions of the settings and the procedures followed in the development of categories and the coding of topics. They also provide a sample of the findings relating to the main themes that characterized healthcare-related web forums in Saudi Arabia. Yeslam and Radwan conclude their chapter by presenting some concluding remarks regarding the value of the method used for researching online forums.

Systemic lupus erythematosus is a chronic autoimmune illness that usually affects women during their childbearing years. In chapter 17, Cindy Mendelson argues that women with lupus must learn to live with a variety of unpredictable symptoms, making a consistent source of support and information important for day-to-day illness management. For many women, the Internet fills this need. The purpose of Cindy's chapter is to discuss Internet listservs as sources of support for women with lupus and as potential sites from which participants with chronic illness can be recruited for participation in qualitative research. In the course of this discussion, Cindy presents some of the ethical and methodological challenges facing researchers pursuing this type of research. Throughout this chapter, Cindy refers to her experiences in conducting an ethnographic study of women with lupus that included an Internet component.

Barbara Thomas, in chapter 18, argues that for a person seeking access to information and support about breast cancer, the Internet may be just the spacecraft needed to guide them through the galaxy of resources. As the fastest growing health information source, the Internet has become an important tool for patients, their families, health care providers and researchers. Since breast cancer web sites are among those most frequently visited, in this article, Barbara examines a variety of applications of this evolving medium, using breast cancer as the example. She outlines a guide to evaluating health information on the Internet. She also reviews studies that address women's preferences about receiving online breast cancer information, that identify where women find medical information about their illness and tracks changes over and compares the needs of breast cancer patients with those of prostate cancer patients. Evaluations of community-based cancer support groups, including both face-to-face groups and Internet groups are also examined. Indications are that such interventions will have more impact on psychosocial functioning and /or health-related quality of life than on survival. Although art and aesthetics have not been the traditional mode of providing health information, they provide an alternative view among the galaxy of breast cancer resources. They have been effectively used to give vision and voice to women experiencing breast cancer. As a form of expression and communication, they can effectively convey health messages and potentially influence health practices through the medium of the Internet. Barbara presents some issues to consider in evaluating the aesthetic quality of web sites on the Internet and discusses a specialized application of the Internet, the monitoring of the quality of cancer care in a region in this chapter. The Internet allows for public accountability so that progress being made in cancer care can be demonstrated and the areas needing improvement can be identified. She addresses a number of innovative research and educational uses along with some practical issues, difficulties and personal experiences in using the internet as a research tool. While the plethora of breast cancer websites may be overwhelming, this chapter provides some guidance for the "hitchhiker" navigating the multifaceted resource of the Internet.

Lastly, I attempt to close the book by pointing out to some of the salient issues we need to think in doing our cyber research in the future. I argue that technology will move very fast and we, as qualitative researchers, will move along with this rapid development. The rapid advance of technology has great ramifications for us as cyber qualitative researchers. But whatever happens in the future, we should not lose sight of the interpretive and reflexive nature of qualitative research.

Like any book, it will never be published without the assistance of "Others". I wish to thank Nova Science for taking up this book. I am grateful to all contributors; many have become my good friends and a community of support from a distance. Without you, I would not have been able to bring this book to life. I thank Rosemary Oakes for editing my chapters and my children Zoe Sanipreeya Rice and Emma Inturatana Rice, who always have to put up with my busy working life, to which they see as endless.

Pranee Liamputtong
Melbourne, June 2005

In: Health Research in Cyberspace
Editor: Pranee Liamputtong, pp. 1-24
ISBN 1-59454-819-6

Chapter 1

QUALITATIVE CYBER RESEARCH: AN INTRODUCTION

Pranee Liamputtong

The growth of the Internet is one of the greatest cultural phenomena of our time, impacting almost all areas of life".

(Wittel, 2000: 1)

There were twenty people sitting in the hot-tup when I arrived late on a Saturday night. One man had spent the day surfing waves in South Africa while another had surfed the library at the University of Nebraska. Without leaving their favourite chair at home, people can be transported across cyberspace by modems and phone lines so that they may visit an art exhibit in Moscow, go on a tour of the White House, or chat with a friend in Ireland. In cyberspace, people are falling in love with others that they have never seen in person or touched with their own hands. Our traditional ideas of distance, friendship, love, and sex (amongst other things) are being challenged by what people are doing in cyberspace.

(Hamman, 1996: 1)

INTRODUCTION

We now ever before in human existence not only are able to reach out to other human beings but also to obtain knowledge rapidly, as new global technology such as the use of computer and the Internet has intruded into our lives more and more (Brodie et al., 2000; Cotton, 2003; Broad and Joos, 2004; Plant, 2004; Cotton and Gupta, 2004; Herring, 2004; Pitts, 2004; Ziebland, 2004; Ziebland and Chapple, 2004). As our lives and societies are being transformed by new technology, there are new forms of data for qualitative researchers to collect and new ways for us to obtain and analyse the data (Jones, 1999; Cotton, 2001; Gibbs et al., 2002; Mann and Stewart, 2002; Johns et al., 2004; Markham, 2004, 2005). I argue that, as researchers, we need to engage in what Murray (1995: 11) refers to as "the fourth revolution" in "the production of knowledge", which is "vital to our understanding of how language, society and technology intersect". Qualitative researchers cannot ignore considering the electronic communication as a research resource and tool (Strickland et al., 2003; Broad and Joos, 2004; Markham, 2004, 2005). As Markham (2005: 794) succinctly puts, "we are saturated in technologies". And "Internet technologies have the potential to shift the ways in which qualititative researchers collect, make sense of, and represent data". This is particularly so for social scientists who, as O'Dochartaigh (2002: 7) argues, are "concerned with understanding different aspects of collective human behaviours".

In this chapter, I shall point to several salient issues concerning doing qualitative health and social science research in cyberspace. I will first look at the definition of online qualitative research and then discuss some positive aspects of going online. This follows with its pitfalls. I then proceed to examine the private and pubic issues of online information, as these have implications for ethics in cyber research. The rest of the chapter discusses ethical issues in conducting cyber research. It is noted that I use the words online research and cyber research interchangeably when I refer to what I am about to discuss in the sections that follow in this chapter.

WHAT IS CYBER RESEARCH AND WHY SHOULD WE GO FOR IT?

Cyber qualitative research, according to Denzin (2004: 4) is:

> An interdisciplinary, transdisciplinary, and sometimes counterdisciplinary field. It cross-cuts the humanities, the social sciences, and the physical sciences. Online qualitative research is many things at the same time. It is multiparadigmatic in focus. Its practitioners are sensitive to the value of the multimethod approach. They are committed to the naturalistic perspective and to the interpretive understanding of human experience. At the same time, the field is inherently political and shaped by multiple ethical and political positions.

Denzin (2004: 5) contends that online qualitative has its own tensions and contradictions both in terms of the methods and interpretations of the findings. Nevertheless, cyber researchers have the tendency to commit themselves to "modern postmodern, postexperimental sensibilities and the approaches to social research that these sensibilities imply". These are reflected in the writing of many contributors in this volume.

Why should qualitative researchers adopt cyber research? Lincoln and Denzin (2000) argue that we are living in the postmodern world and dealing with "the seventh moment of inquiry". This seventh moment, Denzin (2004: 1) asserts, "is a period of ferment and explosion". This period "is defined by breaks from the past, a focus on previously silenced voices, a turn to performance texts, and a concern with moral discourse, with critical conversations about democracy, race, gender, class, nation, freedom, and community" (see also Gubrium and Holstein, 2001; Plummer, 2001; Broad and Joos, 2004). These characteristics essentially lend themselves to cyber research, as we will see throughout in this book.

Researching online offers many advantages over more conventional research methods. In this section, I suggest several points.

Its Speed and Immediacy

In practical terms, the salient features of using electronic communication technology as research tools are the speed and immediacy offered. Cyber research offers an almost instantaneous exchange between the researcher and the researched (Smith and Leigh, 1997: Selwyn and Robson, 1998; see also Parker, 1992; Kenney, 2000; Sweet, 2001; Im and Chee, 2003 and this volume). Email, according to Parker (1992: 52), "is fast and easy to use... One of its major advantages is the obliteration of time-zone hassles... Respondents all over the world would be able to answer during their normal working hours". The immediacy of online interaction allows the researchers to prompt their participants quickly if they feel that their entries are not forthcoming or insufficient (Hessler et al., 2003, this volume). In Hessler and colleagues study (2003), they were able to read entries daily and respond to them while they were still new. The researchers were able to keep track of the participants' responses and remind them if they had not sent detailed descriptions of their daily lives. They were successful in getting the participants' daily entries from almost all of them except one case (see also Chapter 6 in this volume). Lindlof (1995: 210) too contends that the researcher's "contextual memory" can be best used due to a quick turn around of data. This means a more comprehensive understanding of the research interaction can be achieved with quick access to the data. Also, as Lindlof (1995) points out, with the delays of the transcripts researchers may change their perceptions of who said what and the context in which something was discussed.

Practical and Cost Effective Way

Online communication is a practical and cost-effective way of undertaking research, and it can reach a large number of people from different geographical and socio-cultural boundaries (Parker, 1992; Bennett, 1998; Hahn, 1998; Selwyn and Robson, 1998; Dunne, 1999; Punathambekar and Fraley, 2000; Thomas et al., 2000; Sweet, 2001; Hessler et al., 2003; Strickland et al., 2003; Molone et al., 2003). As Mann and Stewart (2002: 607) contend, the most powerful advantages of cyber research is its lower cost. For researchers who can access the Internet within their institutions, the cost is minimal, as illustrated in Thomas and colleagues' study (2002) on breast health education and screening. Hessler and colleagues (2003) adopted email as a research tool for their cyber research on risky behaviours with young people precisely due to their limited research budget. Selwyn and Robson (1998: 3) contend that "interviewing by electronic mail is not constrained by geographical location or time-zone; the need for proximity between the interviewer and interviewee is no longer an issue". Mann and Stewart (2000: 80) too argue that "the global range of the Internet opens up the possibilities of studying projects which might not have seemed impracticable before". Dunne (1999), for example, was able to conduct in-depth interviews with gay fathers from different international boundaries including the UK, New Zealand, Canada and the USA. Stewart et al. (1998) too undertook their virtual focus group with young women from Fiji, China, Malaysia and Australia. And Bennett (1998) managed to talk online with men from the United States, the United Kingdom and Australia.

Producing Instantaneous Text File

The production of a text file is instantaneous in cyber research (Selwyn and Robson, 1998; Chen and Hinton, 1999; Brown, 2002; Hessler et al., 2003; Im and Chee, 2003; Strickland et al., 200; Liehr et al., 2004; see also Couch and Liamputtong in this volume). There is no need to set aside a budget for tape recorders, transcribing machines or transcription costs. The immediate production of a text file also eliminates delays caused by transcription (Mann and Stewart, 2000; Sweet, 2001; Strickland et al., 2003). In cyber research, researchers work with digital data. The data can be saved, and stored on computer diskettes or compact discs. Cyber research also benefits data analysis process as the data can be moved directly into qualitative analysis software packages (Creswell, 1998; Fielding and Lee, 1998; Selwyn and Robson, 1998; Ezzy, 2002; Moloney et al., 2003). Selwyn and Robson (1998: 4) state that "as well as saving the researcher time and money this also eliminates any errors introduced through incorrect transcription. With email interviewing the data that is eventually analysed is exactly what the interviewee wrote". According to Hessler et al. (2003), email works well to transfer large text files quickly and accurately to other researchers on the research team. Stewart, in her role as a facilitator in virtual focus group research on women's perceptions of tobacco use (1998), transferred data to other researchers in Beijing and Australia via email. This is similar to what Liehr and colleagues (2004) did in their studies on the meaning of health for Japanese elders and the experience of take care of patiens with severe acute respiratory syndrome (SAR) among Chinese nurses.

Enhancing Rapport and Interaction

Some researchers suggest that rapport and interaction between the researcher and the researched can be better enhanced through online communication (Parker, 1992; Janney, 1996, Kawaura et al., 1999; Ferri, 2000; O'Connor and Madge, 2001; Mann and Stewart, 2002; Hessler et al., 2003). Selwyn and Robson (1998: 4) also suggest that "the problem of interview effect, whether resulting from visual and non-verbal cues or status differences between interviewee and interviewer" can be reduced in cyber research. Especially, in online focus groups, problems caused by dominant and shy participants can be reduced, or even eliminated. Due to this, as Roberts et al. (1997) suggest, online interviewing potentially reduces some of the interpersonal problems that researchers using conventional interviewing techniques tend to experience.

"Democratisation of Exchange"

Selwyn and Robson (1998: 2) elucidate that cyber research offers a "democratisation of exchange" more than orthodox research methodologies (see also Ferri, 2000). Bosshier (1990: 51), for example, suggests that online communication such as email "provide a context for the kind of non-coercive and anti-hierarchical dialogue that Habermas claimed constitutes an 'ideal speech situation', free of internal or external coercion, and characterised by equality of opportunity and reciprocity in roles assumed by participants". More importantly, as Spender

(1995) argues, when communicating electronically, race, gender, age and sexuality are not necessarily applicable. Grimaldi and Goette (1999) and Seymore (2001) too contend that online communication has benefited individuals with disabilities in the way that other users will not know that the person they are communicating with has a disability. Hence, the marginalities of people with disabilities are eliminated in their interaction with others. The characteristic nature of online communication technologies indeed reduces the traditional biases that occur with face-to-face research methods. Participants can respond when they feel comfortable or decide how they will respond. In short, the primary advantage of online communication, particularly email, is its "friendliness" to the participants (Thach, 1995; Selwyn and Robson, 1998).

Reaching a Range of Participants

Cyber research provides possibilities to reach a wide range of participants, such as mothers at home with small children, shift workers, people with disabilities, older people, and members of socially marginalised groups such as gay and lesbians and ethnic minorities, who may not be easily accessed in face-to-face research methods (Kennedy, 2000; Seymour, 2001; Gajjala, 2002; Madge and O'Connor, 2003; Mann and Stewart, 2002; Flicker et al., 2004; Broad and Joos, 2004; Davis et al., 2004; Nip, 2004; Seymour and Lupton, 2004). These people can connect with others from their familiar and physically safe environments (see Correll, 1995; Spender, 1995; Hoffman and Novak, 1998; Edworthy, 1999; Brodie et al., 2000; Fridman, 2000; Greenberg, 2000; Sweet, 2001; Adler et al., 2002; Thomas et al., 2002; Merkes, 2003; Im and Chee, 2003; Pandey et al., 2003). Finn (1999) suggests that online communication offers the option for participating in research for those who are unable to leave the home for health reasons. People with disabilities can have access to email and necessary online information and respond without having to leave home or be mobile (Grimaldi and Goettte, 1999; Seymour, 2001; Seymour and Lupton, 2004). Cyber research also offers researchers a possible means of connecting with people located within restricted access like hospitals, government offices, the military, schools, cult and religious groups, bikers, surfers, punks and so on.

Possibilities of Researching Sensitive or Dangerous Areas

Cyber research, Mann and Stewart (2002: 606) assert, provides the possibilities of carrying out research within politically sensitive or dangerous areas. Both the researchers and the researched are protected due to the anonymity and physical distance (see Coomber, 1997, Fleitas, 1998; and Chapters 5, 6, 7, 8, 9, 10, 11, 13, and 16 in this volume for example). Some highly sensitive and vulnerable participants, such as political and religious dissidents or human rights activist, will be more likely to participate in cyber research without excessive risk. Censored, politically or militarily sensitive data can be accessed without needing to be physically in the field. People living or working in war zones, or sites of corruption or criminal activity, or places where diseases abound can be reached without needing to grapple with the danger involved in actually visiting the area. Online communication also allows researchers to distance themselves physically from ideological camps. This helps to reduce the likelihood of suspicion that might alienate some participants. Also communication with both police and criminals can be conducted without being seen or without leaving themselves open to charges of spying.

Preserving the Anonymity of the Participants

Some researchers argue that conducting their research online has helped them to preserve the anonymity of the participants (Fleitas, 1998; Morahan-Martin, 2000; Punathambekar and Frawley, 2000; Sweet, 2001; Madge and O'Connor, 2002). The anonymity of the technology indeed has assisted some researchers to access members of socially marginalised communities including gay fathers (Dunne, 1999), men who avoided discussing emotions if interviewed face-to-face (Bennett, 1998), young people engaging in risky behaviours such as sex, drinking, drugs, and fast driving (Hessler et al., 2003; Flicker et al., 2004; see also Hessler in this volume), and women (Morahan-Martin, 2000). Indeed, Morahan-Martin (2000: 683) asserts that:

> On-line anonymity and lack of face-to-face interaction frees individuals of social and physical constraints, and has allowed women to express parts of themselves that they might not have otherwise in a safe environment, enabling them to explore new identities, heal inner wounds and express sexuality.

Stones and Perry (1998) have utilised the Internet to access and interview vulnerable individuals with specific disorders including panic attacks. The email journal approach which was used in the work of Hessler and colleagues with young people (2003), was sufficiently anonymous to allow these young people to share sensitive thoughts and activities with adult researchers. Hessler et al. (2003) contend that this situation would have been difficult to achieve with orthodox face-to-face research methods. Punathambekar and Frawley (2000) undertake an online synchronous focus group and show that their participants openly expressed their opinion much more than in a face-to-face situation. In particular, opinions considered not politically correct would not be easily said in a face-to-face method were in fact expressed. Fleitas (1998), Punathambekar and Frawley (2000), and Flicker et al. (2004) too suggest that the anonymous nature of online interaction helps to elicit viewpoints on sensitive topics and issues that conventional focus groups may have difficulty obtaining. Thomas et al. (2002) used the Internet to examine women's knowledge and perceptions about breast health education and screening and the support that influence their participation in these practices. Thomas et al. (2002) argue that due to the anonymity of their participation, women across North America took part in this sensitive research. Similarly, as Illingworth (2001: par. 7.1) points out in her research on women's perceptions of assisted reproductive technologies, "because of the sensitive nature of this research, a number of respondents emphasized their reluctance to participate had this research been conducted in a more conventional, face-to-face setting". Indeed, Illingworth argues, "online participation offered personal anonymity in a very emotive field".

Problems with Going Online

What I have thus far discussed, is not to say that conducting research online has no drawbacks. As any other research methods, researching online is problematic in some ways.

Absence of Face-To-Face Interaction

The absence of face-to-face interaction, according to Berg (2004: 60) "could be considered as a loss of potential data (in the various forms of visual cues and symbolic information contained in grimaces, winces, body movements)" commonly used in qualitative approach. Hessler and colleagues (2003: 123) state that online data collection "precluded observation of the research settling in conducting fieldwork". Hessler et al. (2003: 123) regrettably admit in their online study that "we probably would have handled the problems we had with educators in the field better if we had spent some time on site and therefore had a better sense of the optimal entry strategies to use". Holge-Hazelton (2002: 9) too concedes in her study with young people living with diabetes that "I could not see what went on in the room where the individual young person sat and wrote to me, or what went on in their minds after they sent me their e-mails". However, she also acknowledges that "I do not consider this any different than my lack of knowledge of what happens when I leave the house of one of my other informants". See also Couch and Liamputtong in this volume.

Lack of Verbal Interaction

Lack of verbal interaction in cyber research is another salient limitation of its use as a research tool (Selwyn and Robson, 1998; DeLorme et al., 2001; Strickland et al., 2003). This lack of non-verbal communication can be problematic for both the researcher and the researched. Selwyn and Robson (1998: 4) contend that much of tacit information that could be observed in a face-to-face research is lost. Although cyber research is seen to gain in accuracy, the valuable non-verbal data are lost. But Selwyn and Robson (1998: 4) argue that "the fact remains that e-mail interaction is not comparable to verbal interaction in many ways. Online discussion requires different skills from both the interviewer and the subject… Indeed, the language of all computer-mediated communication tends toward a simplified register due to the space and time constraints of the medium, in effect making e-mail messages a hybrid of oral and written language" (see also Murray, 1995). Although verbal interaction is now possible, this will require suitable computer software and equipment. Hence, the cost of data collection will increase (Strickland et al., 2003).

Access to the Internet and Social Structures

Access to the Internet is bounded by a number of social structures and personal circumstances (see Warf, 2001; Davis, 2002; Skinner et al., 2003). It has been suggested that access to the use of the Internet can be limited for economic reasons (Loader, 1998; White et al., 2001; Thomas et al., 2002). But, as Riva (2001), Mann and Stewart (2000) and Kerka (1995) suggest, individuals' social locations including gender, culture, ethnicity and language may limit access for many others. Selwyn and Robson (1998:.2) too contend that "the fundamental failing of using e-mail is the extremely self-selective, limited and therefore biased population that it covers. E-mail is limited to those individuals with access to a computer". Riva (2001) suggests that people who tend to participate in cyber research are self-selected. They are usually those belonging to the high end of the socio-economic and educational status (Han and Belcher, 2001; Hewson, 2003). Graham and Marvin (1996), Kendall (1999), ACNielsen (2000) and Hewson (2003) too note that people who have access to a computer either at home or at work have a higher household income and come from a higher socio-economic background. Men, historically, dominate the use of electronic communication although there have been more women making use of the technology (Herring, 1994, 1996; Tannen, 1994; Cherny and Weise, 1996; Savicki et al., 1996; Kendall, 1999, 2000; Merkes, 2003; Ferganchick-Neufang, 2004). Additionally, Lockhard (1996) notes that the virtual world is a "Euro-American whiteness" phenomenon. As Thomas et al. (2002) point out in their study, people from outside North America had low responses. This may be due in part because they have less access to computers (see also Kenway, 1996; Kendall, 2000; Han and Belcher, 2001; Cotton, 2003; Im and Chee, 2003; Orbuch and Fine, 2003). Lastly, young people are at present the consumers of the Internet (Kendall, 1999), although the numbers of older generations making use of the technology are increasing. These current patterns have great ramifications for recruiting research participants. As a result, as Schmidt (1997) suggests, online methodologies can only be considered for researches which target specific, and narrowly defined, populations with easy access to the online world.

Breaching of Ethical Issues

Researchers have raised the ethical issue regarding researching online like the Internet, as it is perceived that ethical issues are easily breached on the Web (Jones, 1994; Murray, 1995; Shields, 1996; Thomas, 1996; Coomber, 1997; Smith and Leigh, 1997; Thimbleby, 1998; Thomas et al., 1998; Stanton and Rogelberg, 2001; Mann and Stewart, 2002; Holge-Hazelton, 2002; Thomas et al., 2002; Hessler et al., 2003; Im and Chee, 2003). In their study with young people, Hessler et al. (2003: 123) tell us that, "a significant negative aspect of our e-mail methodology stemmed from the inherent security problems all e-mail systems have at present". Despite some safeguards that Hessler and colleagues attempt to do, there is a possibility to match the email entries with the actual participants. Hessler et al. (2003: 123) contend, "several respondents had put themselves on the line, so to speak, and if their teachers, parents, or friends found out what they had written, it might have been very difficult for all concerned". But Thomas (1999) argues that, egregious violations of ethics in online communication are low. Berg (2004: 59) comments that despite problems have been identified and a number of solutions have been found, the potential use and misuse of online communication continues to be a concern among researchers (see Schneier, 2000; Frankel and Siang, 2004; Thomas, 2004). Attempts to find means to maintain ethical integrity in research when using online communication as a research tool are continued (Binik et al.,

1999; DeLorme et al., 2001; Cotton, 2003; Im and Chee, this volume; Jones, 2004; Thomas, 2004).

SUSTAINING ONLINE INTERACTION

In most cases, it may be difficult to sustain online interaction over time. This may be due to "Internet churn (loss of access to the technology) or the participants disappear into cyberspace" (Mann and Stewart 2000: 607). Bennett (1998) contends that the participants might disengage because of pressures of time and other commitments. Selwyn and Robson (1998: 3) too suggest that as online communication becomes more common, people will be dealt with "information overload". Research via email, for example, may be seen as "junk mail". People will be bombarded with email to the extent that attending to every mail message will be burdensome (Berge and Collins, 1995; Moloney et al., 2003). Attempts by researchers to obtain data online, such as via email, may be simply ignored or, worse, the message deleted before being read (Selwyn and Robson, 1998). Robinson (2001: 713) also asserts that "Internet data can be ephemeral". A site may be closed down or merged with others. Researchers may find that a site that they have just visited several days before are gone when they re-visit it. This type of problem may have to be considered when attempting to examine narratives on the Internet.

DATA IN CYBERSPACE: PRIVATE OR PUBLIC ISSUE?

Are postings on an internet community "private" or "public" data? This has certainly raised a heated debate among researchers and it has implications for research ethics (Bromseth, 2002; Barnes, 2004; see also Chapters 2 and 5 in this volume). Some will argue that discussions or messages posted on the Internet are public document, but others may disagree (Pitts, 2004). Eysenbach and Till (2001: 1104) contend that what people post on the Internet may resemble letters or stories published in newspapers, but "there are important psychological differences and people participating in an online discussion group cannot always be assumed to be 'seeking public visibility'". As Barnes (2004: 203) tells us, people who post their stories online would see that their stories are private and these people are "often outraged by the ideas of researchers using their messages in studies". Thomas (2004: 208) too argues that support groups in particular see their exchanged messages among group members private as the function of support groups is to "enable people to share their intimate feelings". People may confess some intimate issues or secrecy online. Hence, their secret stories should not be used for research or other purposes.

How do we know then that the groups and their discussions are intended to be private of pubic? According to Barnes (2004: 208), the welcoming introductory statements can indicate the private or public nature of a group. Eysenbach and Till (2001: 1104) suggest the following concerns as important.

- The group is likely to regard itself as private if a subscription or registrations is required to gain access to the discussion group.
- If the numbers of users of the group are small (say around 10), then it is more likely that the group will regard itself as private than a mailing list of say 1000 subscribers.
- If there are norms, codes, target audiences or aims which are laid down in the "Frequent Asked Questions" of the group, then it is likely to be a private group.

Bromseth (2002: 39, original emphasis) takes a similar view to Eysenbach and Till (2001) when she contends that when people sign up for a membership on the Internet community, this "signals a sense of privacy to the outside world, drawing a boundary around the group of people that is considered belonging to the group as separate from the great mass of net-users". In this sense, if researchers wish to undertake their research within the private discussion groups, particularly in highly sensitive areas such as disability, victim of violence or abuse, drug uses and crime, extreme care must be ensured. As Bromseth (2002: 40) puts, researchers must "'handle with care', no matter how accessible the information is" to them. Informed consent from individual member of the group is also needed.

There have been some transgressions of this issue in cyber research (see for example, King, 1996; Reid, 1996). In political journalism, private exchanged between support group members were published in newspapers. A member of an online support group told others that he/she had committed a murder via an email exchange and this was leaked to the press. It was later published in The New York Times (Harmon, 1998). In social science research, a similar transgression has also occurred. In the books written by Rheingold (1993), Hertz (1995), and Seabrook (1997), names of the participants and their direct quotations from email messages were cited and these authors did not show any concern about people they write about. Hafner (1997) also portrayed an individual called Tom Mandel who was addicted to the Internet negatively. Finn and Lavitt (1994) examined messages posted on the support group for survivors of sexual abuse bulletin board, without asking permission from the group or individuals. They also published the group's original names, dates and times of the messages sent. The main reason for doing so was that messages posted on a BBS (bulletin board system) by the members were perceived as public information. King (1996) argues that it was unnecessary to name the group in this instance. Instead, it placed strain to the group members as they can be identified and it violated the function of the group; that is to provide a supportive environment to group members. See also a good example of this line of argument in Reid (1996).

Ethical Concerns of Reseaching Online

Mann and Stewart (2000: 39) contend, "the online world is seen as a place for the transgression of cultural rules and the breaking of taboos which raises issues of self-regulation and responsibility for the qualitative researcher" (see also Murray, 1995; Allen, 1996; Reid, 1996; Shields, 1996; Thomas et al., 1998; Hsiung, 2000; DeLorme et al., 2001; Eysenbach and Till, 2001; Sixsmith and Murray, 2001; Walther, 2001; Cotton, 2003; Im and Chee, 2003; Flicker et al., 2004; Frankel and Siang, 2004; Jones, 2004; Thomas, 2004; Markham, 2005). Numerous ethical issues have been raised and these include the breaches of confidentiality due to the nature of online communications such as lurking on the Internet, the loss of unauthorised access, and the right to access personal data among the participants (see Mann and Stewart, 2000; Sixsmith and Murray, 2001; Barnes, 2004; Jones, 2004; Pitts, 2004; Thomas, 2004). For example, if people discuss criminal activity online, the line may be tapped by law keepers, and the researchers might be under pressure or legally forced to disclose the identities of their participants (see Frankfort-Nachmias and Nachmias, 1992; Coomber, 1997; Hudson, 2004).

Additionally, "netiquette" - appropriate etiquette on the Internet (Babbie, 1996; Danielson, 1996; Scheuermann and Taylor, 1997; Sharf, 1999; Mann and Stewart, 2000; Hall et al., 2004) is another ethical concern for online communication and cyber research. Sharf (1999: 244-245) refers to netiquette as "rules of thumb, to encourage politeness, civility, and enhanced understanding among participants". Babbie (1996: 68) contends that netiquette will become "a template for relationships on the net". Mann and Stewart (2000: 48) argue that "appropriate netiquette depends upon context of use". This is clearly the case for researching online. This is what Danielson (1996: 70) refers to as "artificial morality". Danielson argues that "it is not the technological change but the social changes it enables". Hence, according to Danielson (1996), "an ethical breach is seen as a socially irresponsible use of the common resources available on the Internet" (Sharf 1999: 245). Nevertheless, Hall et al. (2004: 243-244) argue that "consideration of a clear 'netiquette' that may help clarify proper research conduct on the Net seems both appropriate and necessary".

In this section, I shall focus my discussions on the following two issues which are more relevant to the carrying out of research: confidentiality and risks to participants. See Sharf (1999: 253-255) and Flicker et al. (2004) for their insightful and practical ethical concerns and conduct that researchers should consider in the undertaking of their cyber research.

Confidentiality: How to Ensure This?

Confidentiality is more problematic in cyber research than conventional ones. Data collected online can have multiple risks. Sharf (1999: 246) points out that online communication such as email "is analogous to a letter or phone call, ostensibly private but capable of interception", as email may be copied or forwarded to others without the knowledge of a sender. Living in a postmodern world, there are many vulnerable people, who may be in acute stages of loss and grief, or confronted with sexual dysfunctions, life-threatening illnesses, or addictions, who find interaction through cyberspace is the only or main source of information and social support. Sharf (1999: 246) contends, "in the spirit of therapeutic alliance and human catharsis, they may pour out their very deeply held feelings to one another". What if the "Others" intercept or access this highly confidential information? Would the participants be in a dangerous or embarrassing situation, which is perceived as "harm" in the undertaking of research? Sharf (1999: 257-248) suggests that people, who respond to the researchers' requests to participate in cyber research, have made a conscious choice to do so. They are able to change their identities with user names which will not reveal their true identities or locations. These participants are able to decide how much information they want to share. These participants may not then be in a vulnerable situation as those whose life stories are used for discourse analysis. These people are not able to choose to exercise the same sorts of control as those mentioned above (see King, 1996; Reid, 1996; Sixsmith and Murray, 2001; Bromseth, 2002; Barnes, 2004; Flicker et al., 2004).

Mann and Stewart (2000: 43) argue that despite the fact that researchers may promise confidentiality in the way the data are used, they cannot give a guarantee to their participants that the information will not be accessed by others. Researchers need to be cautious about assuring confidentiality to their participants (Reid, 1996; Im and Chee, 2003 and in this volume). Mann and Stewart (2000: 57) suggest that “the most honest response may be for researchers simply to make clear to potential participants that they are unable to ensure total confidentiality. At the same time, they could emphasise that they would take every precaution within their power to act ethically (that is, ensure confidentiality) in their research undertakings”. Reid (1996: 173) too strongly suggests that, “it is not simply a question of researchers doing their best to respect subjects’ sensibilities and wishes-on the Internet, where perceptions of interpersonal affect and effects may be obscured by the nature of the medium itself, we must be very careful to ensure that our subjects are aware of the potential consequences of agreeing to participate in our studies”.

As in social science qualitative research, a researcher may make use of pseudonyms as a means to preserve the identities of participants in cyber research reports or other publications. In research using email, for example, real names, user names, domain names, signatures can be adjusted to disguise the true identity of the participants (Dibbell, 1998; Reid, 1996; Sharf, 1999; Im and Chee, 2003; Flicker et al., 2004). For example, the real names can be replaced with “nicknames”, or “pseudonyms”. In Stewart et al. study (1998), participant’ names include for example “Red Beijing, Red Australia, Yellow Beijing”. Paccagnella (1997) called his participants names like SweetBabe. In Kendall’s study (1999), she changes “all names in the research including the name of the forum and people’s online pseudonyms”. Turkle (1995: 324) too tells us that when she reports cases of people who have been part of research on the Internet, “I protect confidentiality by disguising identities. This means that among other things, I change MUD names, character names, and city names”. But when she refers to data obtained online from publicly archived materials, “I simply indicate the sources”. Allen (1996: 178) too tells us that in her writing about identity practices in a virtual reality community of MOO (Mud, Object Oriented), she called the four participants by their LambdaMOO names (i.e., their pseudonyms) in the writing. And the participants were never be identified by their “real-life” names (cf. Pitts, 2004; see also Mendelson and Couch and Liamputtong in this volume).

Another way to protect the confidentiality of the participants is not to cite their direct quotes in our publications, even though we have changed their names or remove their personal information (King, 1996; Reid, 1996). Eysenbach and Till (2002: 1105) contend that the identity of the person who provide the quote can be identified by a powerful search engine, such as Google, as this machine can retrieve the original message which includes the email address of the person (see also Pitts, 2004). If this occurs then surely the confidentiality of the participant is breached. Eysenbach and Till (2001) suggest that if researchers need to use direct words of the participants, they should be informed clearly about potential consequences, and explicit consent to use their quotes must be done.

Risk to Participants

Flicker and colleagues (2004) contend that the researchers have a responsibility to protect their research participants from any unintentional risk and harm. When the researcher examines the Internet communities by lurking on the Internet, this can damage the researched communities in some ways (see Reid, 1996). King (1996), for example, documented a quote of a group member who withdrew from a mailing list because he/she realised that his or her community has been 'watched' by a researcher. And this is what he or she remarked:

> When I joined this, I thought it would be a *support* group, not a fishbowl for a bunch of guinea pigs. I certainly don't feel at this point that it is a 'safe' environment, as a support group is supposed to be, and I will not open myself up to be dissected by students of scientists (King, 1996: 122)

The ethical dilemma in this case is that due to the attempt of a researcher to do research on this community, the community lost its member as a result. This may have even further implications for the community if the community is a small group which members really have to rely on the existence of other members.

For researchers who attempt to post a notice of their research and obtain informed consent from their research participants, this may also pose some distress to the participants (see King, 1996 and Reid, 1996 for example). In her attempt to obtain informed consent from a Breast Cancer list, Sharf (1999: 250) tells us that one woman was "hostile" toward her. She assumed that the researcher "had behaved voyeuristically, taking advantages of people in distress". To many members of this list, "the idea of using the conversations as data had not occurred to many members, including this woman". Eysenbach and Till (2001) did a search on the Google to see how people respond to request from researchers, they found negative comments. One interesting comment which serves to illustrate the point I am making here is that:

> The researcher isn't familiar with newsgroup culture – problem akin to those occasionally experienced by anthropologists when they try to interpret the behaviour of cultures they really don't understand. And on the rare occasions when I've seen someone who's part of that culture attempt to study the group he/she is part of, it resulted in a rippling sense of resentment and betrayal among those who find such things underhanded (cited in Eysenbach and Till, 2001: 1104).

In sensitive research that may involve highly personal information, Sharf (1999) suggests, researchers need to be particularly cautious about "public exposure" of their participants. Researchers may not be able to protect participants who stray into dangerous zones in cyberspace. As Coomber (1997) notes, people may think that the Internet is an uncensored, unpoliced environment and they may be more willing to tell other online users about their use of illegal drugs or crimes they have committed (as aforementioned story). In conventional qualitative research, researchers are able to warn the participants, turn off the interviewed tape or decline to transcribe the sensitive parts. But these cannot be done in online interviews. Even if the researcher attempts to delete the message on the screen, a total deletion is not possible. A good example from a highly controversial case was of Monica

Lewinsky's case. Her deleted important email messaged was recovered from her computers both at home and at work (Barnes, 2004).

Hiltz and Turoff (1993) note that people tend to treat online communications in an unguarded way. They compare the attempt as "a conversation on a train". Despite the fact that the electronic medium is inherently impersonal, there has been evidence of intimate exchanges between people who have never met face-to-face, and probably never will. Hiltz and Turoff (1993: 28) point out "revelations about personal inadequacies, deviant preferences, past love affairs, and serious personal problems ... have passed through the [computer conferencing] system as private messages to strangers who were 'met' on the system".

In online focus groups, participants may come across harassment and abuse (Mann and Stewart, 2000; Moloney et al., 2003). The harassment and abuse among research participants may be prevented by making it clear to all participants about netiquette and the need to respect confidentiality in research. The moderator may have influence on this and needs to be able to control the groups. Conducting focus groups through the conferencing site can also prevent outsider's harassment and abuse as only the researched participants can access the conference site. In addition, all participants should be told not to share the information outside the researched groups. This harassment and abuse can also occur within Internet communities. The group members may post messages that attack other individuals or groups, contain sexual overtones, and violate community tenets (Flicker et al., 2004). In this case, as Flicker and colleagues have done, research staff had to monitor the board daily. If there are violations in whatever form, the messages will be edited or deleted and replaced with a new message explaining the change, so that members understood what was happening on their board.

Deception is easily done on online communication. Often the deception emerges from the part of the participants as it is difficult to tell if the participants are telling the truth of who they actually are (Nosek and Banaji, 2002; Flicker et al., 2004; Markham, 2005). How do we know if our participants are actually females representing intimate sexual encounters that we are researching? We cannot be sure about this. More importantly, as Mann and Stewart (2000: 80) suggest, virtual researchers are able to "camouflage aspects of personal identity such as class, age, gender and ethnicity in order to make previously limited or proscribed access possible" (see Schneier, 2000). Bennett (1998: 69) concedes in her study with men that "I cannot give an iron-clad guarantee that these people are really men, even though I have gone to some lengths to make sure this is so". In her study of content analysis of personal web pages on breast cancer, Pitts (2004: 40) tells us too that:

> I can make no claims about the off-line identities of the authors who wrote the web sites, and I do not assume that cybersubjects' online identities are necessarily identical to their off-line identities. Nonetheless, throughout this analysis, I operate under the assumption that the web pages are indeed, as they claim, authored by someone who has breast cancer or knows someone with breast cancer, and that the issues they raise are real to the writers themselves.

The deception will have great impact not only on the researchers, but also among the researched participants themselves. Van Gelder (1991) tells us about the case that the psychiatrist disguised himself as a severely handicapped woman in order to obtain intimate confessional stories from women online. The psychiatrist discovered that women were much more open and intimate with him when they thought that his identity was female and so he invented a female person named Joan. When the women discovered his real identity as an "able-bodied male", they described their experiences as "mind rape, pure and simple - a cheat and a fraud" (Mann and Stewart, 2000: 55). This is what Janne Bromseth (Chapter 5 in this volume) has also encountered in her research with lesbian and bisexual women.

What can researchers do then to prevent such things as I have just pointed out? Mann and Stewart (2000: 55) suggest that it is the ethical responsibility of researchers to ensure that the potential participants are aware of the public nature of online communications prior to giving out consent form and during the study. They contend, "participants must be allowed to protect themselves, by considering carefully whether they are prepared for each message to be made public before they send it" (p. 55). In Im and Chee's study (2003, and in this volume) with cancer patients, some participants used their real names when sending their messages. Although this was an intention of the participants, Im and Chee (2003: 294) suggest that researchers may need to change "the security measures". Therefore, rather than the participants' anonymity is ensured, confidentiality and privacy of the discussion need to be guarded against.

Here, perhaps I can refer to King's excellent suggestions of some strategies to ensure that no harm will occur to group members in our examination of any Internet group. King (1996: 127) strongly advocates that we should remove: all references to the name and to the type of the group such as email or BBS and so on; all headers and signatures of the members; and all references to any member's name or pseudoname. He also suggests that researchers should not make reference to the type or location of forum studied.

Although researchers may make particular attempts to ensure that their participants will receive no harm, in reality, there may still be some risk to our participants, whatever risk that may be. As Reid (1996: 173) contends:

> In all social research involving human subjects there is the potential for harm to come to those subjects. Guidelines for ethical behaviour can never eliminate that potential; all they can do is attempt to minimize the risk. It would be disingenuous of researchers to pretend that such risk was nonexistent. We must face our moral and ethical dilemmas rather than side-stepping them… Try as we might to act with consideration and responsibility, we can never eliminate all risk.

Conclusion

In this chapter, I have provided readers with some salient issues in doing research online. As all research methods, cyber research offers some valuable and practical means that we may not be able to do so with our conventional offline research. But cyber research also has its pitfalls. Ethical issues are more problematic in cyber research; more so than that of offline ones. Because it is easy to reach people across the world or to lurk on what people have written in cyberspace does not mean that we can do whatever and however we like to do. There are issues of privacy and risk of the research participants that we, as researchers, need to take into account. The many salient issues I have raised in this chapter, I hope, will prompt readers to be more cautious about doing research in cyberspace.

ACKNOWLEDGEMENT

This chapter is based on a chapter in my book, Qualitative Research Methods, 2nd edition, published by Oxford University Press, 2005. Permission is granted by Oxford University Press.

REFERENCES

[1] ACNielsen, 2000, 'ACNielsen Survey Finds Nearly Two Thirds of U.S. Population Age 12 or Older are Online.' *<http://www.acnielsen.com.news.american/us/2000/20000508.html>*

[2] Adler, C.L., and Zarchin, Y.R., 2002, 'The "Virtual Focus Groups": Using the Internet to Reach Pregnant Women on Home Bed Rest', *Journal of Obstetrics, Gynaecologist and Neonatal Nursing*, vol. 31, pp. 418-427.

[3] Allen, C., 1996, 'What's Wrong with the "Golden Rule"? Conundrums of Conducting Ethical Research in Cyberspace', *The Information Society*, vol. 12, pp. 175-187.

[4] Babbie, E. 1996, *The Practice of Social Research*, 6th edition, Wadsworth, Belmont, CA.

[5] Barnes, S.B., 2004, 'Issues of Attribution and Identification in Online Social Research', in M.D. Johns, S-L.S. Chen, and G.J. Hall (eds.), *Online Social Research: Methods, Issues, and Ethics*, pp. 203-222, Peter Lang, New York.

[6] Bennett, C., 1998, Men Online: Discussing Lived Experiences on the Internet, Unpublished honours dissertation, James cook University, Townsville, Queensland, Australia.

[7] Berg, B.L., 2004, *Qualitative Research Methods for the Social Sciences*, Pearson, Boston.

[8] Berg, Z.L. and Collins, M., 1995, 'Computer Mediated Scholarly Discussion Groups', *Computers and Education*, vol. 24, no. 3, pp. 183-189.

[9] Binik, Y.M., Mah, K., and Kiesler, S., 1999, 'Ethical Issues in conducting Sex Research on the Internet', *Journal of Sex Research*, vol. 36, pp. 82-90.

[10] Bosshier, R., 1990, 'Socio-Psychological Factors in Electronic Networking', *International Journal of Lifelong Education*, vol. 9, no. 1, pp. 49-64.

[11] Broad, K.L. and Joos, K.E., 2004, 'Online Inquiry of Public Selves: Methodological Considerations', *Qualitative Inquiry*, vol. 10, no. 6, pp. 923-946.

[12] Brodie, M., Flournoy, R.E., Altman, D.E., Blendon, R.J., Benson, J.M. and Rosenbaum, M.D., 2000, 'Health Information, the Internet, and the Digital Divide', *Health Affairs*, vol. 19, no. 6, pp. 255-265.

[13] Bromseth, J.C.H., 2002, 'Public Places – Public Activities?: Methodological Approaches and Ethical Dilemmas in Research on Computer-Mediated Communication Contexts', in A. Morrison (ed.), *Researching ICTs in Context*, pp. 33-61, InterMedia Report, University of Oslo, Oslo.

[14] Brown, D., 2002, 'Going Digital and Staying Qualitative: Some Alternative Strategies for Digitizing the Qualitative Research Process', *Forum qualitative Social Research* [on-line journal], vol. 3, no. 2. *<http://www.qualitative-research.net/fgs/fqs-eng.html>*

[15] Chen, P. and Hinton, S.M., 1999, 'Realtime Interviewing Using the World Wide Web', *Sociological Research Online* [on-line journal], vol. 4, no. 3. <*http://www.socresonline.org.uk/socresonline/4/3/chen.html*>

[16] Cherny, L. and Weise, E.R., (eds.), 1996, *Wired Women: Gender and New Realities in Cyberspace*, Seal Press, Seattle.

[17] Coomber, R., 1997, 'Using the Internet for Survey Research', *Sociological Research Online*, vol. 2, no. 2. < *http://ww.socresonline.org.uk/socresonline/2/2/2.html*>

[18] Correll, S., 1995, 'The Ethnography of an Electronic Bar: The Lesbian Café', *Journal of Contemporary Ethnography*, vol. 24, pp. 270-298.

[19] Cotten, S., 2001, 'Implications of Internet Technology for Medical Sociology in the New Millennium', *Sociological Spectrum*, vol. 21, pp. 319-340.

[20] Cotten, S.R. and Gupta, S.S. 2004, 'Characteristics of Online and Offline Health Information Seekers and Factors that Discriminate between them', *Social Science and Medicine*, vol. 59, pp. 1795-1806.

[21] Cotton, A.H., 2003, 'The Discursive Field of Web-Based Health Research: Implication for Nursing Research in Cyberspace', *Advances in Nursing Science*, vol. 26, no. 4, pp. 307-319.

[22] Cresswell, J., 1998, *Qualitative Inquiry and Research Design: Choosing Among Five Traditions*, Sage, Thousand Oaks, CA.

[23] Danielson, P., 1996, 'Psuedonyms, Mailbots, and Virtual Letterheads: The Evolution of Computer-Mediated Ethics', in C. Ess (ed.), *Philosophical Perspectives on Computer-Mediated Communication*, pp. 67-93, State University of New York Press, Albany.

[24] Davis, J.J., 2002, 'Disenfranchising the Disabled: The Inaccessibility of Internet-Based Health Information', *Journal of Health Communication*, vol. 7, pp. 355-367.

[25] Davis, M., G. Bolding, Hart, G., Sherr, L and Elford, J, 2004, 'Reflecting on The Experience of Interviewing Online: Perspectives From the Internet and HIV Study in London', *AIDS Care*, vol. 16, no. 8, pp. 944-52.

[26] DeLorme, D.E., Zinkhan, G.M. and French, W., 2001, 'Ethics and the Internet: Issues Associated with Qualitative Research', *Journal of Business Ethics*, Vol. 33, pp. 271-286.

[27] Denzin, N.K., 2004, 'Prologue: Online Environments and Interpretive Social Research', in M.D. Johns, S-L.S. Chen, and G.J. Hall (eds.), *Online Social Research: Methods, Issues, and Ethics*, pp. 1-12, Peter Lang, New York.

[28] Dibbell, J., 1998, *My Tiny Life*. Henry Holt, New York.

[29] Dillman, D.A., 2000, *Mail and Internet Surveys. The Tailored Design Method*, 2nd ed., John Wiley and Sones, New York.

[30] Dunne, G., 1999, *The Different Dimensions of Gay Fatherhood: Exploding the Myths*, Report to the Economic and Social Research Council, London School of Economics, London.

[31] Edworthy, S.M., 1999, 'World Wide Web: Opportunities, Challenges, and Threats', *Lupus*, vol. 8, no. 8, pp. 596-605.

[32] Eysenbach, G. and Till, J.E., 2001, 'Ethical Issues in Qualitative Research on Internet Communities', *British Medical Journal*, vol. 323, no. 7321, pp. 1103-1105.

[33] Fielding, N.G. and Lee, R.H., 1998, *Computer Analysis and Qualitative Research*, Sage Publications, Thousand Oaks, CA.

[34] Finn, J., 1999, 'An Exploration of Helping Processes in an Online Self-Help Group Focusing On Issues of Disability', *Health and Social Work*, vol. 24, pp. 220-231.

[35] Ferganchick-Neufang, J.K., 2004, 'Virtual Harassment: Women and Online Education', *Firstmonday: Peer-Reviews Journal on the Interne*. *<http://www.firstmonday.dk/issues/ issue3_2/fergan/index.html>*

[36] Ferri, B., 2000, 'The Hidden Cost of Difference: Women with Learning Disabilities', *Learning Disabilties: A Multidisciplinary Journal*, vol. 10, no. 3, pp.129-138.

[37] Finn, J. and Lavitt, M., 1994, 'Computer Based Self-Help Groups for Sexual Abuse Survivors', *Social Work with Groups*, vol. 17, pp. 21-46.

[38] Fleitas, J., 1998, 'Spinning Tales from the World Wide Web: Qualitative Research in an Electronic Environment', *Qualitative Health Research*, vol. 8, pp. 283-292.

[39] Flicker, S., Haans, D. and Skinner, H., 2004, 'Ethical Dilemmas in Research on Internet Communities', *Qualitative Health Research*, vol. 14, no. 1, pp. 124-134.

[40] Frankfort-Nachmias, C. and Nachmias, D., 1992, Research Methods in the Social Sciences, 4th edition, Edward Arnold, London.

[41] Frankel, M.S. and Siang, S., 2004, 'Ethical and Legal Aspects of Human Subjects Research on the Internet.' *http://www.aaas.org/spp/dspp/sfrl/projets/intres/report.pdf*

[42] Fridman, S., 2000, 'Money, Not Race, Underline Digital Divide', *Newsbytes*, June 19.

[43] Gaiser, T., 1997, 'Conducting On-Line Focus Groups', *Social Science Computer Review*, vol. 15, pp. 135-144.

[44] Gajjala, R., 2002, 'An Interupted Postcolonial/Feminist Cyberethnography: Complicity and Resistance in the "Cyberfield"', *Feminist Media Studies*, vol. 2, no. 2, pp. 177-193.

[45] Gibbs, G.R., Friese, S. and Mangabeira, W.C., 2002, 'The Use of New Technology in qualitative Research: Introduction to Issue 3(2) of Forum Qualitative Social Research, *Forum qualitative Social Research*, vol. 3, no. 2. *<http://www.qualitative-research.net /fgs/fqs-eng.html>*

[46] Graham, S. and Marvin, S., 1996, *Telecommunications and the City: Electronic Spaces, Urban Places*, Routledge, London.

[47] Grimaldi, C. and Goette, T., 1999, 'The Internet and the Independence of Individuals with Disabilities', *Internet Research: Electronic Networking Applications and Policy*, vol. 9, no. 4, pp. 272-280.

[48] Greenberg, P.A., 2000, 'Digital Divide Not Race-Based', *E-Commerce Times*, April 17.

[49] Gubrium, J.F. and Holstein, J.A. (eds.), 2001, *Institutional Selves: Troubled Identities in a Postmodern World*, Oxford University Press, New York.

[50] Hafner, K., 1997, 'The Epic Saga of the Well', *Wired*, May Issue, pp. 98-142.

[51] Hahn, K., 1998, 'Qualitative Investigation of an E-Mail Mediated Help Service', *Internet Research: Electronic Networking Applications and Policy*, vol. 8, no. 2, pp. 123-135.

[52] Hall, G.J., Frederick, D. and Johns, M.D., 2004, '"NEED HELP ASAP!!!": A Feminist Communitarian Approach to Online Research Ethics', in M.D. Johns, S-L.S. Chen, and G.J. Hall (eds.), *Online Social Research: Methods, Issues, and Ethics*, pp. 239-252, Peter Lang, New York.

[53] Hamman, R., 1996, 'One Hour in the eWorld Hot Tub: A Brief Ethnographic Project in Cyberspace'. *<http://www.socio.demon.co.uk/project.html>*

[54] Han, H.R. and Belcher, A.L., 2001, 'Computer-Medicated Support Group Use among Parents of Children with Cancer - An Exploratory Study', *Computer in Nursing*, vol. 19, pp. 27-33.

[55] Harmon, A., 1998, 'On-line Trail to an Off-Line Killing', *The New York Times*, April 30, A1, A30.

[56] Herring, C. S., 1994, 'Posting in a Different Voice: Gender and Ethics in Computer-Mediated Communication, in C. Ess (ed.), *Philosophical Perspectives on Computer-Mediated Communication*, pp. 115-146, State University of New York Press, Albany.

[57] Herring, C. S., 2004, Slouching Toward the Ordinary: Current Trends in Computer-Mediated Communication', *New Media and Society*, vol. 6, no. 1, pp. 26-36.

[58] Hewson, C., 2003, 'Conducting Research on the Internet', *Psychologist*, vol. 16, pp. 290-293.

[59] Hertz, J.C., 1995, *Surfing the Internet: A Nethead's Adventures On-Line*. Little, Brown and Company, New York.

[60] Hessler, R.M., Downing, J., Beltz, C., Pelliccio, A., Powell. M. and Vale, W., 2003, 'Qualitative Research on Adolescent Risk Using E-Mail: A Methodological Assessment', *Qualitative Sociology*, vol. 26, no. 1, pp. 111-124.

[61] Hiltz, S. and Turoff, M., 1993, *The Network Nation: Human Communication via Computer*, MIT Press, Reading, MA.

[62] Hoffman, D. and Novak, T., 1998, 'Bridging the Racial Divide on the Internet', *Science*, vol. 280, pp. 390-391.

[63] Holge-Hazelton, B., 2002, 'The Internet: A New Field for Qualitative Inquiry?', *Forum qualitative Social Research* [on-line journal], vol. 3, no. 2. < http://www.qualitative-research.net/fgs/fqs-eng.html>

[64] Hsiung, R.C., 2000, 'The Best of Both Worlds: An Onine Self-Help Group Hosted by a Mental Health Professional', *CyberPsychology and Behavior*, vol. 3, no. 6, pp. 935-950.

[65] Hudson, P., 2004, 'Email, SMS Bugging for Crime Fight', the Age Sunday, April 11, p. 1.

[66] Illingworth, N., 2001, 'The Internet Matters: Exploring the Use of the Internet as a Research Tool', *Sociological Research Online*, vol. 6, no. 2. *<www.socresonline.org. uk/6/2/illingworth.html>*

[67] Im, E-O., and Chee, W., 2003, 'Feminist Issues in E-Mail Group Discussion among Cancer Patients', *Advances in Nursing Science*, vol. 26, no. 4, pp. 287-298.

[68] Janney, R.W., 1996, 'E-Mail and Intimacy', in B. Gorayska (ed.), *Cognitive Technology: In Search of a Humane Interface*, pp. 201-211, Elsevier Science Publishing Company, Amsterdam.

[69] Johns, M.D., Chen, S-L.S. and Hall, G.J. (eds.), 2004, *Online Social Research: Methods, Issues, and Ethics*. Peter Lang, New York.

[70] Jones, R.A., 1994, 'The Ethics of Research in Cyberspace', *Internet Research: Electronic Networking Applications and Policy*, vol. 4, no. 3, pp. 30-35.

[71] Jones, S. (ed.) 1999, *Doing Internet Research: Critical Issues and Methods for Examining the Net*. Sage Publications, Thousand Oaks, CA.

[72] Jones, S., 2004, 'Introduction: Ethics and Internet Studies', in M.D. Johns, S-L.S. Chen, and G.J. Hall (eds.), *Online Social Research: Methods, Issues, and Ethics*, pp. 179-185, Peter Lang, New York.

[73] Kawaura, Y., Yamashita, K. and Kawakami, Y., 1999, 'What Makes People Keep Writing Web Diaries?, *Japanese Journal of Social Psychology*, vol. 14, pp. 133-143.

[74] Kendall, L., 1999, 'Recontexualizing Cyberspace: Methodological Considerations for On-Line Research', in S. Jones (ed.) 1999, *Doing Internet Research: Critical Issues and Methods for Examining the Net*, pp. 53-74, Sage Publications, Thousand Oaks, CA.

[75] Kendall, L. 2000, '"Oh No! I' m a Nerd!": Hegemonic Masculinity on an Online Forum', *Gender and Society*, vol. 14, pp. 256-274.

[76] Kennedy, T.L.M., 2000, 'And Exploratory Study of Feminist Experiences in Cyberspace', *Cyberpsychology and Behavior*, vol. 3, pp. 707-720.

[77] Kenway, J., 1996, 'The Information Superhighway and Post-Modernity: The Social Promise and the Social Price', *Comparative Education*, vol. 32, no. 2, pp. 217-231.

[78] Kerka, S., 1995, *Access to Information: To Have and Have Not, Centre on Education and Training for Employment*, Colombus, Ohio.

[79] King, S.A., 1996, 'Researching Internet Communities: Proposed Ethical Guidelines for the Reporting of Results', *The Information Society*, vol. 12, pp. 119-127.

[80] Liehr, P., Takahashi, R., Liu, H., Nishimura, C., Ito, M. and Summers, L.C., 2003, 'Bridging Distance and Culture with a Cyberspace Method of Qualitative Analysis', *Advances in Nursing Science*, vol. 27, no. 3, pp. 176-186.

[81] Lincoln, Y.S. and Denzin, N.K., 2000, 'The Seventh Moment" Out of the Past', in N.K. Denzin and Y.S. Lincoln (eds.), *Handbook of Qualitative Research*, 2nd edition, pp. 1047-1065. Sage Publications, Thousand Oaks, CA.

[82] Lindlof, T., 1995, *Qualitative Communication Research Method*, Sage, Thousand Oaks, CA.

[83] Loader, B.D., (ed.), 1998, *Cyberspace Divide: Equality, Agency and Policy in the Information Society*, Routledge, London.

[84] Lockard, J., 1996, Virtual Whiteness and Narrative Diversity, Undercurrent [Online Journal], vol. 4. < *http://darkwing.uoregon.edu/~ucurrent/uc4/4-lockard.html*>

[85] Madge, C. and O'Connor, H., 2002, 'On-Line with E-Mums: Exploring the Internet as a Medium for Research', *Area*, vol. 34, no. 1, pp. 92-102.

[86] Mann, C. and Stewart, F., 2000, *Internet Communication and Qualitative Research: A Handbook for Researching Online*, Sage Publications, London.

[87] Mann, C. and Stewart, F., 2002, 'Internet Interviewing', in J.F. Gubrium and J.A. Holstein (eds.), *Handbook of Interview Research: Context and Method*, pp.603-627, Sage Publications, Thousand Oaks.

[88] Marcus, G.E., 1995, 'Ethnography in/of the World System: The Emergencies of Multisited Ethnography', *Annual Review of Anthropology*, vol. 24, pp, 95-117.

[89] Markham, A.H., 1998, *Life Online: Researching Real Experience in Virtual Space*, AltaMira Press, Walnut Creek, CA.

[90] Markham, A.H., 2004, 'Internet as a Tool for Qualitative Research', in D. Silverman (ed.), *Qualitative Research: Theory, Method, and Practice*, pp. 95-123, Sage Publications, London.

[91] Markham, A.H., 'The Methods, Politics, and Ethics of Representation in Online Ethnography', in N.K. Denzin and Y.S. Lincoln (eds.), *Handbook of Qualitative Research 3rd edition*, pp. 793-820, Sage Publications, Thousand Oaks, CA.

[92] Merkes, M. 2003, *A Longer Working Life for Australian Women of the Baby Boom Generation? – Women's Voices and the Social Policy Implications of an Ageing Female Workforce*, unpublished doctoral thesis, School of Public Health, La Trobe University, Melbourne.

[93] Moloney, M.A., Dietrich, A.S., Strickland, O.L. and Myerburg, S., 2003, 'Using Internet Discussion Boards as Virtual Focus Groups', *Advances in Nursing Science*, vol. 26, no. 4, pp. 274-286.

[94] Morahan-Martin, J., 2000, 'women and the Internet: Promise and Perils', *Cyberpsychology and Behavior*, vol. 3, pp. 683-692.

[95] Murray, E.E., 1995, *Knowledge Machines: Language and Information in a Technological Society*, Longman, London.

[96] Nip, J.Y.M., 2004, 'The Relationship between Online and Offline Communities: The Case of the Queer Sisters', *Media, Culture and Society*, vol. 26, no. 3, pp. 409-428.

[97] Nosek, B.A. and Banaji, M.R., 2002, 'E-Research: Ethics, Security, Design and Control in Psychological Research on the Internet', *Journal of Social Issues*, vol. 58, no. 1, pp. 161-176.

[98] O'Connor, H. and Madge, C., 2001, 'Cyber-Mothers: Online Synchronous Interviewing using Conferencing Software', Sociological Research Online, vol. 5, no. 4. *<http://www.socresonline.org.uk/5/4/oconnor.html>*

[99] O' Dochartaigh, N., 2002, *The Internet Research Handbook: A Practical Guide for Students and Researchers in the Social Sciences*, Sage, London.

[100] Orbuch, T.L. and Fine, M.A., 2003, 'The Context of Race/Ethnicity in Interpersonal Relationships: Crossing the Chasm', *Journal of Social and Personal Relationship*, vol. 20. no. 2, pp. 147-152.

[101] Paccagnella, L., 1997, 'Getting the Seats of Your Pants Dirty: Strategies for Ethnographic Research on Virtual Communities', *Journal of Computer Mediated Communication*, vol. 3, no. 1, pp. 1-17. *<http//www.ascusc.org/jcmc/vol3/issue1/ paccangella.html>*

[102] Pandey, S.K., Hart, J.J. and Tiwary, S., 2003, 'Women's Health and the Internet: Understanding Emerging Trends and Implications', *Social Science and Medicine*, vol. 56, pp. 179-191.

[103] Parker, L., 1992, 'Collecting Date the E-Mail Way', *Training and Development*, vol. 46, no. 7, pp. 52-55.

[104] Pitts, V., 2004, 'Illness and Internet Empowerment: Writing and Reading Breast Cancer in Cyberspace', *Health*, vol. 8, no. 1, pp. 33-59.

[105] Plant, R., 2004, 'Online communities', *Technology in Society*, vol. 26, no. 1, pp. 51-65.

[106] Plummer, K., 2001, *Document of Life 2: An Invitation to a Critical Humanism*, Sage Publications, London.

[107] Punathambekar, A. and Fraley, T. 2000, 'Virtual Focus Groups: A Methodological Assessment', paper presented at the Conference of the Midwest Association of Public Opinion Research, November.

[108] Reid, E., 1996, 'Informed consent in the Study of On-Line communities. A Reflection on the Effects of Computer-Mediated Social Research', *The Information Society*, vol. 12, no. 2, pp. 169-174. < *http://www.slis.indiana.edu/TIS/abstracts/ab12-2/reid.html>*

[109] Rheingold, H., 1993, *The Virtual Community: Homesteading on the Electronic Frontier*, Addison-Wesley, Menlo Park, CA.

[110] Riva, G., 2001, 'The Mind over the Web: The Quest for the Definition of a Method for Internet Research', *CyberPsychology and Behavior*, vol. 4, no. 1, pp. 7-16.

[111] Roberts, L.D., Smith, L.M. and Pollack, C., 1997, *'"U R a lot Bolder on the Net": The Social Use of Text-Based Virtual Environments by Shy Individuals'*, paper presented to First International Conference on Shyness and Self-Consciousness, Cardiff University, July.

[112] Robinson, K.M., 2001, 'Unsolicited Narratives from the Internet: A Rich Source of Qualitative Data', *Qualitative Health Research*, vol. 11, no. 5, pp. 706-714.

[113] Ross, M.W., Mansson, S-A., Daneback, K., Cooper, A. and Tikkanen, R., 2005, 'Biases in Internet Sexual Health Samples: Comparison of an Internet Sexuality Survey and a National Sexual Health Survey in Sweden', *Social Science and Medicine*, vol. 61, pp. 245-252.

[114] Savicki, V., Lingenfelter, D. and Kelley, M., 1996, 'Gender Language Style and Group Composition in Internet Discussion Groups', *Journal of Computer Mediated Communication*, vol.2, no. 3, pp. 1-12. *<http//www.ascusc.org/jcmc/vol2/issue3/savicki.html>*

[115] Scheuermann, L. and Taylor, G., 1997, 'Netiquette', *Internet Research: Electronic Networking Applications and Policy*, vol. 7, no. 4, pp. 269-272.

[116] Schmidt, W., 1997, 'World-Wide Web Survey Research: Benefits, Potential Problems and Solutions', *Behaviour Research Methods, Instruments and Computers*, vol. 29, pp. 274-279.

[117] Schneier, B., 2000, *Secret and Lies: Digital Security in a Networked World*, Wiley, New York.

[118] Schrum, L., 1995, 'Framing the Debate: Ethical Research in the Information Age', *Qualitative Inquiry*, vol. 1, pp. 311-326.

[119] Seabrook, J., 1997, *Deeper: My Two-Year Odyssey in Cyberspace*. Simon and Schuster, New York.

[120] Selwyn, N. and Robson, K., 1998, 'Using E-Mail as a Research Tool', Social Research Update 21. < *http://www.soc.surrey.ac.uk/sru/SRU21.html*>

[121] Seymour, W.S., 2001, 'In the Flesh or Online? Exploring qualitative Research Methodologies', *Qualitative Research*, vol. 1, no. 2, pp. 147-168.

[122] Seymour, W.S. and Lupton, D., 2004, 'Holding the Line Online: Exploring Wired Relationships for People with Disabilities', *Disability and Society*, vol. 19, no. 4, pp. 291-305.

[123] Sharf, B.F., 1999, 'Beyond Netiquette: The Ethics of Doing Naturalistic Discourse Research on the Internet, in Jones, S. (ed.) 1999, *Doing Internet Research: Critical Issues and Methods for Examining the Net*, pp. 243-256, Sage Publications, Thousand Oaks, CA.

[124] Shields, R. (ed.), 1996, *Cultures of the Internet: Virtual Spaces, Real Histories, Living Bodies*, Sage, London.

[125] Sixsmith, J. and Murray, C.D., 2001, 'Ethical Issues in the Documentary Data Analysis of Internet Posts and Archives', *Qualitative Health Research*, vol. 11. no. 3, pp. 423-432.

[126] Skinner, H., Biscope, S. and Poland, B., 2003, 'Quality of Internet Access: Barrier Behind Internet Use', *Social Science and Medicine*, vol. 57, 875-880.

[127] Smith, M.A. and Leigh, B., 1997, 'Virtual Subjects: Using the Internet as an Alternative Source of Subjects and Research Environment', *Behavior Research Methods, Instruments, and Computers*, vol. 29, pp. 496-505.

[128] Spender, D., 1995, *Nattering on the Net: women, Power and Cyberspace*, Spinifex, Melbourne.

[129] Spender, D. 1997, The Position of Women in Information Technology – Or Who Got There first and With What Consequences? *Current Sociology*, vol. 45, no.2, pp.135-147.

[130] Stanton, J. and Rogelberg, S.G., 2001, 'Using Internet/Intranet Web Pages to Collect Organizational Research Data', *Organizational Research Methods*, vol. 4, no. 3, pp. 199-216.

[131] Stewart, F., Eckerman, E. and Zhou, K., 1998, 'Using the Internet in Qualitative Public Health Research: A Comparison of Chinese and Australia Young Women's Perceptions of Tobacco Use', Internet Journal of Health Promotion, December 29 [On-line]. *<http://www.monash.edu.au/health/IJHP/1998/12>*

[132] Strickland, O.L., Moloney, M.F., Dietrich, A.S., Myerburg, S., Cotsonis, G.A. and Johnson, R.V., 2003, 'Measurement Issues Related to Data Collection on the World Wide Web', *Advances in Nursing Science*, vol. 26, no. 4, pp. 246-256.

[133] Sweet, C., 2001, 'Designing and Conducting Virtual Focus Groups', *Qualitative Market Research: An International Journal, Research in Cyber Space*, June, pp. 1-10. *<casey@focusgroupsonline.net>*

[134] Tannen, D., 1994, 'Gender Gap in Cyberspace', *Newsweek*, May 16, p. 54.

[135] Thach, E., 1995, 'Using Electronic Mail to Conduct Survey Research', *Educational Technology*, March-April, pp. 27-31.

[136] Thimbleby, H., 1998, 'Personal Boundaries/Global Stage', *First Monday: Peer-Reviewed Journal On the Internet. <http://www.firstmonday.dk/issues/issue3_3/thimbleby/index.html>*

[137] Thomas, J., 1996, 'Introduction: A Debate about the Ethics of Fair Practices for Collecting Social Science Data in Cyberspace', *The Information Society*, vol. 12, no. 2, pp. 107-117.

[138] Thomas, J., 1999, 'Balancing the Ethical Conundrums of Internet Research-An Existential View from the Trenches', *Iowa Journal of Communications*, vol. 31, Spring, pp. 8.20.

[139] Thomas, J., 2004, 'Reexamining the Ethics of Internet Research: Facing the Challenge of Overzealous Oversight', in M.D. Johns, S-L.S. Chen, and G.J. Hall (eds.), *Online Social Research: Methods, Issues, and Ethics*, pp. 177-201, Peter Lang, New York.

[140] Thomas, D.S., Forcht, K. and Counts, P., 1998, 'Legal Considerations of Internet Use: Issues to Be Addressed', *Internet Research: Electronic Networking Applications and Policy*, vol 8, pp. 70-74.

[141] Thomas, B., Stamler, L.L., Lafreniere, K. and Dumala, R., 2000, 'The Internet: An Effective Tool for Nursing Research with Women', *Computers in Nursing*, vol. 18, pp. 13-18.

[142] Thomas, B., Stamler, L.L., Lafreniere, K., Out, J. and Delahunt, T.D., 2002, 'Using the Internet to Identify Women's Sources of Breast Health Education and Screening', *Women and Health*, vol. 36, no. 1, pp. 33-48.

[143] Turkle, S., 1995, *Life on the Screen: Identity in the Age of the Internet*, Simon and Schuster, New York.

[144] Van Gelder, L., 1991, 'The Strange Case of the Electronic Lover', in C. Dunlop and R. Kling (eds.), *Computerization and Controversy: Value Conflicts and Social Choices,* pp. 364-375, Academic Press, New York.

[145] Walther, J.B., 2001, 'Research Ethics in Internet-Enabled Research: Human Subjects Issues and Methodological Myopia', Internet Research Ethics. *<http://www.nyu.edu/projects/nissenbaum/projects_ethics.html>*

[146] Warf, B., 2001, 'Segueways into cyberspace: Multiple Geographies of the Digital Divide', *Environment and Planning B, Planning and Design*, vol. 28, pp. 3-19.

[147] White, J., Carey, L. and Dailey, K., 2001, 'Web-Based Instrumentation in Educational Survey Research', *WebNet Journal*, vol. 3, no.1, pp. 46-50.

[148] Wittel, A., 2000, 'Ethnography on the Move: From Field to Net to Internet', *Forum qualitative Social Research* [on-line journal], vol. 1, no. 1. < http://qualitative-research.net/fgs/fqs>

[149] Ziebland, S., 2004, 'The Importance of Being Expert: The Quest for Cancer Information on the Internet', *Social Science and Medicine*, vol. 59, pp. 1783-1793.

[150] Ziebland, S. and Chapple, A., 2004, 'How the Internet Affects Patients' Experience of Cancer: A Qualitative Study', *British Medical Journal*, vol. 328, pp. 564-570.

In: Health Research in Cyberspace
Editor: Pranee Liamputtong, pp. 25-47
ISBN 1-59454-819-6

Chapter 2

CYBER RESEARCH: FOCUSING ON METHODOLOGY

Pranee Liamputtong

Qualitative inquiry is a name for a 'reformist movement that began in the early 1970s in the academy'... Qualitative online, Internet research is a movement within this larger movement. Online research uses the methods, technologies, and languages of the Internet and its complex cultures. Online research molds traditional qualitative research methods to the Internet environment.

(Denzin, 2004: 1)

Researchers in the 21st century are challenged by the simultaneously familiar yet mysterious worlds that lie 'behind the screen' of the computer... Sitting at a computer, using the Internet, researchers can interview disembodied people from across the earth and also the personae who frequent the imagined environments of cyberspace.

(Mann and Stewart, 2002: 603)

INTRODUCTION

In chapter one, I have discussed salient issues relating to cyber research. In this chapter, I will point to some practical ways in conducting research in cyberspace. In particular, I will first examine some important issue in conducting research online. Second, I will suggest some practical ways to access research participants in cyber research and third how to obtain informed consent is given. I then proceed to provide some discussions on qualitative research methods which are commonly employed in online research as well as some detailed examples from exiting literature.

RESEARCH IN CYPERSPACE

Online communication embraces different forms of computer-mediated communication. Terms such as "online communication, computer-mediated communication (CMC), Internet (or Net), and cyberspace" have been interchangeably used (Markham, 1998: 19), and I adopt a similar stance in this chapter.

Online communication, and particularly the Internet, has become a part of the fabric of many people's daily lives and an essentially important part of social groups, professionals and institutions in most societies (Robinson, 2001; Kummervold et al., 2002; Mann and Stewart, 2002; O'Neil, 2002; Zahir et al., 2002; Cotton, 2003; Newman, 2003; Pandey et al., 2003; Cotton and Gupta, 2004; Ziebland, 2004). Evans and Wurster (1999: 18) contend that the Internet has the potential to "unbundle information from its physical carriers". For Light (2001: 1179), the Internet is able to "foster democratic discourse and participation". Pandey et al. (2003: 180) too suggest that "the democratic imperative of the Internet can bring about decentralised and participatory decision-making structures in which citizens will be able to participate more fully in meeting health care needs of their communities".

Cyberspace - the environment created by online communication - is "a social and cognitive space" (Riva, 2001: 8; Chin, 2003). As Riva (2001: 8-9) suggests, online communication "experience as a process by which a group of social actors in a given situation negotiate the meaning of the various situations that arise between them within an electronic environment". According to Merkes (2003: 131), when people or communities are connected via electronic network, a social network is created. People are "connected by a set of social relations, such as friendship, co-working, or information exchange". Chin (2003: 239) too contends that "cyberspace is where new communities are being formed and it is where new human values are being forged". To Sade-Beck (2004: 3), "cyberspace, or cybernetic space, through which users move, does not imitate the real world, but rather creates a rapid, new, immediate, multi-layered world".

Sharf (1999: 244) points out that online discussions generated through a chat room, bulletin boards, listservs and conferences centring around particular issues bring people with shared interests and relevant experiences and expertise from graphically dispersed locations. Eysenbach and Till (2001: 1103) too suggest that material posted on these channels is "a rich source for researchers interested in understanding the experiences and views of people". Because of this, online communication like the Internet is increasingly seen as an excellent source of information. Communication online is seen as "naturalistic interpersonal communication", online discourse, therefore, lends itself well to various analytic and methodological discourses, including content and discourse analysis, and participant observation (Sharf, 1999: 244), as I shall show in later section.

In the last decade and following on from trends in market research (Mehta and Sivadas, 1995; Sweet, 1999, 2001; Sweet and Walkowski, 2002), we have seen more social science research making use of computer-mediated communication (CMC) as a research tool (Mann and Stewart, 2000, 2002; Illingworth, 2001; Robinson, 2001; Merkes, 2002, 2003; Berg, 2004; Markham, 2004, 2004). Survey research has made use of CMC to reach wider research participants and expand the time for their data collection (see Kehoe and Pitkow, 1996; Coomber, 1997; Smith, 1997; Couper et al., 1999; Jones, 1999; Dillman, 2000; Jerome et al., 2000; Dillman and Bowker, 2001; Koch and Emrey, 2001; Thomas et al., 2000, 2002; Eysenbach and Wyatt, 2002; Powell et al., 2003; Tingling et al., 2003; see also Chapter 7 in this volume). Qualitative research has also benefited from the use of this new global technology (Sweet, 2001; Berg, 2004), but has not extensively made use of the technology as in survey research (Selwyn and Robson, 1998; Hessler et al., 2003). The increased use of communication technologies, as Selwyn and Robson (1998: 2) point out, occurs in parallel with an increased popularity of qualitative research methods like phenomenology and grounded theory relying on textual data (see Foster, 1994).

In social science research, online communication emerges as an essential channel because it allows the researcher and the researched to interact directly using text via keyboards. The most commonly utilised text-based modes are email and online or real-time chat (Mann and Stewart, 2002; Im and Chee, 2003). Online communication includes both semiprivate and public domains. The semiprivate domains encompass email, one-to-one discussion and conference/forums discussion. Unlike the public domains, the semiprivate areas allow the researcher and participants some direct control over the nature and content of interaction (Mann and Stewart 2002: 604; Im and Chee, 2003). And this is the focus of my discussion in this section.

There are two distinct types of online communication: synchronous and asynchronous (Riva, 2001). Synchronous communication, or real-time 'chat', is "an interchange of messages between two or more users simultaneously logged on at different computer terminals" (Mann and Stewart 2000: 2), while asynchronous communication which is the characteristics of most email messaging systems, "allows users to type extended messages which are electronically transmitted to recipients who can read, reply, print, forward or file them at their leisure" (Mann and Stewart 2000: 2). Individual interviews can be done via email or real-time one-to-one chat software. Email enables asynchronous one-to-one interviews (see also Parker, 1992; Im and Chee, 2003; see also Im and Chee, Hessler, and Couch and Liamputtong this volume). There are software like AOL's Instant Messager and ICQ that enables users to chat in real time one-to-one or in groups. For focus group interviews, often referred to as "cyber groups, e-groups, or virtual groups" (Sweet 1999: 1), there are options including real-time many-to-many chat and asynchronous many-to-many conferencing options (see O'Connor and Madge, 2001; Madge and O'Connor, 2002; Strickland et al., 2003; Moloney et al., 2003). With real-time many-to-many chat, messages are typed and read at the same time, but in different locations. All users on the same channel will see the message typed by other users. A chat program usually contains a conversation flow area, where users are able to read all contributions and a separate composition area, where all participants write their own messages. Similar to email, the asynchronous many-to-many conferencing allows users to respond to messages from others at a time later. It is, however, undertaken at a "conference site". Unlike individual email address, this type of online communication is an effective channel for doing non-real-time online focus groups. See also Sweet (1999, 2001) for focus group online methodologies used in market research.

Accessing Potential Participants in Online Research

As in offline research, researchers have to have strategies to recruit their potential participants. There have been some strategies that social science researchers adopt to gain access to their potential participants. So far, email seems to be the most adopted method of accessing potential research participants. Mann and Stewart (2000: 81) argue that email "permits direct access to individuals without the use of intermediaries". This is particularly so if researchers are undertaking research with groups with whom they are already familiar or have contacts. Special interest sites where users can make contact with each other provide access to potential participants. Ferri (2000) accessed her participants through existing email discussion groups that targeted people with disabilities. Im and Chee (2003, also this volume) too recruited their research participants through email lists of Internet Cancer Support Groups. Hodkinson, in his personal email to Mann and Stewart (2000: 81) elaborated on his recruitment strategies in his research concerning the goths in the UK that:

> I used a combination of Web-searches and hypertext links, to collect the e-mail addresses of several Goth bands from various parts of the world, and then sent them all an e-mail which introduced my research, and requested an online interview. In fact, finding e-mail addresses was one of the most convenient aspects of using the net. Every Web-site and every e-mailing list post contains the address of the individual responsible for it, making it possible to make contact instantly.

Accessing potential research participants can be done via the Internet. It can be done by including email contact or Web site when advertising the research via leaflets and journals as in conventional recruiting methods. In her study with gay fathers, Dunne (1999) placed her email address in brochures and journals as a way to access an "invisible population marginalised in both mainstream and gay culture". Advertisements in relevant newsgroups or mailing lists have also assisted researchers to access their research participants. Bennett (1998) recruited her male respondents by placing advertisements in newsgroups like "soc.men" and "alt.acadia" making clear that she sought to conduct a confidential one-to-one interaction for an extended period with interested participants. Existing participants can also help with recruitment. Using email software, this can be done by 'snowballing' messages using the 'forwarding' options (Hodkinson, 2000). Another possibility is to post a request for contacts or information when logging onto appropriate Internet sites (Kehoe and Pitknow, 1996; Sweet, 2001; Mann and Stewart, 2000; Merkes, 2003). Participants may also be recruited from those who happen to 'surf' or 'lurk' around the site pre-existing chat rooms, conference groups and listservs (Mann and Stewart, 2000).

Sweet and Walkowski (2002: 11) suggest the following means for recruiting potential participants: email recruiting, telephone recruiting and email/phone combination. Sweet (2001: 2) also advices us that potential participants can be "recruited electronically from established panels, compiled online lists, targeted Web sites, or client-provided lists. Sometimes, telephone recruiting is utilised to recruit audiences less likely to respond online, highly valued audiences where 'high touch' interactions are necessary, or to confirm and obtain e-mail addresses".

The experience of Coomber (1997) in his research into the practices of drug dealers and their drug adulteration/dilution practices provides an excellent and practical example of how to access hard-to-reach participants, although it must be said that his study is largely positivist (using survey on the Internet and WWW). Coomber (1997: 3) contends that "drug dealers, by the very nature of their activities, are a very difficult group to access". Coomber (1997) points out that his previous work on drug dealers using conventional research methods proved that snowball sampling technique was unsuccessful. Therefore, he attempted to recruit his potential participants via the Internet and WWW. Coomber (1997: 7-8) writes:

> In my research, I decided to exploit those areas where it was self evident that those interested in drugs, and those who use or have used drugs, spend some of their cyberspace

time – the drug related newsgroups. A rough of drug related newsgroups turned up 23 main groups… My request to take part in the research was posted to each of the many drug related groups".

Coomber (1997: 9) also suggests that his posting needed to be interesting to catch the eyes of potential participants. Coomber (1997: 9) hence constructed the heading to advertise his posting as: "Have You Ever Sold Powdered Drugs? If So, I Would Like Your Help". He said "if people's curiosity was raised by this heading then a simple 'click' on it would take them to the posting which explained in more detail what the research was and why it was being carried out. If still interested, a click on the posting then whisked people to my Web page and questionnaire". Catchy headings would certainly attract readers' attention. This was also adopted by Galegher et al. (1998) with postings reading as "My Story – My Pain – No Answers". This approach, we believe, can be adopted in accessing potential participants in conducting qualitative research online. In Bennett's research with men online (1998: 79), she posted an advertisement on the 'Pathfinder' Message Board System with a title "Masculinity in the 1990's, what is it like to be a man?" See also Couch and Liamputtong for their posting message to recruit participants to take part in their sex, risk and health in this volume.

In Thomas et al.'s study (2002), they employed several means to recruit their potential participants. Initially, Thomas and colleagues recruited their participants by telling friends and colleagues about the web site and encourage them to participate. Adapting a snowball approach, the participants were then asked to share the information about the web site with others and encourage them to participate. A number of web sites related to women's health and women's issues were approached in order to list the questionnaire web sites at their location. Cards with their names as well as information about the study and the web site address were distributed within the regional community and at some national and international conferences. In their study, Hessler and colleagues (2003) asked severa; trustworthy adults who resided in the same areas as the participants to be recruiters to access young people in their study. These adults were mostly high school teachers who recruited the participants and processed the consent and payment forms. The researchers knew only email pseudonyms of the participants. See also Chapter 6 in this volume.

As in conventional research approaches, researchers may need to access their potential participants through formal "gatekeepers" (Eysenbach and Till, 2001). Gatekeepers, as Mann and Stewart (2000: 81) note, may grant or withhold permission to conduct research within their responsible locations and places. Foster (1996) points out that gatekeepers may refuse access or restrict access to particular areas, times or events if they feel that they need to protect people under their responsibility or for any reasons (Im and Chee, 2003 and in this volume). Foster (1994: 94), in his attempt to access potential participants through mailing lists and interest groups, some gatekeepers (in this case it was the moderators who "intercept and decide on the legitimacy of messages" sent to a mailing list and newsgroups), blocked the survey as it was perceived that his research tool "was not germane to the main business of the group". Im and Chee (2003) contacted 100 Internet Cancer Support Groups and asked if they could send a message about the study to their email lists. Only four agreed to post the study through their Web site or email lists free of charge. But Cole (2000) managed to gain permission from the Web site manager of the "Promise Keepers" movement in the US to follow up email addresses for his potential participants. I would suggest, researchers need to plan carefully if their recruitment has to be done through a formal gatekeeper. If there are other potential channels, they might need to look into these.

Informed Consent: How to Obtain this Online?

Informed consent is an essential part of research endeavour; that the participants are given a comprehensive and correct information about the research, their participations, the promise of confidentiality, and their rights prior to signing their consent to take part in it. Online research is no exception, and due to its nature, it is even more important than when using conventional research methods (Barnes, 2004). In conventional research, the participants can give their consent by signing a consent form, but with online research, how they give their consent is ambiguous and still a debated issue. However, to what follows, I outline some of the points that Mann and Stewart (2000), Sharf (1999) and others have raised.

With email interviewing, Mann and Stewart (2000: 49) suggest the following:

- Information regarding the study and the consent form may be emailed as an attachment or included in the body of an email to potential participants.
- A Web site containing details of the research including consent form may be constructed and posted on the Internet. The potential participants are directed to download the consent form and then email back to the researcher.
- Information of the study and consent form can be sent by conventional "snailmail" (conventional mail) to participants and returned to the researcher via snail-mail.

Obtaining consent from potential participants who participate in online chat in focus groups or online participant observation in mailing lists or newsgroups may be adopted by the strategies outlined above; that is informed consent must be obtained prior to online focus group discussions or online observation (see Reid, 1996; Paccagnella, 1997; Markham, 1998; Denzin, 1999; Strickland et al., 2003; Moloney, 2003).

But how do we secure a signature on informed consent from our participants? Perhaps Seymour et al's study (1999) helps to clarify this. Seymour and colleagues asked their participants to indicate their consent by typing a 'YES' or 'NO' response on the consent form. If problems arose, the participants were asked to sign a consent form that they obtained online and it could then be faxed or sent by a snail-mail back to the researcher. In the research using email group discussion with cancer patients conducted by Im and Chee (2003), potential participants were asked to click the button of "Yes, I agree to participate" contained in the research Web site. Mann and Stewart (2000: 49) remark that "whichever method is adopted, the key question for the researcher is whether an actual signature is required, or whether a tick in a box or typed 'YES' response is an acceptable substitute". See Chen et al. (2004) for some responses from prospective online participants on the attempt of researchers to secure an informed consent for their online research. As Chen et al. (2004) suggest, the researched may not only feel ambivalent about it, but also feel hostile toward this attempt too.

Obtaining informed consent online can be problematic within some institutional ethic committees, as these committees typically require a signed consent form from participants (Jones, 2004). Bennett, in her personal email to Mann and Stewart (2000: 51) points out that obtaining informed consent online is unfamiliar to many research ethics committees. Researchers must strongly argue for their choices. She cleverly elaborates on this that:

> Back up your decision to use email, to obtain consent, with examples of other studies that have done so. Point out that 'traditional' methods of obtaining informed consent do not guarantee any more 'security', reliability or validity than emailed methods.

Bennett (2000) also contends that researchers need to show the research committees their strategies to ensure the return of consent forms from their participants. Bennett (in Mann and Stewart 2000, p. 51) suggests:

> Demonstrate how you intend to ensure that the emailed consent form is in fact returned by 'the participants'... by setting up a code word that only he/she can know, or a set of questions to which only they know the answer to (and which you can return to and clarify throughout the study as a security measure).

Most importantly, Bennett (in Mann and Stewart 2000: 51) suggests, researchers need to identify any weaknesses in using email as a means for obtaining consent in their proposal and "back them up fiercely". See also Couch and Liamputtong for their experience with securing consent form in their research in Chapter 11 in this volume.

Qualitative Research Methods in Cyber Research

Qualitative research methods which have been adopted in research in cyberspace have included in-depth interviewing, focus groups, ethnography, observation and document analysis of life histories or archives. Due to space limitation, I will not discuss each method in detail. Rather, I urge readers to consult other good qualitative texts for extensive coverage of qualitative methods (see Pop and Mays, 2000; Ritchie and Lewis, 2003; Marvasti, 2004; Seale et al., 2004; Silverman, 2004; Denzin and Lincoln, 2005, and Liamputtong and Ezzy, 2005, to name a few). In what follows, I will present some empirical examples of online research making use of different qualitative research methods.

In-Depth Interviewing Method

As in conventional offline research, in-depth interviewing method is by far the most popular approach among online researchers. Most often too is that the interviews are being conducted via email or real-time chat. Bennett's work with men on line (1998) made use of in-depth interview technique using real-time chat (one-to-one). Bennett's research aimed to examine how lived experiences have contributed to the formation and development of men's masculine identities as well as how the men in her study respond to the use of online communication as a means of conveying their lived experiences. Bennett generated her data solely via online communication over seven months of extensive online interaction. She chose real-time chat over email as it established an equitable research balance from the onset of the research. The immediacy of the real-time chat allowed Bennett and her participants to address the issues instantaneously. Bennett argued that it also allowed her and her "co-researchers" (the men) to negotiate the meaning of their discussion. Bennett (1998) confidently argued that online interaction indeed provides new avenues for men to discuss their emotions and feelings openly and with confidence. Bennett (1998: 68) remarked: "I feel that my co-investigators were able to express their thoughts and feelings about themselves, as men, in a way which did not cause or inflict any undue stress or concern. Rather it provided them with a venue to reflect upon their lives in ways not previously available, with a technology and research process which locates them as central and active, reflexive beings". In her conclusion, Bennett (1998: 69) pleaded that "if the electronic environment can assist in the promotion of a new awareness, or a new sense of self, then it is within our means to do so, as social researchers. The technology is here, the desire to utilise it is evident and it should therefore be welcomed".

Seymour and Lupton (2004) recently published their study that examined disability, risk and technology in Adelaide, South Australia. In stage one of the research, 15 in-depth offline interviews were conducted with people with a range of disabilities. An additional 20 participants were recruited from a disability list server; an Internet site concerning people with disabilities. Eight men and twelve women took part in their online research. Seymour and Lupton (2004) utilised a threaded discussion online site which allowed participants to carry out their asynchronous online discussions. Seymour and Lupton (2004: 293) stated that "participants could enter the site as often as they wished, enabling both researcher and researched to extend on a particular topic, to delete or qualify a point, or to clarify their responses over time". Although the researchers had a pre-prepared question to prompt in each interview, "the openness of the medium encouraged discursive, rather than didactic communication. The ongoing exchange offered the participants a significant opportunity to influence the research outcomes". Because the participants were able to respond at the time that suited them, the researchers obtained a large amount of data. The shortest interview was done over 22 days and the longest one extended over 75 days. On average, the duration of interviews was 42.6 days. This might also indicate that people with disabilities found communication online benefiting. In their conclusion, Seymour and Lupton (2004: 303) contended that cyberspace "can be re-positioned to work in the interests of people with disabilities… Text-based, interactive, virtual performance provides the means for people with disabilities to actively engage in the task of breaching the divide" of "the able-bodied-disabled distinction". As such, "techno-sociality and virtual participation promise new avenues for personal fulfilment and political action, and point to new ways of being and having a body" among people with disabilities. See also Davis et al. (2004) and Elford et al. (2004) for their online interviews with gay men regarding seeking sexual partners and its implications for HIV/STD risk behaviours in London. See Al-Saggaf and Kharabsheh, Couch and Liamputtong, Hessler, and Merkes in this volume.

FOCUS GROUP INTERVIEW METHOD

Despite resistance from some focus group researchers (see Greenbaum, 2001), focus group interviews have also been utilised and become more popular in online research. Online focus groups can be carried out in "real time" (synchronous) context or in "non-real time" (asynchronous) conducted through a conference site, and in some cases, the two methods can be combined (Rezebek, 2000; Williams and Robson, 2004). Data collection can be done among small groups of participants from different distant and locations simultaneously (Berg, 2004: 59; see also Gaiser, 1997; Murray, 1997; Stewart et al., 1998; Robson, 1999; Ferri, 2000; Mann and Stewart, 2000; Rezebek, 2000; O'Connor and Madge, 2001; Sweet, 2001; Adler and Zarchin, 2002; Madge and O'Connor, 2002; Moloney et al., 2003; Strickland et al., 2003; Williams, 2003; Williams and Robson, 2004). Stewart and colleagues (1998), for example, undertook virtual focus groups involving young female participants from the Fiji Islands, China, Malaysia and Australia on a range of health issues and practices including smoking, alcohol, drugs, nutrition, stress and sexuality. Their online focus group research was conducted in parallel to face-to-face interviews in all the countries involved. The study was carried out in synchronous or real time chat on 21 March 1998. The parent conference site called RiskStudy was constructed and within the site, four sub-conference chat rooms (Red, Blue, Yellow and Green) were created. Using a conference software, participants in all countries were able to enter the sites and participate in any one of four chat rooms. The chat rooms allowed quick responses from the participants, as whatever was typed by one person it would appear on the screen. Stewart et al. (1998: 8) said that although the virtual focus group was planned for one hour, the group went for almost two hours. This is because online communication and discussion is "eminently suited to the conversation of young women" (see also Spender, 1997).

Ferri (2000) conducted a participatory action research via email discussion group with women with learning disabilities. The women were recruited from existing email discussion groups targeting women or individuals with disabilities. Prior to online discussion, all participants were interviewed by phone to document their biographical data and to explain about the study, their involvement in the study, and logistic processes in accessing electronic mail. Ferri daily collected messages from each participant in her 'closed' discussion list four days a week for eight weeks. She then forwarded everyone's responses after all identifying material had been removed. The responses were sent in "a digest format" (p. 132). Ferri (2000: 132) contended, "this method allowed responses to be collected and sent out to participants in one group message per day. My comments and questions followed the flow of the discussion, as I attempted to draw connections among their different voices, and facilitate a dialogue". Having based her research on participatory action research methodology, one of Ferri's objective of this study was to "explore the potential of electronic mail to transgress boundaries between the researcher and the researched", and "the product and the process of constructing knowledge" (p. 130). As the women in the study could access the daily flow of conversation, this allowed them to respond to, comment on and challenge the responses of others in the group. As a result, the online discussion yielded an interactive and rich data. Ferri (2000: 131) found that "electronic communication afforded greater flexibility than arranging face-to-face or phone contacts, especially for a group discussion". In the middle of the data collection period, a summary of themes emerging from the group discussion was sent to all women and they were asked to respond to Ferri's analysis. The same process was repeated at the end of the project. The women had opportunities to reflect on any of the themes and elaborate on their experiences in participating in this online research. Ferri (2000: 131) also argued that the use of online research "facilitated collaboration, as all participants are able to communicate with one another and assist in the analysis as it unfolded".

Recently, Strickland et al. (2003; see also Moloney et al., 2003) conducted a virtual focus group in their study of perimenopausal women with migraines. In the study, the data were collected through a series of discussion boards which were created during the recruitment period. Each discussion board, which was planned to be a virtual focus group, was assigned its login name and password and these were given to participants after they agreed to take part in the research. Each board had between 4 to 8 participants. Strickland and colleagues believed that these numbers were suitable to encourage interaction and communication between the participants. There were 22 participants, comprising 18 White, 3 African American and 1 English Indian women who were living in different parts of the US, and who were involved in the study. The participants were recruited by word of mouth, flyers posed in the actual community and via the Internet. The boards were conducted in non-real time focus groups, this meant that participants were able to log in and out at their convenience. The boards were kept active for 3 to 5 weeks. For each board, the moderator initially posted a welcome message and a number of questions to act as beginning "threads" in order to encourage discussions within the group. Depending on the discussions, other new threads were posted. Often, a new thread emerged from the group discussion. Apart from responding to the moderator's questions, the participants were also encouraged to begin their own new threads. Strickland et al. (2003: 254) told us that "it was possible to have an ongoing discussion board/focus group with women from diverse geographical locations. Women who otherwise could not have found a common time to meet were able to participate at different times of the day and night". See also Madge and O'Connor (2002) for their interesting online focus group research with mothers of young children in the United Kingdom, and good descriptions of virtual focus groups on the employment experiences of inflammatory bowel disease sufferers and deviance and harm within online environments of Williams and Robson (2004).

ETHNOGRAPHY

The emerging concept of "global ethnography" (Burawoy et al. 2000), or "virtual ethnography" (Hine, 2000) and "cyber community" (Rheingold, 1993; Thomsen et al., 1998; Baym, 1999, 2000) renders new ways of doing ethnographic fieldwork in cyberspace (see also Dicks and Mason, 1998; Thomsen et al., 1998; Wittel, 2000; Clegg Smith, 2004; Markham, 2004; Sade-Beck, 2004; Markham, 2005). Burawoy et al. (2000) contend that the present day ethnographers have a "privileged insight into the lived experience of globalisation". They argue for "a need for rethinking the meaning of fieldwork from solitary confinement and from being chained to a specific time and place towards a more flexible concept adjustable to time and space" (in Holge-Hazelton 2002: 2). This idea renders the necessity of conducting ethnography online. Hine (2000) strongly advocates ethnographic research online, in which she coins the method as "virtual ethnography". Hine argues that ethnography has encountered "crisis" in the postmodern world (see also Denzin, 1997; Marcus, 1995, 1998; Dicks and Mason, 1998; Sade-Beck, 2004). This "crisis" facing ethnography, however, as Hine contends (2000: 43), is "an opportunity for making a form of ethnographic enquiry suited to the Internet, involving a different kind of interaction and ethnographic object from those with which ethnography has traditionally been concerned.".

Hine (2000: 64) argues that the interactive media such as the Internet "provides a challenge and an opportunity for ethnography, by bringing into question the notion of a site of interaction". To Hine (2000: 64), cyberspace is not a space which is separated from "any connections to 'real life' and face-to-face interaction. It has rich and complex connections with the contexts in which it is used. It also depends on technologies which are used and understood differently in different contexts, and which have to be acquired, leant, interpreted and incorporated into context". And this, Hine contends, is essentially ethnographic principles. See Hine (2000) for an excellent and provocative ethnography of the Louise Woodward case on the Internet (Louise Woodward is a British nanny who was charged for murdering a child in her care in the US).

Participation observation, an essential part of ethnography, has been adopted in literature in online research (Correll, 1995; Turkle, 1995; Hamman, 1996; Paccagnella, 1997; Horn, 1998; Markham, 1998; Thomsen et al., 1998; Kendall, 1999, 2002, 2004, Sharf, 1999; Baym, 2000; Hine, 2000; Hodkinson, 2000; Eichhorn, 2001; Holge-Hazelton, 2002; Clegg Smith, 2004; LeBesco, 2004: Sade-Beck, 2004). Hamman (1996) contends that participant observation is suitable for carrying out research that researchers have little knowledge about including cyberspace. Hamman (1996: 4) remarks, "it allows the researcher to gain insights and contacts that would elude them if other methods were chosen". Hamman (1996: 4) also acknowledges in her work that, "had I not used participant observation to do this research, I would not have located Sarah, nor would I have understood the 'insider' vocabulary she used. I never would have thought to ask some of the questions that I asked in the interview had I not spent many hours participating in on-line chat rooms myself". Hamman (1996: 4) strongly suggests that participant observation "is a valuable tool for sociologists researching those who inhibit cyberspace". Kendall (1999: 57) strongly advocates for including participation in online research. She succinctly puts: "I would never have the audacity to suggest that all social research projects ought to include participant observation. Yet with regard to research on interactive online forums, I recommend just that". Kendall suggests that even if researchers wish to utilise other methods, "participant observation can provide information important to the successful implementation of online research". See also her recent and fascinating book "Hanging out in the virtual pub" (2002) and her most recent writing on online ethnography and identity (2004).

Markham (1998) undertook an ethnographic study of a lived experience of what it means to go and be online. She wished to understand the way of life in a virtual community by participating online. Markham (1998: 16) contended, "I wanted to know why people spent so much time online. I wondered what cyberspace meant to them, how it affected or changed their lives. I wanted to know how they were making sense of their experiences as they shifted between being in the physical world and being in these textual worlds created by the exchange of messages, where they could re-create bodies, or leave them behind". To do so, Markham became involved in creating and negotiating the very context that became the object of analysis by immersing herself as one of the users. She pointed out "to be in cyberspace is to learn how to be embodied there. To be embodied there is to participate. To participate is to know enough about the rules for interaction and movement so that movement and interaction with and within this space is possible" (p. 23-24). She argues that this point is "the heart of her ethnography" (p. 18). By participating in online research, Markham established an ethnographic site for examining the meanings of life online; a site where the social transformation of "meanings of identity, intimacy, and community" can be observed. It took three years for Markham to complete her study. Markham (1998: 18) contended, "in the end, this is a study of a place I helped create". Markham raised the question of what it means to have, or to be, a self in the disembodied spaces of life online. She pointed out, "although cyberspace is nothing more or less than a network of computer system passing digitized strings of information back and forth through copper or fiber-optic cables, people who connect to this network often feel a *sense of presence* when they are online. Even in purely text-based online contexts, people establish and maintain intimate friendships, romantic relationships, and stable communities" (p. 17, original emphasis). Ironically, in her conclusion, Markham eloquently put:

> In the end, I think the Internet is both blown completely out of proportion and completely underestimated regarding its capacity to change us and our world. I don't think it will take away our humanity, but I thing it has the capacity to take us away from a grounded, bound-to-the-earth sort of understanding of what it means to live a full and healthy life....This has serious implications for traditional notions of community, family and the environment, but it isn't the technology that does it to us. We engage it. We live it. We use it. We choose.

Paccagnella (1997) provided an innovative example of conducting ethnographic research on virtual communities through his work on the Italian virtual community built around a computer conference named cyber_punk. Paccagnella conducted an eighteen months participant observation in order to "gain an intimate understanding of the culture and the symbolic system of the conference" (p. 9). He recorded and archived all the messages in a separate file every month and managed to collect a total of 10,000 messages from 400 users. Paccagnella contended that in order to prevent him from "going native" in participant observation, he "exploited the possibility of an extremely simple, fast, and effective exploration of the thousands of collected messages: multiple windows showed on the screen the results of searches for particular situations for example the dialogues between specific groups of actors, in a given period, on a particular topic" (p. 10). He also performed some statistical analysis using content analysis program and SPSS. From his "integrated approach", Paccagnella was confident in his interpretation of "the basic social characteristics of this virtual community, including its peculiar slang, the role structure, socialization processes and the evolution over time of the overall social climate of the conference" (p. 10). Paccagnella also told us that it was "possible to understand and describe the expectations related, for example, to the role of leaders, whose linguistic competency is far from being simply that of a *computer nerd* and refers instead to a collective sense of identity" (p. 10). Moreover, Paccagnella suggested that his "analogical communication" analysis reveals "the importance of the use of smileys, interjections, and informal styles of conversation in the building of a strong and culturally vivacious community" (p. 10). See Holge-Hazelton for her participant observation with a group of young people with newly diagnosed diabetes within the "Diabetes a School for Life" study in Denmark and Cindy Mendelson for her experiences in conducting an ethnographic study of women with lupus that included an Internet component in this volume.

Discourse Analysis and Life History

The Internet, according to Eysenbach and Till (2001: 1103), "is the most comprehensive electronic archive of written material representing our world and peoples' opinions, concerns, and desires". It has become a forum of communication for many voiceless people to express themselves through such channels as bulletin boards, guestbooks, Web pages, newsgroups, usenets, listservs (mailing lists), chat rooms and IMs (Robinson, 2001), and recently Web logs (known as "blogs") (Chen et al., 2004). It then provides an excellent site for discourse analysis, one of the commonly employed approaches in unobtrusive methods. How people construct their own meaning of a social situation is a central concern of discourse analysis. Thomsen and others (1998: 12) point out, discourse analysis "is an attempt to recognise patterns, rules, or procedures that occur among participants and the way in which these structures or conventions influence meaning and effect". The method allows researchers to examine "the way meaning is accomplished by everyone involved" in their "ordinary, mundane, naturally occurring talk" (Mann and Stewart, 2000: 86). Researchers may adopt this method by observing "the natural conversations of various kinds of newsgroups, or synchronous conferencing (using real-time chat). By 'lurking' unseen, they are able to watch the interaction without intervening in any way" (Mann and Stewart, 2000: 86; Chen et al., 2004; See also Hardey, 2002; Gillet, 2003; Pitts, 2004; and Chapters by Bradley and Carter, Hardey, Lombardo and Gillet, Mendelson, and Thomas in this volume).

Denzin (1999), for example, conducted discourse analysis to examine the gendered narratives of self in a newsgroup known as alt.recovery.codependency (a.r.c.) on recovery from alcoholism by detailed examination of threads of conversation elaborated by participants. Alt.recovery.codependency (a.r.c.) is "an online Internet newsgroup that draws on the tenets of the Adult Children of Alcoholics (ACOA) and the Co-Dependents Anonymous (CoDA) movements" (p. 107). Denzin (1999: 108) argued that "cybernarratives are grounded in the everyday lives and biographies of the women and men who write them, yet they circulate in the anonymous, privatized territories of cyberspace. The life on the screen that occurs for this, or any other newsgroup, involves struggles over identity, meaning, and the self" (see also Turkle, 1995, Markham, 1998; Baym, 2000; Kendall, 2002; see also Chapters 4 and 5 in this volume). As in any newsgroup, the users participating in the newsgroup post messages to all Internet sites which carry the newsgroup and others may respond to a specific message. From these responses, a "thread or connected series of messages" can be created (Parks and Floyd, 1996: 80). Denzin (1999) performed intensive discourse analyses of two complex threads in this study: "Choices, Holidays and Gifts" and "Help Me Understand Something". Clearly, Denzin adopted lurking in this study. Denzin (1999: 123) admited that, "I never identified myself to the group, nor did I obtain permission to quote from posting, thereby violating many of Schrum's (1995) ethical injunctions for electronic research". However, Denzin (1999: 122) claimed that his observation of online communities help to "make visible the cultural apparatuses and biographical histories that allow such talk to be produced and understood". See also Hardey (2002) for his recent analysis of personal home pages containing individuals' accounts of their illnesses posted on the Internet and Chapter 14 in this volume.

The rise of new technologies which are implicated in postmodern life also renders changes in the way oral history is conducted, archived and retrieved (Plummer, 2001: 98). As

Berg (2004: 59) points out, oral historians can now quickly access archives located on the Web, whereas it might have been taken days or weeks to reach their sources in the past. Plummer (2001: 96) contends that life histories begin to appear in new forms of media. Due to the advance of online communication, Plummer (2001: 99) suggests, "life stories may be put in digital form and made accessible with hypertext allowing the reader access to an electronic document where each page has many buttons which can lead you to further pages". Plummer also points out "we are just at the start of what may be called 'virtual life story documents' – existing in computer memories, but having no tangible form in print. And of course, through a global information highway, much of this can move across vast spaces in a rapid time".

Solomon (2004, and in this volume), for example, conducted an online research on personal stories of people living with Multiple Sclerosis (MS). Solomon (2004: 1) contended "personal stories of tragedy and triumph over illness have turned ordinary citizens into heroes, and celebrities into spokespersons for disease". In this study, Solomon examined "the ways in which members of a social support group for Multiple Sclerosis used narrative resources to accomplish their identities and communicate information and support about their illness experiences with one another in an online support group" (p. 2). Solomon went through a number of MS Web sites but discovered that only one site would agree for the research to be carried out with their members. This site was an active support group for people living with MS and their families and was established by a woman with MS. The information about the study was posted on the message board. Solomon sent an introductory message to the online group members and asked for their permission to use their stories and support they shared online in her research. Solomon (2004: 4) told us that "within twenty minutes of posting my Introductory Message group members began responding with welcoming permission and encouragement". As Solomon attempted to observe the narrative interactions occurring among group members, she did not pose formal interview questions nor initiate online conversations after the initial contact. She maintained her role as an observer. During the eight weeks period, more than 150 stories posted on the message board were collected. Solomon (2004: 12) concluded in the study that "the personal ways in which narrative resources are taken up, and the unique ways that illness experiences are expressed, re-inform available narrative resources indicating to us and to others that our experiences story a unique and authentic identity".

Multi-Methods Approach

It should be noted, though, that there has been an increasing use of a multi-methods approach on online research in a similar way to conventional methods (see for example, Kleinman, 2004; Sade-Beck, 2004). As Denzin (1970), Silverman (1993), Hammersley and Atkinson (1995) and Creswell (2003) suggest, we will not obtain a full story from just one method, online researchers have utilised multi-method for triangulation. For those who decide to use both online and face-to-face interviews, Markham (2005: 809) contends, may "claim that their efforts will add authenticity to their interpretation-by adding paralinguistic or nonverbal cues to the words people speak-and thereby add more credibility to their findings".

Paccagnella (1997) and Sharf (1999), for example, undertook participation observation of groups online, but they also carried out documentary analysis of newsgroup or list materials. Some researchers attempt to access the users of virtual worlds in real life (Turkle, 1995). Baym (1995) too makes clear that her ethnographic study on the performance of humour in cyberspace made use of both observation online and interaction with the participants. Correll (1995) used a three-way methodology to study an online community and its processes. First, she observed the daily traffic between participants at a virtual café, occasionally asking them to explain various actions or conversations. Second, she interviewed 12 participants using semi-structured interviews via private email. Finally, she interviewed 8 participants in two face-to-face focus groups. Kendall (1999) also combined three years of online participant observation, thirty face-to-face interviews, participation in face-to-face gatherings and analysis of online documentary material via newsgroups and email lists in her research on an online forum known as BlueSky. Kendall (1999: 70-71) contends that "nobody lives only in cyberspace… [hence] the ability to access offline environments provides useful information between online and off-line interaction". She concludes that the comparison of participants' narratives of their online behaviour with the actuality of that behaviour helps her to critically examine claims made by participants about the effects of online participation. Kleinman (2004) too, in her case study of an online mailing list (listserv) named OURNET which examined how women in science and engineering use online group as a resource for social support, information, role models and mentors, utilised email message, interphone interviews, online participant observation and the membership roster.

Recently, Sade-Beck (2004) conducted a virtual ethnography about Israeli support communities involved in loss and bereavement. He wanted to examine "the characteristic traits of expression of very painful and difficult emotions of bereavement over the Internet in the Israeli context" (p. 2). Sade-Beck (2004: 2) argued that the advancement of electronic technology and large number of Internet-base studies "offer anthropologist a new and fascinating field for social research" but at the same time they present "a long line of methodological difficulties". How do researchers conduct a fieldwork in cyberspace? How do we observe participants for a long period of time? How do people express their emotions in an alienated virtual world? Can we actually observe this in the written world? Sade-Beck attempted to overcome this problem by combining three methods in the study: online observations, offline interviews, and content analysis of supplementary materials including traditional hard copy press, the online press and Internet databases.

Sade-Beck (2004) contended that only through the use of the mixed-method, rich ethnographic material was collected. For Sade-Beck (2004: 11), the use of three methods, online and offline, helped him to "collect comprehensive information from various realms about the sites and to assemble a complex ethnography". Sade-Beck (2004: 13) also recommended the use of both online and offline for data collection in virtual ethnography so that researchers may be able to obtain the "overflowing description". Sade-Beck (2004: 13) concluded that the use of multi-methods was "to overcome the problematic aspects involved in ethnographic Internet research following the false dichotomy between the virtual world and the actual real world, and the need to redefine fieldwork so as to mediate between the two worlds".

Conclusion

In this chapter, I have provided readers with some practical ways of doing research online. These include discussions on CMC, how to access potential research participants, how to obtain informed consent and qualitative research methods commonly employed in online research with empirical examples. What I hope to achieve in this chapter is that readers may adopt certain aspects I have outlined here to their research projects. We learn from previous mistakes and good things and from this learning we then will be able to carry out our research more efficiently. Some of the examples I have outlined here will do just that: giving readers some practical experiences of doing research in cyberspace.

Acknowledgement

This chapter is based on a chapter in my book, Qualitative Research Methods, 2nd edition, published by Oxford University Press, 2005. Permission is granted by Oxford University Press.

References

[1] Adler, C.L. and Zarchin, Y.R., 2002, 'The "Virtual Focus Groups": Using the Internet to Reach Pregnant Women on Home Bed Rest', *Journal of Obstetrics, Gynaecologist and Neonatal Nursing*, vol. 31, pp. 418-427.

[2] Barnes, S.B., 2004, 'Issues of Attribution and Identifiction in Online Social Research', in M.D. Johns, S-L.S. Chen, and G.J. Hall (eds), *Online Social Research: Methods, Issues, and Ethics*, pp. 203-222, Peter Lang, New York.

[3] Baym, N.K., 1995, The Performance of Humour in Computer-Mediated Communication, Journal of Computer Mediated Communication [on-line journal], vol. 1, no. 2. *<http://shum.huji.ac.il/jcmc/vol1/issue2/baym.html>*

[4] Baym, N.K., 1999, 'The Emergence of On-Line Community', in S.G. Jones (ed.), *Cybersociety2.0: Revisiting Computer-Mediated Communication and Community*, pp. 35-68, Sage, Thousand Oaks, CA.

[5] Baym, N.K., 2000, *Tune In, Log On: Soaps, Fandom, and Online Community*. Sage Publications, Thousand Oaks, CA.

[6] Bennett, C., 1998, Men Online: Discussing Lived Experiences on the Internet, Unpublished honours dissertation, James cook University, Townsville, Queensland, Australia.

[7] Berg, B.L., 2004, *Qualitative Research Methods for the Social Sciences*, Pearson, Boston.

[8] Burawoy, M., Blum, J.A., George, S., Gille, Z. Gowan, T., Haney, L., Klawiter, M., Lopez, S.H., Riain, S.O. and Thayer, M., 2000, *Global Ethnography: Forces, Connections, and Imaginations in a Postmodern World*, University of Los Angeles Press, Berkeley.

[9] Chen, S-L.,S., Hall, G.J., and Johns, M.D., 2004, 'Research Paparazzi in Cyberspace: The Voices of the Researched', in M.D. Johns, S-L.S. Chen, and G.J. Hall (eds.), *Online Social Research: Methods, Issues, and Ethics*, pp. 157-175, Peter Lang, New York.

[10] Chin, P.L., 2003, 'From the Editor', *Advances in Nursing Science*, vol. 26, no. 4, pp. 239.

[11] Clegg Smith, K.M., 2004, '"Electronic Eavesdropping": The Ethical Issues Involved in Conducting a Virtual Ethnography', in M.D. Johns, S-L.S. Chen, and G.J. Hall (eds.), *Online Social Research: Methods, Issues, and Ethics*, pp. 223-238, Peter Lang, New York.

[12] Coomber, R., 1997, 'Using the Internet for Survey Research', *Sociological Research Online,* vol. 2, no. 2. *<http://ww.socresonline.org.uk/socresonline/2/2/2.html>*

[13] Correll, S., 1995, 'The Ethnography of an Electronic Bar: The Lesbian Café', *Journal of Contemporary Ethnography*, vol. 24, pp. 270-298.

[14] Cotten, S.R., and Gupta, S.S., 2004, 'Characteristics of Online and Offline Health Information Seekers and Factors that Discriminate Between Them', *Social Science and Medicine*, vol 59, pp. 1795-1806.

[15] Cotton, A.H., 2003, 'The Discursive Field of Web-Based Health Research: Implication for Nursing Research in Cyberspace', *Advances in Nursing Science*, vol. 26, no. 4, pp. 307-319.

[16] Couper, M.P., Blair, J. and Triplett, T., 1999, 'A Comparison of Mail and Email for a Survey of Employees in US Statistical Agencies', *Journal of Official Statistics*, vol. 15, pp. 39-56.

[17] Creswell, J.W., 1998, *Qualitative Inquiry and Research Design: Choosing Among Five Traditions*, Sage, Thousand Oaks, CA.

[18] Creswell, J.W. 2003, *Research Design: Qualitative, Quantitative, and Mixed Methods Approaches*, Sage, Thousand Oaks, CA.

[19] Davis, M., G. Bolding, Hart, G., Sherr, L and Elford, J, 2004, 'Reflecting on The Experience of Interviewing Online: Perspectives From the Internet and HIV Study in London', *AIDS Care*, vol. 16, no. 8, pp. 944-52.

[20] Denzin, N., 1997, *Interpretive Ethnography: Ethnographic Practices for the 21st Century*, Sage, Thousand Oaks, CA.

[21] Denzin, N.K., 1970, *The Research Act*, Aldine, Chicago.

[22] Denzin, N., 1999, 'Cybertalk and the Method of Instances', in S. Jones (ed.) 1999, *Doing Internet Research: Critical Issues and Methods for Examining the Net*, pp. 107-125, Sage Publications, Thousand Oaks, CA.

[23] Denzin, N.K., 2004, 'Prologue: Online Environments and Interpretive Social Research', in M.D. Johns, S-L.S. Chen, and G.J. Hall (eds.), *Online Social Research: Methods, Issues, and Ethics*, pp. 1-12, Peter Lang, New York.

[24] Danzin, N.K. and Lincoln, Y.S. 2005, *Handbook of Qualitative Research, 3rd edition*, Sage, Thousand Oaks, CA.

[25] Dicks, B. and Mason, B., 1998, 'Hypermedia and Ethnography: Reflections on the Construction of a Research Approach', *Sociological Research Online*, vol. 3, no. 3. *<http://www.socresonline.org.uk/3/3/3.html>*

[26] Dillman, D.A., 2000, *Mail and Internet Surveys. The Tailored Design Method*, 2nd ed., John Wiley and Sones, New York.

[27] Dillman, D.A. and Bowker, D.K., 2001, 'The Web Questionnaire Challenge to Survey Methodologists', in M. Bosnjak (ed.), *Dimensions of Internet Science*, pp. 159-178, Pabst Science Publishers, Lengerich.

[28] Dunne, G., 1999, *The Different Dimensions of Gay Fatherhood: Exploding the Myths*, Report to the Economic and Social Research Council, London School of Economics, London.

[29] Eichhorn, K., 2001, 'Sites Unseen: Ethnographic Research in a Textual Community', *International Journal of Qualitative Studies in Education*, vol. 14, no. 4, pp. 565-578.

[30] Elford, J., Bolding, G., Davis, M., Sherr, L. and Hart, G., 2004, 'The Internet and HIV Study: Design and Methods', *BMG Public Health*, vol. 4, no. 39. *<http://www.biomedcentral.com/bmcpublichealth>*

[31] Evans, P. and Wurster, T.S., 1999, *Blown to Bits: How the New Economic of Information Transforms Strategy*, Harvard Business School Press, Boston, Massachusetts.

[32] Eysenbach, G., and Till, J.E., 2001, 'Ethical Issues in Qualitative Research on Internet Communities', *British Medical Journal*, vol. 323, no. 7321, pp. 1103-1105.

[33] Eysenbach, G. and Wyatt, J., 2002, 'Using the Internet for Surveys and Health Research', *Journal of Medical Internet Research*, vol. 4: e13.

[34] Ferri, B., 2000, 'The Hidden Cost of Difference: Women with Learning Disabilities', *Learning Disabilties: A Multidisciplinary Journal*, vol.10, no. 3, pp. 129-138.

[35] Foster, G., 1994, 'Fishing the Net for Research Data', *British Journal of Educational Technology*, vol. 25, no. 2, pp. 91-97.

[36] Foster, P., 1996, 'Observational Research', in R. Sapsford and V. Jupp (eds.), *Data Collection and Analysis*, pp. 57-93, Sage Publications, London.

[37] Gaiser, T., 1997, 'Conducting Online Focus Groups', *Social Science Computer Review*, vol. 15, pp. 135-144.

[38] Galegher, J., Sproull, L. and Kiesler, S., 1998, 'Legitimacy, Authority, and Community in Electronic Support Grouts', *Written Communication*, vol. 15, pp. 493-530.

[39] Greenbaum, T.L., 2001, 'Online Focus Groups are No Substitute for the Real Thing', Groups Plus. < heet://www.groupsplus.com/pages/qmr0601.html>

[40] Hamman, R., 1996, 'One Hour in the eWorld Hot Tub: A Brief Ethnographic Project in Cyberspace'. *<http://www.socio.demon.co.uk/project.html>*

[41] Hardey, M., 2002, ''The Story of My Illness': Personal Accounts of Illness on the Internet', *Health:*, vol. 6, no. 1, pp. 6-11.

[42] Hessler, R.M., Downing, J., Beltz, C., Pelliccio, A., Powell. M. and Vale, W., 2003, 'Qualitative Research on Adolescent Risk Using E-Mail: A Methodological Assessment', *Qualitative Sociology*, vol. 26, no. 1, pp. 111-124.

[43] Hine, C., 2000, *Virtual Ethnography*, Sage, London.

[44] Hodkinson, P., 2000, *The Goth Scene as Trans-Local Subculture*, Unpublished PhD thesis, Centre for Urban and Regional Studies, University of Birmingham, UK.

[45] Holge-Hazelton, B., 2002, 'The Internet: A New Field for Qualitative Inquiry?', *Forum qualitative Social Research* [on-line journal], vol. 3, no. 2. *<http://www.qualitative-research.net/fgs/fqs-eng.html>*

[46] Horn, S., 1998, *Cyberville: Clicks, Culture and the Creation of an Online Town*, Warner Books, New York.

[47] Illingworth, N., 2001, 'The Internet Matters: Exploring the Use of the Internet as a Research Tool', *Sociological Research Online*, vol. 6, no. 2. <*www.socresonline.org.uk /6/2/illingworth.html*>

[48] Im, E-O., and Chee, W., 2003, 'Feminist Issues in E-Mail Group Discussion among Cancer Patients', *Advances in Nursing Science*, vol. 26, no. 4, pp. 287-298.

[49] Jerome, L.W., Deleon, P.H., James, L.C., Folen, R., Earles, J. and Gedney, J.J., 2000, 'The Coming Age of Telecommunication in Psychological Research and Practice', *American Psychologist*, vol. 55, pp. 407-421.

[50] Jones, S. (ed.) 1999, *Doing Internet Research: Critical Issues and Methods for Examining the Net,* Sage Publications, Thousand Oaks, CA.

[51] Jones, S., 2004, 'Introduction: Ethics and Internet Studies', in M.D. Johns, S-L.S. Chen, and G.J. Hall (eds.), *Online Social Research: Methods, Issues, and Ethics*, pp. 179-185, Peter Lang, New York.

[52] Kehoe, C.M. and Pitkow, J.E., 1996, 'Surveying the Territory: GVU's Five WWW User Surveys', *World Wide Web Journal*, vol. 1, no. 3, pp. 77-84.

[53] Kendall, L., 1999, 'Recontexualizing Cyberspace: Methodological Considerations for On-Line Research', in S. Jones (ed.) 1999, *Doing Internet Research: Critical Issues and Methods for Examining the Net*, pp.57-74, Sage Publications, Thousand Oaks, CA.

[54] Kendall, L. 2000, *Hanging Out in the Virtual Pub: Masculinities and Relationships Online*. University of California Press, Berkeley.

[55] Kendall, L., 2004, 'Participants and Observers in Online Ethnography: Five Stories about Identity', in M.D. Johns, S-L.S. Chen, and G.J. Hall (eds.), *Online Social Research: Methods, Issues, and Ethics*, pp. 125-140, Peter Lang, New York.

[56] Kleinman, S.S., 2004, 'Researching OURNET: A Case Study of a Multiple Methods Approach', in M.D. Johns, S-L.S. Chen, and G.J. Hall (eds.), *Online Social Research: Methods, Issues, and Ethics*, pp. 47-62, Peter Lang, New York.

[57] Koch, N.S. and Emrey, J.A., 2001, 'The Internet and Opinion Management: Surveying Marginalized Populations', *Social Science Quarterly*, vol. 82, pp. 131-138.

[58] Kummervold, P.E., Gammon, D., Bergvik, S., Johnsen, J.K., Hasvold, T. and Rosenvinge, J.H., 2002, 'Social Support in a Wired World: Use of Online Mental Health Forums in Norway', *Nordic Journal of Psychiatry*, vol. 56, no. 1, pp. 59-65.

[59] LeBesco, K., 2004, 'Managing Visibility, Intimacy, and Focus in Online Critical Ethnography', in M.D. Johns, S-L.S. Chen, and G.J. Hall (eds.), *Online Social Research: Methods, Issues, and Ethics*, pp. 63-79, Peter Lang, New York.

[60] Liamputtong, P. and Ezzy, D., 2005, *Qualitative Research Methods, 2nd edition*, Oxford University Press, Melbourne.

[61] Light, D.W., 2001, 'Managed Competition, Governmentality, and Institutional Response in the United Kingdom', *Social Science and Medicine*, vol. 52, pp. 1167-1181.

[62] Madge, C. and O'Connor, H., 2002, 'On-Line with E-Mums: Exploring the Internet as a Medium for Research', *Area*, vol. 34, no. 1, pp. 92-102.

[63] Mann, C. and Stewart, F., 2000, *Internet Communication and Qualitative Research: A Handbook for Researching Online*, Sage Publications, London.

[64] Mann, C. and Stewart, F., 2002, 'Internet Interviewing', in J.F. Gubrium and J.A. Holstein (eds.), *Handbook of Interview Research: Context and Method*, pp. 603-627, Sage Publications, Thousand Oaks.

[65] Marcus, G.E., 1995, 'Ethnography in/of the World System: The Emergencies of Multisited Ethnography', *Annual Review of Anthropology*, vol. 24, pp, 95-117.

[66] Marcus, G.E., 1998, *Ethnography Through Thick and Thin*, Princeton University Press, Princeton.

[67] Markham, A.H., 1998, *Life Online: Researching Real Experience in Virtual Space*, AltaMira Press, Walnut Creek, CA.

[68] Markham, A.H., 2004, "representation in Online Ethographies: A Matter of Context Sensitivities, in M.D. Johns, S-L.S. Chen, and G.J. Hall (eds.), *Online Social Research: Methods, Issues, and Ethics*, pp. 141-156, Peter Lang, New York.

[69] Markham, A.H., 'The Methods, Politics, and Ethics of Representation in Online Ethnography', in N.K. Denzin and Y.S. Lincoln (eds.), *Handbook of Qualitative Research 3rd edition*, pp. 793-820, Sage Publications, Thousand Oaks, CA.

[70] Marvasti, A.B., 2004, *Qualitative Research in Sociology*, Sage, London.

[71] Mehta, R. and Sivadas, E., 1995, 'Comparing Response Rates and Response Content in Mail versus Electronic Mail Surveys', *Journal of the Market Research Society*, vol. 37, no. 4, pp. 429-439.

[72] Merkes, M. 2002, 'BabyBoomWomen@Work2020 – Reflections on the Methodology of a Research Project using Futures Scenarios and Computer Mediated Communication', *Journal of Futures Studies*, vol.6, no. 3, pp. 83-94.

[73] Merkes, M. 2003, *A Longer Working Life for Australian Women of the Baby Boom Generation? – Women's Voices and the Social Policy Implications of an Ageing Female Workforce*, unpublished doctoral thesis, School of Public Health, La Trobe University, Melbourne.

[74] Moloney, M.A., Dietrich, A.S., Strickland, O.L. and Myerburg, S., 2003, 'Using Internet Discussion Boards as Virtual Focus Groups', *Advances in Nursing Science*, vol. 26, no. 4, pp. 274-286.

[75] Murray, P.J., 1997, 'Using Virtual Focus Groups in Qualitative Research', *Qualitative Health Research*, vol. 7, no. 4, pp. 542-554.

[76] Newman, M.A., 2003, 'A World of No Boundaries', *Advances in Nursing Science*, vol. 26, no. 4, pp. 240-245.

[77] O'Connor, H. and Madge, C., 2001, 'Cyber-Mothers: Online Synchronous Interviewing using Conferencing Software', Sociological Research Online, vol. 5, no. 4. *<http://www.socresonline.org.uk/5/4/oconnor.html>*

[78] O'Neil, D., 2002, 'Assessing Community Informatics: A Review of Methodological Approaches for Evaluating Community Networks and Community Technology Centers', *Internet Research: Electronic Networking Applications and Policy*, vol. 12, no. 1, pp. 76-102.

[79] Paccagnella, L., 1997, 'Getting the Seats of Your Pants Dirty: Strategies for Ethnographic Research on Virtual Communities', *Journal of Computer Mediated Communication*, vol. 3, no. 1, pp. 1-17. *<http//www.ascusc.org/jcmc/vol3/issue1/ paccangella.html>*

[80] Pandey, S.K., Hart, J.J. and Tiwary, S., 2003, 'Women's Health and the Internet: Understanding Emerging Trends and Implications', *Social Science and Medicine*, vol. 56, pp. 179-191.

[81] Parker, L., 1992, 'Collecting Date the E-Mail Way', Training and Development, vol. 46, no. 7, pp. 52-55.

[82] Parks, M. and Floyd, K., 1996, 'Making Friends in Cyberspace', *Journal of Communication*, vol. 46, pp. 80-97.

[83] Plummer, K., 2001, *Document of Life 2: An Invitation to a Critical Humanism*, Sage Publications, London.

[84] Pop, C. and Mays, N., 2000, *Qualitative Research in Health Care, 2nd edition*, BMJ Books, London.

[85] Powell, J., McCarthy, N. and Eysenbach, G., 2003, 'Cross-Sectional Survey of Users of Internet Depression Communities', *BioMed Central (BMC) Psychiatry*, vol. 3, no. 19, pp. 1-7. <http//www. biomedcentral.com/1471-244X/3/19>

[86] Reid, E., 1996, 'Informed consent in the Study of On-Line communities. A Reflection on the Effects of Computer-Mediated Social Research', *The Information Society*, vol. 12, no. 2, pp. 169-174. *<http://www.slis.indiana.edu/TIS/abstracts/ab12-2/reid.html>*

[87] Rezebek, R.J., 2000, 'Online Focus Groups: Electronic Discussions for Research', Forum Qualitative Social Research [On-line Journal], vol.1. no. 1. *<http://qualitative-research.net/fqs>*

[88] Rheingold, H., 1993, *The Virtual Community: Homesteading on the Electronic Frontier*, Addison-Wesley, Menlo Park, CA.

[89] Ritchie, J. and Lewis, J., 2003, *Qualitative Research Practice: A Guide for Social Science Students and Researchers*, Sage, London.

[90] Riva, G., 2001, 'The Mind over the Web: The Quest for the Definition of a Method for Internet Research', *CyberPsychology and Behavior*, vol. 4, no. 1, pp. 7-16.

[91] Robinson, K.M., 2001, 'Unsolicited Narratives from the Internet: A Rich Source of Qualitative Data', *Qualitative Health Research*, vol. 11, no. 5, pp. 706-714.

[92] Robson, K., 1999, *Employment Experiences of Ulcerative Colitis and Crohn's Disease Sufferers*. Unpublished PhD thesis, Cardiff University, Cardiff.

[93] Seale, C., Gobo, G., Gubrium, J.F. and Silverman, D. (eds.), 2004, *Qualitative Research Practice*, Sage, London.

[94] Sade-Beck, L., 2004, 'Internet Ethnography: Online and Offline', International Journal of Qualitative Methods, vol. 3, no. 2. Article 4. *<http://www.ualberta.ca/~iiqm/backissues/3_2/pdf/sadebeck.pdf>*

[95] Schrum, L., 1995, 'Framing the Debate: Ethical Research in the Information Age', *Qualitative Inquiry*, vol. 1, pp. 311-326.

[96] Selwyn, N. and Robson, K., 1998, 'Using E-Mail as a Research Tool', Social Research Update 21. *<http://www.soc.surrey.ac.uk/sru/SRU21.html>*

[97] Seymour, W. and Lupton, D., 2004, 'Holding the Line Online: Exploring Wired Relationships for People with Disabilities', *Disability and Society*, vol. 19, no. 4, pp. 291-305.

[98] Seymour, W.W.D., Lupton, D. and Fahey, N., 1999, *Negotiating Disability, Technology and Risk: Towards a New Perspective*, Report, School of Social Work and Social Policy, University of South Australia, Magill Campus.

[99] Sharf, B.F., 1999, 'Beyond Netiquette: The Ethics of Doing Naturalistic Discourse Research on the Internet, in Jones, S. (ed.) 1999, *Doing Internet Research: Critical Issues and Methods for Examining the Net*, pp. 243-256, Sage Publications, Thousand Oaks, CA.

[100] Silverman, D., 1993, *Interpreting Text and Data: Methods for Analysing Talk, Text and Interaction*, Sage, London.

[101] Silverman, D., (ed.), 2004, *Qualitative Research: Theory, Method and Practice, 2nd edition*, Sage, London.

[102] Smith, C.B., 1997, 'Casting the Net: Surveying and Internet Population', *Journal of Computer Mediated Communication*, vol. 3, no. 1, pp. 1-17. *<http//www.ascusc.org/ jcmc/vol3/issue1/smith.htm>*

[103] Solomon, M., 2004, 'Illness Narratives: Sharing Stories and Support Online: A Study of Narrative Resources and Identity in and Online Support Group for Multiple Sclerosis', paper presented at the *10th Annual International Qualitative Health Research Conference*, Banff, Alberta, Canada, April 30 – May 4, 2004.

[104] Spender, D. 1997, The Position of Women in Information Technology – Or Who Got There first and With What Consequences? *Current Sociology*, vol. 45, no. 2, pp. 135-147.

[105] Stewart, F., Eckerman, E. and Zhou, K., 1998, 'Using the Internet in Qualitative Public Health Research: A Comparison of Chinese and Australia Young Women's Perceptions of Tobacco Use', Internet Journal of Health Promotion, December 29 [On-line]. *<http://www.monash.edu.au/health/IJHP/1998/12>*

[106] Strickland, O.L., Moloney, M.F., Dietrich, A.S., Myerburg, S., Cotsonis, G.A. and Johnson, R.V., 2003, 'Measurement Issues Related to Data Collection on the World Wide Web', *Advances in Nursing Science*, vol. 26, no. 4, pp. 246-256.

[107] Sweet, C., 1999, 'Anatomy of an On-Line Focus Group', *Quirk's Marketing Research Review*, December. *<http://www.quirks.com/articles>*

[108] Sweet, C., 2001, 'Designing and Conducting Virtual Focus Groups', *Qualitative Market Research: An International Journal, Research in Cyber Space*, June, pp. 1-10. *<casey@focusgroupsonline.net>*

[109] Sweet, C. and Walkowski, J., 2002, Frequently Asked Questions (FAQs) About Online Qualitative Research, The QRCA Online Qualitative Research Task Force, New York.

[110] Thomas, B., Stamler, L.L., Lafreniere, K. and Dumala, R., 2000, 'The Internet: An Effective Tool for Nursing Research with Women', *Computers in Nursing*, vol. 18, pp. 13-18.

[111] Thomas, B., Stamler, L.L., Lafreniere, K., Out, J. and Delahunt, T.D., 2002, 'Using the Internet to Identify Women's Sources of Breast Health Education and Screening', *Women and Health*, vol. 36, no. 1, pp. 33-48.

[112] Thomsen, S.R., Straubhaar, J.D. and Bolyard, D.M., 1998, 'Ethnomethodology and the Study of Online Communities: Exploring the Cyberstreets', *Information Research* [on-line], vol. 3. no.3. *<http://www.shef.ac.uk/~is/publications/infres/paper50.html>*

[113] Tingling, P., Parent, M. and Wade, M., 2003, 'Extending the Capabilities of Internet-Based Research: Lessons from the Field', *Internet Research: Electronic Networking Applications and Policy*, vol. 13, no. 3, pp. 223-235.

[114] Turkle, S., 1995, *Life on the Screen: Identity in the Age of the Internet*, Simon and Schuster, New York.

[115] Williams, M., 2003, *Virtually Criminal: Deviance and Harm within Online Environments*. Unpublished PhD thesis, Cardiff University, Cardiff.

[116] Williams, M. and Robson, K, 2004, 'Reengineering Focus Group Methodology for the Online Environment', in M.D. Johns, S-L.S. Chen, and G.J. Hall (eds.), *Online Social Research: Methods, Issues, and Ethics*, pp. 25-45, Peter Lang, New York.

[117] Wittel, A., 2000, 'Ethnography on the Move: From Field to Net to Internet', *Forum qualitative Social Research* [on-line journal], vol. 1, no. 1. *<http://qualitative-research.net/fgs/fqs>*

[118] Zahir, S., Dobing, B. and Hunter, M.G., 2002, 'Cross-Cultural Dimensions of Internet Protals', *Internet Research: Electronic Networking Applications and Policy*, vol. 12, no. 3, pp. 210-220.

[119] Ziebland, S., 2004, 'The Importance of Being Expert: The Quest for Cancer Information on the Internet', *Social Science and Medicine*, vol. 59, pp. 1783-1793.

In: Health Research in Cyberspace
Editor: Pranee Liamputtong, pp. 49-66
ISBN 1-59454-819-6

Chapter 3

An Expanding Universe of Symbiotic and Colliding Worlds: Issues and Concerns for Healthcare Professionals Conducting Health Research in Cyberspace

Antoinette H. Cotton

Background

In a society that is seemingly growing more and more dependent on Computer Mediated Communication (CMC) technologies across the realms of health, healthcare, education, economics, politics and daily life, there is currently increasing pressure for healthcare professionals to embrace these new technologies in their healthcare delivery, health promotion, education and research practices. CMC refers to "both the physical layer where the work takes place in the human/computer interface, and the applications that are then possible…in the discovery, search and retrieval of information" (Paulsen, 1994: 1). Thomas et al. (2000:13) suggest the "increased use of electronic networking and collaborative problem solving …may be the hallmark of healthcare professionals in the 21st Century", while Waldo (2000: 99) insists "it's not only time to adopt Internet technology, it's mandatory".

The Internet is the largest global computer network, linking satellites, computer networks and people, seemingly erasing boundaries of time and distance with its multidirectional, transnational, instantaneous communication abilities. The Internet has been promoted as a low cost, easy access, fast response, time-saving, flexible medium in which to conduct both quantitative and qualitative research, enabling potential data collection not only from large and diverse segments of populations across the globe, but also from reluctant and vulnerable groups (Lakeman, 1997; Kaye and Johnson, 1999; Fyfe et al., 2001; Duffy, 2002; Elford et al., 2004).

Although graphical, three-dimensional, virtual worlds with synchronous, rich, multimedia interaction may provide potential innovative modes for data-collection, to date cyber researchers have largely concentrated on text-based systems. Such cyber research data collection methods have been used in studies of diverse health related topics as: anorexia nervosa (Hardin, 2003), functional abilities of girls with Rett Syndrome (Fyfe et al., 2001), online cancer support groups (Sharf, 1997; Klemm et al., 1998; 1999), online support for caregivers of survivors of stroke (Pierce et al., 2002), the lived experiences of pregnant women confined to home rest following a diagnosis of preterm labour (Adler and Zarchin, 2002), experiences of perimenopausal women with migraine headaches (Moloney et al, 2003), and online support to middle-aged rural women living with chronic illness (Cudney and Weinert, 2000).

Given the embeddedness of the phenomena in wider disciplinary, cultural, political and social contexts, the dynamic, multidimensional (including virtual) identities of cyber participants and researchers, power contestations, and the importance of material and discursive contexts in constituting the phenomenon, there is a need for critical evaluation of not only the utility of cyber health research as a data collection method, but also the many ontological, ethical, methodological, professional and political challenges and implications it raises. Hence, this chapter seeks to interrogate the literature related to health research in cyberspace, particularly as it relates to the constitution of the discursive and non-discursive worlds and their relation to other online and offline worlds of embodied cyber participants and cyber researchers, and draw out implications for healthcare professionals conducting health related research in cyberspace.

The Phenomenon in Wider Contexts

Health research in cyberspace is a complex, multifaceted, dynamic phenomenon that varies across multiple dimensions (for example, ontological and experiential), contexts (such as online, offline, socio-cultural), and perspectives (connected, unconnected, cyber participants, cyber researchers, patients, and clinicians). Each view has its own horizons of meanings and understandings, as well as being situated differently in terms of dominant power-knowledge structures.

Hegemonic and Subjugated Knowledges

Health and healthcare discourses are embedded in and informed by a complex array of diverse and often competing discourses (such as scientific, technological, academic, professional, medical, economic, holistic and caring discourses), that dynamically contest for dominance in a "battle about the status of truth and the economic and political role it plays", where 'true' discourses are "centred on the form of scientific discourse and the institutions that support it" (Foucault, 1980a: 131-132). With the emergence of cyber research, new political struggles and "discipline anxiety" (Willcocks, 2004: 273) over what is to be legitimated as scientific knowledge have developed.

According to Foucault (1980b: 106), "disciplines are the bearers of a discourse", aiming to define, describe and delimit what may or may not be possible said, done and thought about a particular area such as cyber health and healthcare. Discourses are historically contingent, institutionally rule-governed " practices that systematically form the objects of which they speak" (Foucault, 1994: 49). Professional healthcare discourses of, in and around cyber health and healthcare have provided sites for new kinds of subjects (such as virtual patients, electronic healthcare professionals, cyber health research participants and cyber healthcare researchers), and constituted not only such new knowledge objects as electronic healthcare and cyber health, but also cyber disorders like cyber sex addiction, Internet Addiction Disorder, compulsive online shopping and gambling (see Young, 1998; Hansen, 2002; Johansson and Gotestam, 2004).

Wajcman (2004: 128) maintains the "juxtaposition of scientific expertise with lay citizens' knowledge has become a mainstream political issue in today's accident-prone world". The current, professional healthcare literature, in the rhetoric of autonomy and devolution, extols the potential democratic, revolutionary and transformative potential of cyberspace, proclaiming cyber health consumers will be able to optimally take charge of their own health. The literature, however, goes on to paint an alarming picture of "patients who surf the Internet…drowning" in the avalanche of health and medical information (Brooks, 2001: 69), hundreds of proliferating pseudoscientific, commercial, and unauthorized health-related websites targeting unsuspecting, potential research participants, and a plethora of outdated, poor quality, inaccurate, even potentially life threatening health information on the Internet, often provided by unqualified individuals. Hence, it is argued, the urgent need for the offline experts in health care and health research (scientists, academics, health and healthcare professionals) to extend their authority, expertise and methods online to prevent or minimize cyber health consumers and potential cyber health research participants making misguided decisions with harmful effect (see Klemm et al., 1998; 1999; Eachus, 1999; Hamilton, 1999; Rodriguez, 1999; Brooks, 2001; Eysenbach et al., 2002; Stanberry, 2002; Terry, 2002).

The healthcare gaze is the authoritative, seeing, hearing, speaking, governing judgemental gaze of the healthcare professional, supported and legitimated by the social institutions of science, the academy and the health professions. Such a gaze is not only therapeutic; it is also "calculating" and aims to dominate the entire field of possible knowledge (Foucault, 1975: 89). This deciphering, rationalist, professional speaking gaze "can understood only by those initiated into true speech" (Foucault, 1975: 115). Whilst there are up to 10,000 languages on earth, fewer than a hundred are spoken by 95% of the population (Ferraro, 1998). The English language, at levels "frequently too high," even for those whose first language is English (Eysenbach et al., 2002: 2694), dominates the content of health-related Internet sites, discriminating against most of the global population who would be unable to read it, even if they had access to it (see also Chapter 1 in this volume). Academic, technological and disciplinary language exacerbates the researcher-participant divide, with potentially serious consequences for health outcomes, research findings and ethical conduct of the research. Nonetheless, hegemonic discourses reconstruct cyber participants as rational consumers and decision makers who can make informed decisions about the benefits and risks of their participation in health research projects, negotiate the considerable power differentials in the research situation, and give valid informed consent, even though the same discourses have made much of their inability to assess the quality of health information online.

The healthcare professions have mirrored the contradictions of the current age that have produced both a global culture and cultural fragmentation, commodifying, homogenizing and internationalising their knowledge objects, whilst fragmenting into ever increasing more localized bodies of control and a plethora of specialities and sub-specialities (Cotton, 1997). Offline, healthcare knowledge production and delivery have been dominated by English language and Western medicine and healthcare delivery systems (Upvall, 1993; Thorne, 1997). Within the health professions, knowledge producers (researchers) are privileged over knowledge users (patients and clinicians) (Chopoorian, 1990). The ascendency of quantitative, evidence-based practice (EBP) research and the sub-discipline of epidemiology have been greatly facilitated by the Internet, since it allows for the collection and use of huge health related data bases, including "valuable epidemiological data about health and illness" (Yellowlees, 2001: 31; see also Chapter 7 in this volume).

Discourses both enable and constrain possibilities for knowledge production and subjectivization, opening up spaces for new ways of talking, thinking, acting and being, as well as for multiple forms of resistance (Foucault, 1994). Resistance may include people avoiding participating in cyber research and electronic healthcare, securing boundaries of what can be known about them, faking acceptable, compliant behaviours, providing false information about their medical and health status, or seeking legal sanctions and remedies (Phelps, 2000; Schneier, 2000; Duffy, 2002). Not all modes of resistance, however, may be effective or conducive to optimal health.

Foucault (1983: 231-232) argues, "my point is not that everything is bad, but that everything is dangerous…then we always have something to do. So my position leads not to apathy, but to a hyper- and pessimistic activism". CMC technologies can multiply the number and range of diverse discourses, where millions can potentially hear even a single speaker, and allow for collective groupings and strategic alliances with those currently marginalized by the powerful discourses in and around cyber health knowledge production. Wajcman (2004: 77) claims, however, that any "emancipatory politics of technology…needs wetware – bodies, fluids, human agency".

Connected and Unconnected Worlds

CMC technologies are claimed to potentially deliver benefits such as enhanced healthcare delivery and improved health outcomes for individuals, communities and populations in cost effective ways (Phelps, 2000; Wooldridge, 2000, Yellowlees, 2001). Tito (2000: 156), however, maintains "there are the many people in our community that are not 'on-line', and who are precluded from access due to poverty or disability". Bell (2001: 121) states there are now "'digital ghettos' that "don't get wired…the spaces of information poverty". Webster and Robins (1998: 39) claim cyberspace has spawned a "cultural apartheid between the mobile elite and the immobile residue of the 'unproductive masses'". Technological proficiency has become the cultural capital of the elite class of technological experts, giving them power, privilege and status over those using cyber information (for example, electronic healthcare professionals, cyber researchers, and cyber participants), as well as over the offline digital underclass (Webster and Robins, 1998; Bell, 2001).

Although the number of people using the Internet cannot be accurately determined, the estimated number of users has surged from 25 million in 1995 (The Pew Research Center for the People and the Press, 1995) to over 600 million in 2002 (NUA, 2003). According to the World Economic Forum (2002), only 10% of the world's population are Internet users, and of these, 88 percent are in developed countries. Recent studies related to Internet use in the United States indicate that while the gender digital divide is narrowing, other digital divides are discriminating against older persons, lower socio-economic groups, some ethnic groups (such as African-American and Hispanic-American groups), and those living in rural areas (Chen and Wellman, 2003; Lenhart et al., 2003; see also Chapter 1). This raises serious questions in relation to the ethical conduct of cyber research by healthcare professionals, since health researchers are required to abide by the ethical principle of justice that involves "the fair distribution of the benefits and burdens of participation in research" in society, and "non-discrimination in selection and recruitment of actual and future participants" (National Health and Medical Research Council [NHMRC], 2002: C5).

RESEARCH IN, OF, AND RELATED TO CYBERSPACE

Early portrayals of cyberspace were largely of a homogeneous mindscape or a singular virtual world, often romanticized in utopian or dystopian visions (Gibson, 1984; Benedikt, 1992). William Gibson, who at the time "did not own or know how to operate a personal computer" (Gunkel and Gunkel, 1997: 134), coined the term 'cyberspace' in his influential cyberpunk novel, *Neuromancer*, to describe "a consensual hallucination...A graphic representation of data abstracted from the banks of every computer in the human system" (Gibson, 1984: 51). According to Polit et al. (2001: 15), qualitative research approaches utilizing naturalistic methods of inquiry "always takes place in the field (that is, in naturalistic settings)". Some health professionals may reject cyberspace as a legitimate research field where relevant, ethical, practice-based research can be conducted. According to Mann and Stewart (2000: 205), cyberspace is a viable research field involving discrete virtual cultures that are "*different from* both real life and each other". Fletcher (1999) points out that online worlds are connected to other online and offline worlds in complex, interrelated ways. Realist approaches to cyber research may adopt standards of authenticity based on a correspondence with facts established in the offline world.

The ontological status of cyberspace has been variously characterized as imagined, virtual, real and actual (see Calhoun, 1991; Woolley, 1992; Heim, 1993; Rheingold, 1993). Traditional scientific approaches have constituted the space of cyberspace in terms of a realist ontology and Cartesian three-dimensional geography (Gunkel and Gunkel, 1997). Coyne (1995) claims cyberspace cannot be an ontological world since it is based on information alone. Others maintain the development of realistic recreations of the human body, surgical simulation, and telepresence have constituted hybrid worlds that are half real and half virtual (see Satava, 1992; Csordos, 1997).

Bell (2001: 187) claims cyber researchers need to consider the issues and concerns arising from using cyberspace in various ways such as: "(i) researching cyberspace, (ii) researching *in* cyberspace, and (iii) researching *cyberspace in cyberspace*". For example, can scientifically rigorous and ethical research be conducted in virtual worlds, by virtual researchers with virtual participants? Fox and Roberts (1999) maintain cyber ethnography has no underlying reality upon which it can be based. Jacobson (1999: 133) states:

> Most research in cyberspace has not obtained and/or does not present data on the off-line (or 'real') characteristics of its participants (respondents or informants), and the conclusions they reach (e.g., in cyberspace, women behave differently in various ways than do men) are unwarranted by the evidence provided.

In most health related research, participants may not only need to verify their identities and consent, but also that they meet particular demographic and health-related criteria. Fyfe et al. (2001: 542) claim cyber researchers must have adequate mechanisms for authenticating "whether online respondents actually have the disorder or condition of interest". Given the difficulties inherent in authenticating identities and pertinent characteristics online, Binik et al. (1999) advise cyber researchers to implement multi-sourced (online and offline) verification procedures (see also Chapter 2 in this volume).

Cyber health research is subject to unique, major methodological, ethical and professional problems that undermine traditional constructions of scientific rigour, as well as ethical and professional standards established offline. These problems include: the open, global, contingent nature of the Internet allowing for possible breaches of anonymity, confidentiality and privacy, population biases, discriminatory sampling practices, very low response rates for online surveys from online samples, inadequate mechanisms for random sampling and calculating response rates, difficulties in validating informed consent and the identities, characteristics and responses of multifaceted, virtual participants in multiple virtual and actual sites, including the number and nature of their submissions, cultural variations in meaning and understanding, issues relating to differences in the scope and standards of professional practice across state, national and transnational boundaries, concerns relating to participant-researcher relationships, and the difficulties inherent in protection of participants, researchers and data in cyber research (see Waskul and Douglass, 1996; Kaye and Johnson, 1999; Brooks, 2001; Couper, 2001; DeLorme et al., 2001; Eyfe et al., 2001; Duffy, 2002; Terry, 2002; Elford et al., 2004; see also Chapter 1).

In the absence of definitive, scientifically sanctioned cyber research methods, and the inherent difficulties of extrapolating offline methods online, healthcare professionals conducting health research in cyberspace appear to have used a variety of ad hoc approaches, eclectically mixing modes of CMC and data collection methods, such as, posting questionnaires on web sites (Thomas et al., 2000; Fyfe et al., 2001), conducting asynchronous virtual focus groups via listserv accounts (Adler and Zarchin, 2002) and online discussion boards (Moloney et al., 2003), or qualitative, online interviews through synchronous, text generated, online chat in private chat rooms (Elford et al., 2004; see also Couch and Liamputtong in this volume). Klemm et al. (1998) downloaded and content analyzed messages from an online (email) colorectal support group, while Hardin (2003) used critical discourse analysis to analyze data collected from message boards of an anorexia support group. In Elford et al.'s (2004) study of the role of the Internet in relation to gay men's sexual practice and HIV prevention, a plurality of methods (quantitative and qualitative) and sources (online and offline) was used. Elford at al. (2004) estimated that the response rate for the online questionnaire completed by the online sample did not even reach 1%. This raises the question of how representative such samples can be, and supports the need for the use of multiple data sources and methods rather than just relying on online methods and samples alone.

LIFE, EMBODIMENT AND IDENTITY

Cyberspace has been described as "a new frontier, a very real one...open to exploration and ultimately settlement" (Woolley, 1992: 122), replicating the patterns of the Enlightenment, Western expansionism, Columbian voyages of discovery and the old West of North America, where the virtual worlds of cyberspace can be conquered, plundered, enlightened and controlled (Sardar, 1996; Gunkel and Gunkel, 1997). Bell (2001: 195) reports "there has been something of an academic land-rush into cyberspace, matching those colonists who want to claim it as a community-space or an economic resource".

Cyber discourses vie in a field of power with other discourses, contesting the notions of embodiment, life, humanity, identity, and what it means to inhabit a world. While Li (2004) claims cyberspace cannot be real because no one can live there, Bell (2001: 2) argues cyberspace is a lived culture and needs to be "understood as it is lived". Others maintain initiatives such as the Visible Human Project (VHP) have resulted in "*flesh made code*" (Bell, 2001: 156), constituting "life *as information*, and information *as life*" (Sandelowski, 2002: 67-68). The VHP data set has been eulogized as the new standard for teaching human physiology to healthcare professionals, as well as for educating surgeons of the future (Satava, 1992; Csordas, 1997). Sardar (1996: 28), however, laments, "our humanity is digested by cyberspace".

Cyber discourses have constituted a bewildering array of new entities such as cyborgs, simuloids (software controlled, virtual entities), avatars (human controlled, virtual entities representing living people) and shades (offline corpses projected and reanimated in cyberspace as virtual persons) (Csordas, 1997), which are claimed to offer opportunities for new posthuman dimensions of being in the 21st Century (Haraway, 1991; Sandoval, 1995; Csordas, 1997; Bell, 2001). Dystopic visions see machine-human composites (like cyborgs and prostheticized humans), evolving to make embodied humans redundant, although the 'brain in the vat' may achieve a type of immortality through its technological and virtual extensions (Bell, 2001). Nonetheless, human bodies are increasingly being constituted as "objects of network power" (Willcocks, 2004: 287), enhanced by communication prosthetics such as the mobile phone and hand held computers. Wajcman (2004: 39) argues the "conception of the non-human as actant...involves a view of society as a *doing* rather than a *being*," where "the material world itself exercises a kind of agency".

Virtual systems may facilitate new subject forms and positions at the expense of excluded others. Gunkel and Gunkel (1997: 131-132), claim cyberspace maintains offline systems of domination as it "insidiously excludes those differentiated by gender, race and class under the guise of inclusion, which in the end, is nothing more than appropriation". Wajcman (2004: 77) argues, "the embodied and situated nature of knowledge has been denied precisely because it is based upon the invisible work of women". Following a review of 101 cyber research studies, Im and Chee (2001: 68) found such research might be supporting predominantly androcentric and ethnocentric views, cautioning "nursing knowledge that is developed based on research using the Internet definitely will mislead nursing practice" (see also their writing in Chapter 9 in this volume). Sardar (1996: 19) maintains that "cyberspace is a giant step towards museumisation of the world, where anything remotely different from Western culture will exist only in digital form".

CMC technologies allow for potentially different ways of situating, dislocating, relocating body and selfhood, such as embodying the self and the 'enselfing' the body (Waskul, 2002). In Waskul's (2002: 199) study of televideo cybersex, cyber participants interacted and presented themselves in real time through digital cameras "as only a body", experiencing "total embodiment" – a condition in which one is embodied within an image of one's own body" (Waskul, 2002: 220).

The dislocated nature of cyberspace interactions, however, is more usually experienced as "ultimate disembodiment" (Waskul, 2002: 220). Cyberspace has been construed as the perfect linkage of minds, with the physical body as devalued or redundant. In *Neuromancer*, Gibson (1984: 10) proclaimed that in the "bodiless exultation of cyberspace…the body was meat". Such constructions draw upon the Cartesian mind-body dualism of Western metaphysics, privileging the solipsistic, rational mind of the knowing subject by the "violent erasure of other bodies and the body of the other" (Gunkel and Gunkel, 1997: 131). Given the somological basis of healthcare knowledge, and the health care professions' societal mandate to care for the health and welfare of embodied individuals and populations, such constructions of cyberspace and their inhabitants are untenable. Waskul and Douglass (1996: 137) caution that "the utter absence of flesh and blood" in online research can "potentially result in extreme objectifications that…will always impair a researcher's ethical judgement".

Phenomenological and material views of corporeality emphasize that cyber selves, no matter how virtual multiple or hybrid they may be, are always connected to the reality of the offline, living embodied self situated in the social and political contexts of daily life through which online participation is perceived and negotiated. Hence, any study of cyber participants' experiences must be ground in everyday embodied practices to be rigorous (Introna and Ilharco, 2004).

In cyberspace, potentially anyone can be anyone or anything, and multiple, dynamic, anonymous, fractured, hybrid, or even fraudulent or malicious identities may be assumed. For example, children may represent themselves online as adults or visa versa. Shared accounts, use of anonymous re-routers, hacking, identity fraud and the like may further complicate matters. This presents cyber researchers with serious problems related to verification of data and sources, credibility of findings, and adequate protection of human subjects (see also Chapters 1 and 5 in this volume).

Private and Public Worlds

Waskul and Douglass (1996) argue online interactions are both public and private. Cyber participants may be alone or with others in a variety of physical settings (such as work, home, cyber cafes, and computer laboratories). These settings may markedly influence their perceived sense of privacy, levels of self-disclosure, and how they negotiate their online research participation (Waskul and Douglass, 1996; Binik et al., 1999; Moloney et al., 2003).

Cyber health knowledge production is coordinated with power, whose purpose is to construct and normalize what is health and healthcare. The technologies and microtechniques of cyber research have effectively permitted private practices of individuals to enter the public sphere, where they become visible and subject to disciplinary gazes of power. Indeed, the healthcare professions have eagerly endorsed the extension and amplification of the clinical gaze to noncorporeal dimensions, so as to better know and care for their clients as 'whole' persons (May, 1992).

Online communities and groups have been enthusiastically promoted as providing plentiful, opportunistic sites for online research generally, and for online qualitative research methods such at cyber ethnography in particular. Much of this enthusiasm appears to hinge on researchers classifying online sites such as bulletin boards, chat rooms and MUDs as public places and therefore, so the argument goes, open for research purposes and excusable from requirements that protect human participants (see Paccagnella, 1997; Smyres, 1999; Hardin, 2003; Chapters 1 and 2 in this volume). Waskul and Douglass (1996: 132) argue, however, that "such a viewpoint can promote a researcher to completely fail to acknowledge participants altogether. Such a perspective is intellectually barbaric and clearly unethical". Munhall (1994: 11) states ethical, qualitative research must acknowledge that "meaning comes from the source" of the subjective experience of the individual, and therefore cannot be "presumed, assumed or assigned".

The Cyber Panopticon

CMC technologies act as an anonymous, invisible, constant, asymmetrical electronic gaze of power amplifying not only the productive, but also the surveillance, control and normalization capabilities of disciplinary technologies. It is important to note that this cyber gaze is fixed upon researchers and health professionals as well as patients and participants. According to Foucault (1975: 39), "the gaze that sees is a gaze that dominates...it dominates its masters". Indeed, economic discourses construct cyber health and research as a means to survey, monitor and improve the quantity, quality and efficiency of health researchers and healthcare professionals' knowledge production and healthcare delivery. Meanwhile, others conducting health research and healthcare online remain largely unregulated (Stanberry, 2002; Terry, 2002).

Invasions of privacy may leave cyber participants open to serious harm from cyber crime, cyber stalking, spying, theft, voyeurism, prosecution, fraud, flaming, spamming and physical harm (Binik et al., 1999; Schneier, 2000; Lubka and Holden, 2001; see also Chapters 1 and 5 in this volume). Bernal (1999: 1) claims the Internet has "the 'Four Horseman of the Infocalypse,' terrorists, drug dealers, paedophiles and organized crime". Spiders, web crawlers, web logs, search engines and other automated systems can link data to persons and create comprehensive profiles on them. Hackers, spyware, government surveillance systems and the like further complicate the picture. Networked computers allow data bases to be traded and sold (Schneier, 2000). Participants in cyber health research studies may leave electronic data trails creating misleading profiles about their health status (Lubka and Holden, 2001).

Confidentiality relates to the prevention of unauthorized reading of data, and ensuring that sensitive personal identification and details of participants are not disclosed to unauthorized persons (Schneier, 2000). Breaches of confidentiality have led to people being "harassed, threatened and fired" (Schneier, 2000: 66; see also Chapter 5 in this volume). Much of health research deliberately gathers information in relation to personal and often sensitive areas, such as HIV status, domestic violence, mental illness and drug taking history.

Alpert (1998: 97) claims the greatest potential to personal privacy in health is from the "trusted insider". Phelps (2000: 39) points out that consumers are becoming increasingly aware that breaches of confidentiality related to their health status have the potential to: "exploit, stigmatise, discriminate and disadvantage an individual in every aspect of their lives: employment, finances, housing, education, access to a range of private and public services and travel".

Health Professionals Researching in Cyberspace

Cyber health research involves multiple cultural practices and technologies used by multidimensional, embodied human beings in multiple (offline and online) locations embedded in wider sociocultural contexts. Virtual worlds, cyber identities and communities do not exist in isolation, but are inextricably linked in complex ways to other virtual worlds of cyberspace, as well as offline worlds. Cyber health research involves the participation of offline, real, embodied, living people who really are in pain, suffering ill health or seeking to enhance their wellness, and whose welfare may be potentially significantly enhanced or harmed by their involvement in online research. Waskul and Douglass (1996: 137) point out that cyber researchers active involvement in researching "sensitive and fragile" online groups, such as self help groups, may not only disrupt the phenomenon being researched, but also could be "disastrous to participant's on-line experiences". Olsen (2003: 126) maintains nurse researchers should adhere to the guiding principle of contextual caring that involves acting "in accord with personal caring concern for the concrete specific other within one's immediate scope". Cyber nurse researchers, therefore, must be careful not to focus on the disembodied, decontextualized, entity of cyberspace, but rather on the holistic, individualized care of the embodied, living person in his or her situated contexts, that includes, but is not reducible to, their virtual selves in cyberspace.

Cyber health research also involves real, situated, embodied researchers who may be vulnerable from attacks from fraudulent, or malicious respondents and hackers, as well as on their privacy, identity, credentials and intellectual property. Moreover, health professionals conducting research are subject to ever increasing surveillance, classification and regulation via a plethora of a state, national, international laws and professional and ethical codes of conduct, both online and offline, and their professional reputation may be enhanced or hindered by online research activities. De Lorme et al. (2001: 282) caution those researching in cyberspace that "reputation is the currency of trade for legitimate researchers…slow to be built, but easily destroyed".

Healthcare professionals involvement in cyber research may be both research and practice based, involving "a unique set of roles, responsibilities and risks that must be appropriately planned for, carefully executed and routinely evaluated" (Cudney and Weinert, 2000: 42). Rodriguez (1999) advises healthcare professionals to develop appropriate communication and privacy policies, as well as disclaimers and legal waivers on their Internet sites. Researchers, Institutional Review Boards, Human Research Ethics Committees and Privacy Committees involved in cyber research should consult with information technology security experts to ensure confidentiality, availability and integrity of health research data. Adequate liability cover as well as adequate representation of online legal and information technology expertise on these committees is essential for the protection of online researchers and participants (Hamilton, 1999; Rodriguez, 1999; Duffy, 2002). Phelps (2000: 38) insists that:

> Government has an obligation to ensure health providers are given clear and consistent guidelines on their responsibilities under law...[and] such law is consistent with the ethical and philosophical foundations of their profession.

The healthcare professions need to keep up to date with the rapid developments of CMC technologies, consider their professional responsibilities and accountabilities to their members and the public they profess to serve, and provide clear and consistent ethical and conduct codes to guide cyber researchers and protect cyber participants. Moreover, the health professions need to examine and address their role in the perpetuation of traditional offline and creation of new online oppressive power-knowledge structures that are incongruent with their professed tenets.

Cyber research raises serious questions in relation to the protection of human participants. If the research involves human subjects, then informed consent must usually be obtained. Indeed, health research involving cyber participants from the European community "will generally require 'explicit and unambiguous' consent of the data subject" (Electronic Privacy Information Center and Privacy International, 2002: 10). Cyber researchers need to provide participants with not only information of the benefits, aims, methods, requirements and outcomes of the research, but also the risks and possible harm the research may entail, and ongoing opportunities to voluntarily give or withdraw their informed consent. In addition, to be a valid, informed consent cyber participants' identities and pertinent characteristics, such as being adults, mentally competent and willing to give consent voluntarily, may need to be authenticated (see NHMRC, 1999). Given the ambiguous and open nature of the Internet and the raft of uncoordinated and complex state, national and international laws, and ethical and professional codes of conduct applying to the particular cyber research situation and researcher, healthcare professionals have tended to use offline methods of authentication (alone or in concert with online methods), such as obtaining written consent by mail or in person from cyber participants (see Cudney and Weinert, 2000; Adler and Zarchin, 2002; Pierce et al., 2002; Moloney et al, 2003; Chapter 1 in this volume). Mann and Stewart (2000: 54) note "consent for research involving children should always be obtained from adults in paper form".

Health professionals conducting research in cyberspace should be as honest and trustworthy in their online research endeavours as they are in their clinical practices and relationships offline. This includes respecting the right of individuals to know if they are to be research participants, and avoiding giving assurances of anonymity and confidentiality that they cannot control or guarantee. Cyber researchers should consider the possible serious ethical issues involved in researching in public places in cyberspace where neither notification of their research activities is given nor informed consent of participants is sought. In the context of cyber health and healthcare research, many of these sites involve isolated, ill and vulnerable people. Such research compromises validity of the research findings, professional client and healthcare professional and researcher and participant relationships, and the privacy and dignity of participants. It reproduces power inequalities between researchers and participants, since participants have no actual power to resist or negotiate their so-called participation or how their realities are being interpreted and displayed by the cyber researcher. Waskul and Douglass (1996: 137) "recommend that researchers strive to obtain some degree of informed consent whenever possible", and if researching sensitive online groups such consent "should proceed through key informants".

There are those who advocate the healthcare professional acts as expert coach, mentor or guide for cyber clients and cyber participants (Klemm et al., 1998, 1999). Many healthcare professionals, however, are new to cyberspace, and lack the appropriate technological expertise to take on such a role. Indeed, few healthcare professionals would be information technology security experts. As a consequence, technological experts are increasingly required to assist healthcare professionals as well as cyber participants with their online endeavours. This may seriously impact on the research process, as well as the client and healthcare professional, and participant and researcher relationships. Mohoney (2000) found a 'clash of cultures' between researchers and technology developers led to difficulties with working relationships, time lines, and conduct of rigorous online research.

The NHMRC (2002: C114) maintains "researchers are responsible for ensuring the security of confidential material, including that held in computer systems". The ability for researchers to meet such obligations is markedly compromised by CMC technologies. Electronic mail is commonly used to recruit and communicate with participants, and to transmit research data to other researchers, despite it being a highly insecure form of data transmission that may breach privacy provisions (Schneier, 2000). Encryption of data is an option, but this may alert the interest of hackers, intelligence agencies and law enforcement bodies. Moreover, Mann and Stewart (2000: 44) claim "encryption is still illegal in some countries". Binik et al. (1999: 87) note health researchers dealing with sensitive issues should ensure data is "handled like commercial transactions," although the cost of doing so may prove prohibitive for many types of health research.

Conclusion

Cyberspace has been constructed as a universe brimming with a plethora of multiple, complex, diverse, virtual, sociocultural worlds, offering healthcare professionals unprecedented opportunities to conduct research online. Whilst an online world may operate substantially differently than offline worlds, it is important to note it is inextricably linked to embodied, living, human beings situated in their multiple online and offline worlds. Hence, merging, symbiotic, complementary and colliding relationships between the many different worlds of cyber health research may occur, with not only potential benefits, but also serious risks and substantial costs for either or both cyber participants and cyber researchers.

Health professionals researching in cyberspace need to recognize that research methodologies are context specific, requiring them not only to be reflexive about their ontological perspectives, but also about their use of cyberspace and their participation in the research process and participant-researcher relationships. Given that technologies and methodologies are also affected by the wider socio-political contexts and institutional interests, these situated reflections need to include the paradigmatic assumptions informing the research, the costs and benefits to cyber participants and cyber researchers in the production of such healthcare knowledges, as well as the relevance of the study in relation to the profession and society.

As Phelps (2000: 46) points out, "health is not an area where advances in technology can be simply superimposed". If the enormous revolutionary, transformative, emancipatory potential benefits of CMC technologies are to be harnessed to help the healthcare professions build their knowledge base and meet the dynamic, complex health and healthcare demands of today's society, the major threats they pose, particularly in relation to dignity, privacy, anonymity and confidentiality must be urgently addressed in genuine collaboration with pertinent stakeholders in general, and cyber participants and electronic patients in particular. Research is needed to uncover how the unique and powerful properties of the Internet could be used to develop dialogue, power sharing and collaborative models of participant-researcher relationships, including negotiated modes of informed consent reflective of the ongoing, dynamic clarification of research aims and participants' process consent.

Given the major ontological, epistemological, methodological, legal and ethical problems arising from the unique nature of cyberspace, traditional approaches to scientific research offline cannot be simply extrapolated online. As Lee (2004: 7) contends, "all scholarly knowledge itself " is "a social construction. It is not immutable but under our power as a community of scholars to question, amend, correct and improve". Hence, there is an urgent need to illuminate and explicate practice knowledge embedded in the health and healthcare research and clinical experiences of researchers, clinicians and participants in their actual and virtual settings, so as to provide guidance for health professionals in the conduct of optimal, ethical, and professionally relevant cyber healthcare and health research, so as to enhance possibilities for excellence in healthcare practice and knowledge production. The power knowledge structures and their impact on constraining and enabling meaning related to cyber health and cyber healthcare practice and knowledge production need to be uncovered and critiqued, so as to provide spaces for questioning, challenging and resisting hegemonic constructions, and enhance possibilities for creation and valuing a heterogeneity of perspectives, ways of knowing, being and relating. As Gallagher (1992: 346) points out, there is a need to find ways where we can "encounter each other without violence", and learn from concrete situations the ones that may be justified and are usable in practice.

REFERENCES

[1] Adler, C. L. and Zarchin, Y. R., 2002, 'The "Virtual Focus Group": Using the Internet to Reach Pregnant Women on Home Bed Rest', *Journal of Obstetric, Gynecologic and Neonatal Nursing*, vol, 31, no. 4, pp. 418-427.

[2] Alpert, S. A., 1998, 'Health care information: access, confidentiality, and good practice', in K. W. Goodman (ed.), *Ethics, Computing, and Medicine: Informatics and the Transformation of Health Care*, pp. 75-101, Cambridge University Press, Cambridge.

[3] Bell, D., 2001, *An Introduction to Cybercultures*, Routledge, London and New York.

[4] Benedikt, M., 1992, 'Introduction', in M. Benedikt (ed.), *Cyberspace: First Steps*, pp. 1-26, The MIT Press, Cambridge, Massachusetts and London, England.

[5] Bernal, J., 1999, 'Big Brother is on-line: Public and Private Security in the Internet', *Cybersociology*, no.6. *<http://www.socio.demon.co.uk/magazine/6/enfopol_echelon.html>*

[6] Binik, Y. M, Mah, K. and Kiesler, S., 1999, 'Ethical Issues in Conducting Sex Research on the Internet', *The Journal of Sex Research*, vol. 36, no. 1, pp. 82-90.

[7] Brooks, B. A., 2001, 'Using the Internet for Patient Education', *Orthopaedic Nursing*, vol. 20, no. 5, pp. 69-77.

[8] Calhoun, C., 1991, 'Indirect Relationships and Imagined Communities: Large-Scale Social Integration and the Transformation of Everyday Life', in P. Bourdieu and J. S. Colemen (eds.), *Social Theory for a Changing Society*, pp. 95-120, Westview Press, Boulder CO.

[9] Chen, W. and Wellman, B., 2003, 'Charting and Bridging Digital Divides: Comparing Socio-economic, Gender, Life Stage, and Rural-Urban Internet Access and Use in Eight Countries', The AMD Global Consumer Advisory Board (GCAB). *<http://www.amdgcab.org>*

[10] Chopoorian, T. J., 1990, 'The Two Worlds of Nursing: The One We Teach About, The One That is', in National League for Nursing (eds.), *Curriculum Revolution: Redefining the Student-Teacher Relationship*, pp. 21-36, National League for Nursing, New York.

[11] Cotton, A. H., 1997, 'Power, Knowledge and The Discourse of Specialization in Nursing', *Clinical Nurse Specialist*, vol. 11, no. 1, pp. 25-29.

[12] Couper, M., 2001, *The Promises and Perils of Web Surveys*, Association for Survey Computing, London.

[13] Coyne, R., 1995, *Designing Information Technology in the Postmodern Age: From Method to Metaphor*, MIT Press, Cambridge, MA.

[14] Csordas, T. J., 1997, 'Computerized Cadavers: Shades of Being and Representation in Virtual Reality', After Post-Modernism Conference Papers. *<http://www.focusing.org/apm_papers/compucad.html>*

[15] Cudney, S. A. and Weinert, C., 2000, 'Computer-Based Support Groups: Nursing in Cyberspace', *Computers in Nursing*, vol. 18, no. 1, pp. 35-43.

[16] DeLorme, D. E., Zinkhan, G. M. and French, W., 2001, 'Ethics and the Internet: Issues Associated with Qualitative Research', *Journal of Business Ethics*, vol. 33, pp. 271-286.

[17] Duffy, M. E., 2002, 'Methodological Issues in Web-based Research', *Journal of Nursing Scholarship*, vol. 34, no. 1, pp. 83-88.

[18] Eachus, P., 1999, 'Health Information on the Internet", *International Journal of Health Promotion and Education*, vol. 37, pp. 30-33.

[19] Electronic Privacy Information Center and Privacy International., 2002, 'Privacy and Human rights 2002: An International Survey of Privacy Laws and Developments'. *<http://www.privacyinternational.org/.>*

[20] Elford, J., Bolding, G., Davis, M., Sherr, L. and Hart, G., 2004, 'The Internet and HIV Study: Design and Methods', *BMC Public Health*, vol. 4, no. 39. *<http://www.biomedcentral.com/1471-2458/4/39>*

[21] Eysenbach, G., Powell, J., Kuss, O. and Sa, E-R., 2002, 'Empirical Studies Assessing the Quality of Health Information for Consumers on the World Wide Web: A Systematic Review', *JAMA*, vol. 287, no. 20, pp. 2691-2700.

[22] Ferraro, G. P., 1998, *The Cultural Dimension of International Business*, Prentice Hall, London.

[23] Fletcher, G., 1999, '…Methodological Madness? You, Me and Virtual Ethnography', Paper presented at the annual Australian Anthropological Society Conference, Department of Sociology and Anthropology, University of New South Wales, July 1999. < *http://www.spaceless.com/papers/25.htm*>

[24] Foucault, M., 1975, *The Birth of the Clinic: An Archaeology of Medical Perception*, Vintage Books, New York.

[25] Foucault, M., 1980a, 'Truth and Power', in C. Gordon (ed.), *Power/Knowledge: Selected Interviews and Other Writings 1972-1977*, pp. 109-133, Pantheon Books, New York.

[26] Foucault, M., 1980b, 'Two Lectures', in C. Gordon (ed.), *Power/Knowledge: Selected Interviews and Other Writings 1972-1977*, pp. 78-108, Pantheon Books, New York.

[27] Foucault, M., 1983, 'Afterword (1983): On the Genealogy of Ethics: An Overview of Work in Progress', in H. L. Dreyfus and P. Rabinow (eds.), *Michel Foucault: Beyond Structuralism and Hermeneutics*, 2nd edition, pp. 229-252, The University of Chicago Press, Chicago.

[28] Foucault, M., 1994, *The Archaeology of Knowledge*, Routledge, London.

[29] Fox, N. and Roberts, C., 1999, 'GPs in Cyberspace: The Sociology of a Virtual Community', *The Sociological Review*, vol. 47, no. 4, pp. 643-671.

[30] Fyfe, S., Leonard, H., Gelmi, R., Tassell, A. and Strack, R., 2001, 'Using the Internet to Pilot a Questionnaire on Childhood Disability in Rett Syndrome', *Child: Care, Health and Development*, vol. 27, no. 6, pp. 535-543.

[31] Gallagher, S., 1992, *Hermeneutics and Education*, State University of New York Press, Albany

[32] Gibson, W., 1984, *Neuromancer*, Victor Gollancz Ltd, London.

[33] Gunkel, D. J. and Gunkel, A. H., 1997, 'Virtual Geographies: The New Worlds of Cyberspace', *Critical Studies in Mass Communication*, vol. 14, pp. 123-137.

[34] Hamilton, J. C., 1999, 'The Ethics of Conducting Social-Science Research on the Internet', *The Chronicle of Higher Education*, December, pp. B6-B7.

[35] Hansen, S., 2002, 'Excessive Internet usage or 'Internet Addiction'? The implications of Diagnostic Categories for Student Users', *Journal of Computer Assisted Learning*, vol. 18, no. 2, p. 235-236.

[36] Haraway, D., 1991, *Simians, Cyborgs, and Women: The Reinvention of Nature*, Routledge, New York.

[37] Hardin, P. K., 2003, 'Constructing Experience in Individual Interviews, Autobiographies and On-Line Accounts: A Poststructuralist Approach', *Journal of Advanced Nursing*, vol. 41, no. 6, pp. 536-544.

[38] Heim, M., 1993, *The Metaphysics of Virtual Reality*, Oxford University Press, New York.

[39] Im, E-O. and Chee, W., 2001, 'A Feminist Critique on the Use of the Internet in Nursing Research', *Advances in Nursing Science*, vol. 23, no 4, 67-82.

[40] Introna, L. D. and Ilharco, F. M., 2004, 'Phenomenology, Screens, and the World: A Journey with Husserl and Heidegger into Phenomenology', in J. Mingers and L. Willcocks (eds.), *Social Theory and Philosophy for Information Systems*, pp. 56-102, John Wiley and Sons Ltd, West Sussex.

[41] Jacobson, D., 1999, 'Doing Research in Cyberspace', *Field Methods*, vol. 11, no. 2, pp.127-145.

[42] Johansson, A. and Gotestam, K.G., 2004, 'Internet Addiction: Characteristics of a Questionnaire and Prevalence in Norwegian Youth (12-18 years)', *Scandinavian Journal of Psychology*, vol. 45, no. 3, pp. 223-229.

[43] Kaye, B. K. and Johnson, T. J., 1999, 'Research Methodology: Taming the Cyber Frontier: Techniques for Improving Online Surveys', *Social Science Computer Review*, vol. 17, no. 3, pp. 323-337.

[44] Klemm, P., Reppert, K. and Visich, L., 1998, 'A Nontraditional Cancer Support Group: The Internet', *Computers in Nursing*, vol. 16, no. 1, pp. 31-36.

[45] Klemm, P., Hurst, M., Dearholt, S. L. and Trone, S. R., 1999, 'Cyber Solace: Gender Differences on Internet Cancer Support Groups', *Computers in Nursing*, vol. 17, no. 2, pp. 65-72.

[46] Lakeman, R. 1997, 'Using the Internet for Data Collection in Nursing Research', *Computers in Nursing*, vol. 15, no. 5, pp. 269-275.

[47] Lee, A. S., 2004, 'Thinking about Social Theory and Philosophy for Information Systems', in J. Mingers and L. Willcocks (eds.), *Social Theory and Philosophy for Information Systems*, pp. 1-26, John Wiley and Sons Ltd, West Sussex.

[48] Lenhart, A., Horrigan, J., Rainie, L., Allen, K., Boyce, A., Madden, M. and O'Grady, E., 2003, *The Ever-Shifting Internet Population: A New Look at Internet Access and the Digital Divide*, Pew Internet and American Life Project, Washington.

[49] Li, Y., 2004, 'Architecture in Cyberspace or Cyberspace in Architecture? A Study Into Cyber Technology, Cyber Culture and the Impacts on Man at the Turn of the Millennium. Section 3', *Online Planning Journal. <http://www.casa.ucl.ac.uk/ planning/articles2/cyber3.htm>*

[50] Lubka, W. and Holden, N., 2001, *K.I.S.S. Guide to the Internet*, Dorling Kindersley, St Leonards, NSW.

[51] Mahoney, D. M., 2000, 'Developing Technology Applications for Intervention Research: A Case Study', *Computers in Nursing*, vol. 18. no. 6, pp. 260-264.

[52] Mann, C. and Stewart, F., 2000, *Internet Communication and Qualitative Research: A Handbook for Researching Online*, Sage Publications, London.

[53] May, C., 1992, 'Nursing work, Nurses' Knowledge, and The Subjectification of The Patient', *Sociology of Health and Illness*, vol. 14, no. 4, pp. 472-487.

[54] Moloney, M. F., Dietrich, A. S., Strickland, O. and Myerburg, S., 2003, 'Using Internet Discussion Boards as Virtual Focus Groups', *Advances in Nursing Science*, vol. 26, no. 4, pp. 274-286.

[55] Munhall, P. L., 1994, *Revisioning Phenomenology: Nursing and Health Science Research*, National League for Nursing Press, New York.

[56] National Health and Medical Research Council [NHMRC]., 1999, *National Statement on Ethical Conduct in Research Involving Humans*, Commonwealth of Australia, Canberra.

[57] National Health and Medical Research Council [NHMRC]., 2002, *Human Research Ethics Handbook: Commentary on the National Statement on Ethical Conduct in Research involving Humans*, Commonwealth of Australia, Canberra.

[58] NUA., 2003, 'How many Online?' *<http://www.nua.com/surveys/how_many_online/ index.html>*

[59] Olsen, D. P. (Chair), Working Group for the Study of Ethical Issues in International Nursing Research., 2003, 'Ethical Considerations in International Nursing Research: A

Report from the International Centre for Nursing Ethics', *Nursing Ethics*, vol. 10, no. 2, pp. 122-136.

[60] Paccagnella, L., 1997, 'Getting the Seats of Your Pants Dirty: Strategies for Ethnographic Research on Virtual Gommunities', *Journal of Computer-Mediated Communication*, vol. 3, no. 1. *<http://www.ascusc.org/jcmc/vol3/issue1/paccagnella. html>*

[61] Paulsen, D., 1994, 'CyberSpace and Computer Mediated Communications', *Dave Paulsen and Computer Link Magazine*. *<http://www.reststop.net/dave/c11.html>*

[62] Phelps, K., 2000, 'Enhancing Privacy and Confidentiality in The World of E-Health', in *National Health Information Management Advisory Council: Proceedings from the National Health Online Summit*, Adelaide, 3-4 August, 2000, pp. 38-46, Commonwealth Department of Health and Aged Care, Canberra.

[63] Pierce, L. L., Steiner, V. and Govoni, A. L., 2002, 'In-home Online Support for Caregivers of Survivors of Stroke: A Feasibility Study', *CIN: Computers, Informatics, Nursing*, vol. 20, no. 4, pp. 157-164.

[64] Polit, D. F., Beck, C. T. and Hungler, B. P., 2001, *Essentials of Nursing Research: Methods, Appraisal, and Utilization*, 5th edition, Lippincott, Philadelphia.

[65] Rheingold, H., 1993, *The Virtual Community: Homesteading on the Electronic Frontier*, Addison-Wesley, New York.

[66] Rodriguez, J. C., 1999, 'Legal, Ethical, and Professional Issues to Consider When Communicating via The Internet: A Suggested Response Model and Policy', *Journal of the American Dietetic Association*, vol. 99, no. 11, pp. 1428-1432.

[67] Sandelowski, M., 2002, 'Virtual Humans, Vanishing Bodies, and Virtual Nursing; Complications of Life, Presence, Place, and Identity', *Advances in Nursing Science*, vol. 24, no. 3, pp. 58-70.

[68] Sandoval, C., 1995, 'New Sciences: Cyborg Feminism and the Methodology of the Oppressed', in C. H. Gray, assisted by H J. Figueroa-Sarriera and S. Mentor (eds.), *The Cyborg Handbook*, pp. 407-421, Routledge, New York and London.

[69] Sardar, Z., 1996, 'alt.civilizations.faq: Cyberspace as the Darker Side of the West', in Z. Sardar and J. R. Ravetz (eds.), *Cyberfutures: Culture and Politics on the Information Superhighway*, pp. 14-41, Pluto Press, London.

[70] Satava, R., 1992, 'Robotics, Telepresence and Virtual Reality: A Critical Analysis of the Future of Surgery', *Minimally Invasive Therapy*, vol. 1, pp. 357-363.

[71] Schneier, B., 2000, *Secret and Lies: Digital Security in a Networked World*, John and Wiley and Son, Inc., New York.

[72] Sharf, B. F., 1997, 'Communicating Breast Cancer Online: Support and Empowerment on The Internet', *Women and Health*, vol. 26, no. 1, pp. 65-84.

[73] Smyres, K. M., 1999, 'Virtual Corporeality: Adolescent Girls and Their Bodies in Cyberspace', *Cybersociology*, no. 6. *<http://www.socio.demon.co.uk/magazine/6/ smyres.html>*

[74] Stanberry, B.A., 2002, 'Commentary: Legal Aspects of Health on The Internet: A European Perspective', *British Medical Journal*, vol. 324, pp. 605-606.

[75] Terry, N., 2002, 'Regulating health information: a US perspective', *British Medical Journal*, vol. 324, pp. 602-605.

[76] The Pew Research Center for the People and the Press., 1995, Americans Going Online... Explosive Growth, Uncertain Destinations-Technology in the American Household. < *http://people-press.org/reports/display.php3?ReportID=136*>

[77] Thomas, B., Stamler, L.L., Lafreniere, K. and Dumala, R., 2000, 'The Internet: An Effective Tool for Nursing Research with Women', *Computers in Nursing*, vol. 18, no. 1, pp. 13-18.

[78] Thorne, S., 1997, 'Global Consciousness in Nursing: An Ethnographic Study of Nurses with an International Perspective', *Journal of Nursing Education*, vol. 36, no. 9, 437-442.

[79] Tito, F., 2000, 'Building a Better Evidence Base for Health Care and Delivery – A Consumers' Perspective', in *National Health Information Management Advisory Council: Proceedings from the National Health Online Summit*, Adelaide, 3-4 August, 2000, pp. 150-157, Commonwealth Department of Health and Aged Care, Canberra.

[80] Upvall, M. J., 1993, 'Therapeutic Syncretism: A Conceptual Framework of Persistence and Change for International Nursing', *Journal of Professional Nursing*, vol. 9, no. 1, pp. 56-62.

[81] Wajcman, J., 2004, *TechnoFeminism*, Polity Press, Cambridge, UK.

[82] Waldo, B. H., 2000, 'Redefining the Health Care Landscape with The Internet', *Nursing Economics*, vol. 18, no. 2, pp. 99-100.

[83] Waskul, D. D., 2002, 'The Naked Self: Being a Body in Televideo Cybersex', *Symbolic Interaction*, vol. 25, no. 2, pp. 199-227.

[84] Waskul, D. and Douglass, M., 1996, 'Considering the Electronic Participant: Some Polemical Observations on the Ethics of On-line Research', *The Information Society*, vol. 12, no. 2, pp. 129-139.

[85] Webster, F. and Robins, K., 1998, 'The iron cage of the information society', *Information, Communication and Society*, vol. 1, pp. 23-45.

[86] Willcocks, L. P., 2004, 'Foucault, Power/Knowledge and Information Systems: Reconstructing the Present', in J. Mingers and L.Willcocks (eds.), *Social Theory and Philosophy for Information Systems*, pp. 238-296, John Wiley and Sons Ltd, West Sussex, UK.

[87] Wooldridge, M., 2000, 'Opening Address', in *National Health Information Management Advisory Council: Proceedings from the National Health Online Summit*, Adelaide, 3-4 August, 2000, pp. 13-15, Commonwealth Department of Health and Aged Care, Canberra.

[88] Woolley, B., 1992, *Virtual Worlds*, Penguin, New York.

[89] World Economic Forum., 2002, *Annual Report of the Global Digital Divide Initiative*, World Economic Forum, Geneva.

[90] Yellowlees, P., 2001, *Your Guide to E-Health: Third Millennium Medicine on The Internet*, University of Queensland Press, Queensland, Australia.

[91] Young, K., 1998, *Caught in the Net. How to Recognize the Signs of Internet Addiction and a Winning Strategy for Recovery*, John Wiley, New York.

In: Health Research in Cyberspace
Editor: Pranee Liamputtong, pp. 67-84 ISBN 1-59454-819-6

Chapter 4

PRODUCING CYBER-SELVES THROUGH TECHNOSPATIAL PRAXIS: STUDYING THROUGH DOING[1]

Radhika Gajjala and Melissa Altman

[A]n appraisal of identity that does not simply look to what is seemingly new about the self in the 'virtual age' but looks backward and forward in seeking to provide insights about identity, one that asks what was and what if.

(Nelson et al., 2001: 3-4)

PART I – INTRODUCTION

In this chapter, we discuss the production of subjectivities in virtual (learning) environments through an engagement with the contexts, and a methodology, we term as epistemologies of doing. We, therefore, suggest that researchers studying the production of identity in cyberspace must engage in the production of culture and subjectivity in the specific context while interacting with others doing the same in order to gain a nuanced understanding of how identities form and are performed in such online spaces. This enables us to really talk about the meaning-making that goes on there. For, as has been observed by several researchers who have inhabited online spaces for an extensive period of time, the "hit and run" method of studying online "data" that several researchers adopt provides only partial understanding of how communities are shaped around technologies. The research described in this chapter shows how embodied our engagement with online environments really is. Thus, where you put your body in relation to technospaces – local, global, transnational, "old", "new", "virtual" or "real" – and how you choose to negotiate such spaces within socio-

[1] We wish to thank members of the courses – Computer-mediated Communities (Spring 2002) and Humanistic Research Methods (Spring 2003) for permission to use their assignments, discussions and insights. We also thank Christopher Bollinger and Yahui Zhang (RG's graduate advisees and collaborators and co-authors on projects and papers related to the focus of this chapter) for their valuable work connecting to the larger project of which this chapter is a part.

economic and cultural contexts that are inextricably shaped through various historically and politically formed hierarchies of race, gender, geography, caste and class does indeed matter.

Although analyses of static texts are proliferating, fewer scholars are actually observing the processes of production of culture within such online spaces. This is what this project focuses on—the actual production of cultural experience and materiality of virtuality, as it is experienced by participants in online environments.

Even in these virtual environments, participants do not leave their bodies behind.

Hence, the virtual/real distinction sets up a false binary that cannot be substantiated when we analyze engagement with online environments. Part of what our analysis does is to try to unravel the dichotomy between the virtual and the real. Physicality of the body is expressed through everyday material practices, even when those practices involve online production of self. The practice of *engaging* such a technological environment produces the subject/agent. Meaning, therefore, is made through doing—doing in this case is coding, programming, typing oneself into existence and building objects.

Race in a global cyberspace is nuanced and complex. We are, therefore, concerned with the designing of diverse, embodied and dialogic encounters for the effective use of virtual learning environments in order to study complex processes of meaning making in digital/analogue contexts that shape and are shaped through post 1990s globalizing processes. Thus, this chapter is an extension of the work on race in cyberspace and is based on research examining the production of techno-mediated subjectivities at various interfaces both in traditional classroom pedagogical settings and other online settings.

Virtual learning environments are implicitly and explicitly based in globalization processes that bring together workers, educators, students and employers from multiple socio-cultural, geographical and economic histories and with varying personal histories as well as skills and literacies in relation to digital work. We examine these in the context of digital technology use and consumption. In this chapter, we argue that, between the presences and absences of such raced bodies - produced through layered, nuanced and contradictory workings of class, interpersonal culture, literacy and language - "race in cyberspace" can benefit from a much more complex analysis and response than what has been pursued thus far by scholars studying race in cyberspace.

Further, in previous work examining South Asian and Asian Techno-mediated subjectivities (Gajjala 2004) - which will inform the present piece - one of us has argued that race, class, caste, gender, geography and specific located histories of colonization INTERSECT with specific place-based configurations of access to various literacies associated with the communities of production (within which the Internet becomes important), to shape constructs of identity and ignorance. These constructs of identity and ignorance, in turn, re-produce existing socio-cultural patterns of inclusion and exclusion, thus intersecting with geographically, culturally, historically and nationally produced *place-based* configurations of race to produce contradictory manifestations of racism and acts of silencing online.

This chapter is based on efforts to interrogate these issues through controlled environments in classrooms, and is exploratory. It is part of a larger project that we are working on in an effort to open up different ways for examining issues of race in cyberspace and to provide a variety of possible pedagogic interventions and practices to engage the problem of racialization within cyberspace that is clearly situated in unequal power relations manifested within current "global" economies.

The methodology is illustrated through examples from production of identities within classroom settings. The research, thus, simultaneously sheds light on pedagogical techniques for the understanding of cyberculture as well as on the process of how selves are produced in interpersonal interaction in digitally mediated environments.

Part II of this chapter describes the environments and assignments referred to and Part III analyses selected instances and intersections to produce an understanding of how - in the specific instances described - literacies and offline material practices interact with online cultures to produce virtual/real situations for reflection leading to an understanding of how various complex everyday practices and socio-cultural hierarchies contribute to the formation of online identities. Part III concludes the chapter by discussing how the lenses provided through this kind of methodology can contribute to the understanding of race, gender, sexuality, class and geography in relation to cyberspace while shedding light on how the situated design of technological environments prevents cyberculture from being universally accessible, thus, leading to socio-cultural issues of access in addition to the material problems of physical and monetary access to computer technology that feed into digital divides the world over.

Digitally mediated environments cannot be understood unless the observer/user enters these spaces and tries living in them, working with them, doing things with and in them. Based on such a premise, our methodology draws on ongoing debates in cultural anthropology, feminist epistemology, postcolonial theory and feminist ethnography and combines them with debates regarding the problematics of studying online spaces. The approach emphasizes the doing of technology, building of cyberspatial environments and sustained interaction and "being" online in order that the researcher may understand the everyday practices associated with the context, as well as begin to engage the specifics of such a an engagement. Living online, thus, emphasizes immersion so that there are relational links between the ethnographer and the subject(s) being studied and so that the ethnographer understands how the spatio-temporal praxis of being in such environments might shape her subjectivity. As such, the researcher not only inhabits such spaces, s/he also learns to code herself into existence within such spaces by building, interacting and collaborating within them. Thus, s/he dialogically produces cyberselves.

In other words, academic analyses of techno-mediated subjectivities must self-reflectively engage and observe the Self (and the Other within the Self) "inside" technospaces. "At the momentary intersection of the human being and the machine," writes Munt (2001: 1), "there is spatial praxis: there is technospace." Through acts of building and inviting of participants as well as of inhabiting various online forums and communities, we have been immersed in studying such spatial praxis.

Sally Munt (2001: 11) asks "How is habitus experienced in technospace? What forms of embodiment are practiced in technospace?". It is widely acknowledged by most well known cybertheorists such as Steve Jones, Lisa Nakamura and T.L. Taylor (to name just a few), that "virtual" and "real" in the context of cyber living, are not mutually exclusive. The effects of cyberspacial praxis are real. Real people from real communities form "virtual" community to pursue real relationships, real collaborations and these activities have real goals and consequences. There is indeed accountability to "real life" within such spaces. Real people, after all, lose jobs to so-called virtual workers who in their turn are very real in the way that they contribute to society and the economy.

While the notion that there is no race or gender in cyberspace has long been contested (see works by Lisa Nakamura, 2002, Alondra Nelson 2001) by critical scholars and inhabitants of online spaces, the examination of cyberspatial praxis through the experience of habitus in cyberspace allows us to see how specific socio-culturally and linguistically situated practices of literacy and interpersonal sharing contribute to the production of hierarchies online. Within such hierarchies (intricately interwoven into everyday cultural practices within communities of production) are produced raced, gendered and classed virtual/real subjects online. Although analyses of static[2] texts are proliferating, fewer scholars are actually observing the processes of production of culture within such online spaces. Even in these virtual environments, participants do not leave their bodies behind. Hence, the virtual/real distinction sets up a false binary that cannot be substantiated when we analyze engagement with online environments. Part of what our analysis does is to try to unravel the dichotomy between the virtual and the real. Thus, this project focuses on the actual production of cultural experience and materiality of virtuality, as it is experienced by participants in online environments.

Everyday material practices, even when those practices involve online production of self, are shaped through socio-economic location and cultural literacies. While in the case of offline environments, certain practices and activities have been quite clearly socially coded, in online environments the social coding is different. For instance, in offline environments, the practice of chopping wood might be identified within a certain kind of social hierarchy as manual labor, and the practice of writing is identified within certain hierarchies as an advanced form of literacy, and so on. In online environments, interpersonal codes for ethics and for "netiquette" have been developed and continue to be further developed. Thus, for instance, the practice of "flaming" refers to rude or personal attacks and is generally considered to be socially unacceptable, while the practice of "lurking" refers to people who subscribe to online interactive spaces but do not reveal their presence by visibly communicating. The practices of typing/coding/imaging one's self into existence within various digital environments produces the subjects/agents of differing socio-cultural purchase based on hierarchies of literacy and socio-cultural meaning-making. Meaning is made through coding, programming, typing, one's self into existence through building objects and interacting digitally (through image, audio, text), socially but it is also made in relation to and in the context of larger socio-cultural and economic practices of everyday life.

Scholars such as Marvin (1988), Slack (1989) and Sterne (2003)have pointed out how social ideological struggles are negotiated in relation to technologies and how various practices produce hierarchies around the use, consumption, production, design, reproduction and circulation of such technologies. Jennifer Daryl Slack (1989: 339, italics mine) argues:

> Technology is not simply an object connected in various ways to the institutionaland organizational structures from within which it emerges to be reconnected in a new context, but . . . it is *always an articulated moment of interconnections among the range of social practices, discursive statements, ideological positions, social forces, and social groups within which the object moves.*

[2] In online contexts, text can be static and frozen in time on website and blogs and listproc archives, while during interaction, whether synchronous or asynchronous, the same texts appear "live" and dynamic to users. This is why we use the notion of static text as opposed to text in production in this instance, see Gajjala 1998 and 2004 for more on this.

Material practices within and in relation to digitally mediated environments, therfore, provide a new arena "for negotiating issues crucial to the conduct of social life; among them, who is inside and outside, who may speak, who may not, and who has authority and may be believed" (Marvin,1988: 4). Through a focus on examining practices of production of selves in and around digital technologies and digitally mediated spaces methodologically, we begin to observe more than just how the technology works, thus getting beyond the fascination with the "newness". Therefore, on the one hand, as Marvin (1988: 4-5) states:

> The focus of communication is shifted from the instrument to the drama in which existing groups perpetually negotiate power, authority, representation, and knowledge with whatever resources are available. New media intrude on these negotiations by providing new platforms on which old groups are projected onto new technologies that alter, or seem to alter, critical social distances. New media may change the perceived effectiveness of one group's surveillance of another, the permissible familiarity of exchange, the frequency and intensity of contact, and the efficiency of customary tests for truth and deception .... New practices do not so much flow directly from technologies that inspire them as they are improvised out of old practices that no longer work in new settings.

On the other hand, as Jenny Sunden (2003) notes, a distance—both spatial/physical and between the mind/body—is created between the typist/programmer and subject typed into existence in encounters with digital interfaces such as computers. Writing about the production of selves within online text-based environments known as "MOO", Sunden (2003:4) writes:

> This distance is on one level introduced in text-based online worlds through the act of typing, and further reinforced by the mediating computer technology itself. By actively having to type oneself into being, a certain gap in this construction is at the same time created. The mediation between different realms, the very creation of texts by the means of computers, makes the interspace that always exists between myself and the understanding of this self particularly clear. Following the idea of a subject that can never have a direct and unmediated access to herself, that the I writing and the I written about can never be seen as one, cyber subjects are always at least double.

The action of *producing oneself* in such an environment is enacted through typing, however, the particular participant's agency is produced both through the act of typing and the programming that results as well as through her/his embodied negotiations of socio-cultural literacies, memories, histories, patterns and negotiations in relation to the "old groups" that Marvin (1988) mentions.

In what follows, we draw from several pedagogical scenarios to illustrate the framework explained above. All these scenarios are based in university undergraduate and graduate classrooms where students work on various versions of what we call the "MOO project".

PART II

In this chapter, we will focus on how projects, journals and observations from two specific classes using the MOO shed light on how literacies, culture and offline identities interacted with student experience of the MOO to analyse and reveal specific understandings of cyber-identities as produced through the typing one's self into existence through designing and programming environments and through interpersonal interaction.

Production Of Identity And Cultural Literacies On The Moo

Variations of the MOO project have been assigned in several classes taught by Radhika over the past several years at both the undergraduate and graduate level. This project was used in courses focused on the understanding of processes of meaning making and the production of cultures and identities. Several of the courses that introduced this project were directly offering instruction regarding digital technologies within society with a focus on knowing a certain amount of hands on skills in order to understand how identities, cultures, transnational organizations and processes of globalization are shaped by the introduction of the computer into society. Therefore, in such courses, students came expecting to do some hands on computer work (classes were often held in a computer lab). However, in the case of one specific graduate seminar, the MOO project was explicitly used as a site for all class members to implement a chosen qualititative /critical methodology, drawing from theories introduced to them in class. This was a course on research methods, and students had to choose theories and methods that they considered appropriate for the study of the online MOO environment to which they were introduced in class.

In all these classes, the basic requirements for the MOO project involved exploring the MOO environment, interacting with objects already built and writing narratives and journals based on the understandings that came out of such explorations.

In some classes, students were taken a step further and given "programmer" status while being required to build an environment based on concepts and reading material introduced as part of the course content.

In laying out the context for the specific examples used in this chapter, we must explain how what one of us had begun as a MOO exercise in her undergraduate courses on "new technologies" developed into an exercise for students to examine cyberselves in production. The moo exercise started out with just the instructor, building environments and objects were for students to explore and examine as cultures for communication online. The students participated in the interface as guests, a way of interacting which granted them only opportunities to interact with existing structures and objects, not the capability to build their own objects and spaces. Thus, the students were more like tourists/voyeurs, and their experience was shaped by a limited ability to code and shape the interface. However, we were unsatisfied by their understanding of how online cultures were produced – they still seemed to have what might be called an "outside gaze" perspective where they were still feeling the disembodiedness of online existence as being outside of "real" based in a binary that simplistically categorizes the "virtual" (being online) and "not real". The real goal of the exercise was to to make students understand the nature of DWELLING in cyberculture (granted this was very ambitious considering the short span of a semester), therefore, the next time, the moo exercise was developed for a class students were assigned more extensive abilities to build rooms and objects by requesting the wizards at Lingua MOO[3]. In both undergraduate and graduate classes thereafter students were to build objects that would illustrate their understanding of theoretical concepts and scenarios in class.

The excerpts included below - though seemingly cryptic form scenario's of engagement with cyberculture that lead to understanding of subject formation in such a space. The samples in the text boxed that follow are from a student group. The first text box is from their journal commenting on wrap up activity in an undergraduate class on Performing Digitally Mediated Identities The second and third are from the actual online events that they are referring to. This activity happened on a MUD space that was developed temporarily for this course project – it did not happen on Lingua MOO. Below, a sample is included to give the reader an idea of the form of the interface in which they type. However, since it is a static capture, it cannot adequately give a sense of identity FORMATION as a process in such spaces. Therefore, in later parts of the chapter we analyse specific examples chosen from a variety of such engagements.

> We first started our room and designed it as a computer lab because of the versatility of the environment. We could have a great deal of different objects because of all the things that "belong" in a computer lab (for instance, the beer, the clock, the computers, the instructor, the windows). Many of these objects lend themselves well to having a gender—something we spent a great deal of time looking at during the start of the semester. And, some of the objects didn't have genders, which was something we explored briefly in our last encounter on the MUD.
>
> We built a pretty fair number of objects in the room, but some are more important and more relevant to the project than others. For instance, we built a virtual instructor in the likeness of our own R (instructor). She wandered around the room giving us virtual advice and seeing how we virtually interacted, just like she does in "real life." We also started describing our own characters, where C was a virtual smoker and had a virtually raspy voice, and A was a suck-up and a lab consultant in the virtual lab. We also created virtual animals to run around the lab. This made the environment unique in that it wasn't quite a computer lab (real computer labs don't have beer and cats), but instead was clearly a creation of how we view our class (the disjointedness that we sometimes feel from interacting with group members via teleconferencing and instant messaging was manifest in the chaotic and random atmosphere of the lab).
>
> This activity was, essentially, a culmination of all of our class readings and discussions during the semester. We incorporated elements of gender identity (and gender ambiguity), virtual identities (which were radically different from our "real life" identities), we created a virtual place where we could meet as a group, even though one of our group members wasn't in the classroom with us, and we had a great time personalizing our online lab/classroom in that we made it an environment that was unique to our needs and personalities as college students and people (and cats).

---

[3] We wish to thank Cynthia Haynes for patiently helping me out in this regard each semester! Lingua MOO can be

"ANDY's HOT LAB"
andy's hot lab(#39JL)
Contents:
megan's bud light
wind
Moo Computer(#176)
yellow paper towels
Kitty Treats(#169)
Sadie
a full bar
cheese and crackers
School Counselor
a large open window
Air Condition
Asian People
confused student
Keg
Andy's Newport Lights
Radhika's 6-pack(#102)
radhika
Chelsea's Beer
Radhika(#94)
megan wants a beer
Nerds(#92)
heater
Sweet Clock(#81)
Andy's Computer
Desk
MAC coumputer
computer

look heater

Large steam heater that BGSU uses to try and force Andy to quit working in the labs, but he stays irrespective of the temperature, simply so he can stalk Chelsea from Lab to Lab to Lab...

look Nerds

Nerds(#92)

Several nerds sit in the computer lab, sweating, creating objects in their lovely MUD room. Don't disturb... they're hard at work.

look #94

Radhika(#94)

The instructor wanders around, asking for journals, giving ambiguous and cryptic instructions, seeing how students learn.

---

accessed from http://lingua.utdallas.edu:7000

"Chelsea, Jason, and I say 'Don't let the virtual cat pee on your leg! Thanks for a great class and a bunch of new experiences! Have a great break!

Description of Assignment as Made Available to Students on the Mud

MUD Log:
Trying 69.64.38.199...
Connected to giggle.mudmagic.com.
Escape character is '^]'.
This world is Pueblo 1.0 enhanced

Welcome to TinyMUSH

"connect <name> <password>" connects you to an existing character.
"create <name> <password>" creates a new character.
"WHO" tells you who is logged in to the game (case sensitive).
"QUIT" exits the game and saves your character.
"news" informs you about recent program changes and items of interest.
"help" gives help on the commands, "help commands" for a list.

Note to MOO users and those of you "trained" via other diva projects
- commands here a slightly different from what you maybe used to so type help
frequently. When you feel too lost, type home (not @home)
to get back to where you started. Type "examine" not "@examine"
to examine ...etc

Everything you do is being logged by Wizard Gajjala and she will know
what you did and when. And you will be graded accordingly.

You will build for about 45 minutes and then each individual will
email me (at radhika@cyberdiva.org) a journal describing the
rationale for why your group built the environment, who built
which object and why,
and what were you as a group and as individuals in the group
trying to express by doing so. How does this activity draw on
readings, discussions and
activities done throughout the semester.

Have fun! I look fwd to viewing your projects and reading your journals.

end of messages

MOTD: hello

In another class - a Graduate level Research Methods course in Communications (spring 2004), the MOO project was intended to help entry level graduate students learn the importance of situating themselves and to problematize subject-object relations in Research Methods. For the MOO Ethnography and Research Methods assignment, students were asked to build rooms and explore the MOO. The site was LinguaMOO. At various stages of the MOO ethnography, students were asked to program objects and items to illustrate theoretical concepts and personal location in relation to their objects of inquiry. After the exploration and building stages were done, students were to form groups and write research proposals based on their examination of the MOO and understanding of various methodologies introduced in the course. The rationale for the use of the MOO in this manner was explained using the following quote from Jenny Sunden:

> Even though the border between physical and virtual locations is continuously crossed in online experiences, there is also a separating distance between the two. This distance is on one level introduced in textbased online worlds through the act of typing, and further reinforced by the mediating computer technology itself. By actively having to type oneself into being, a certain gap in this construction is at the same time created. The mediation between different realms, the very creation of texts by the means of computers, makes the interspace that always exists between myself and the understanding of this self particularly clear.
>
> Following the idea of a subject that can never have a direct and unmediated access to herself, that the I writing and the I written about can never be seen as one, cyber subjects are always at least double. This distance can in a similar way be used for methodological purposes, to form a reflexive understanding of research procedures and of the way that oneself as a researcher is always intertwined with these processes. It can be used to create room for reflection on how I, the researcher, am not only a producer of texts, such as this one, but also always a co-producer of the reality that is being written (Sunden, 2003:21).

Along with the MOO assignment students were reading essays on communication and critical theory, critical ethnography, feminist epistemologies, postcolonial theory, and the books "Virtual Materialities" by Jenny Sunden (2003) and "Object Stares Back" by Elkins (1996).

Part III

The MOO has three important attributes. First, it is a text-based environment. It is also a multi-user domain and an object oriented space. This means that the MOO is not merely a chat space like AOL Instant Messenger. The MOO interface is predicated on building text-based virtual locations and objects to serve as the context of interactions between users. Although LinguaMoo (http://lingua.utdallas.edu) allows for some images that can be used as backgrounds or character or object icons, the space is navigated primarily by text entered by the user.

It should be noted that the text-based MOO is a comparatively older technology (even though Lingua MOO has a more current web-interface, it is important to note that most of the object building/programming and interaction with objects usually takes place in the text-based, text-coded environment). MOOs are used consistently in English classes that teach writing skills, however, students in both communication studies classes were unfamiliar with it and did not understand why we were using it. This lack of familiarity with the software or the specific LinguaMoo interface is important to the production of the self in a particular online context. The lack of familiarity produces a contested dynamic techno-mediated space, unsettling notions of digital technology as fostering immediacy and efficiency in a world defined by the rhetoric of "Progress". Not only are these in-between and dynamic information spaces in the way they are used, in allowing for uncertainty of participant experience and encounter, they are also sites for the explicit contestation and negotiation of co-produced and technologically mediated meaning-making processes and of the pseudo-binaries of "Virtual" and "Real". Further the fact that MOOs require the user to establish an avatar and description for their character creates, as Beth Kolko and colleagues (2000: 214) point out, "explicit engagement with identity… [that] makes them fertile ground for exploring how identity and interface interact".

Theorists such as Kali Tal (1996:1) have suggested that cyberspaces usually suffer from an "unbearable whiteness of being". Because most online environments (including LinguaMOO) do not explicitly include race as an avatar characteristic (unlike gender), race is not an automatic character attribute. The following explanation of gender on a MOO is taken from Lingua MOOs help menu. Note that there are various possible "genders" offered.

> Syntax: @gender <gender>
> @gender
> The first form, with an argument, defines your player to have the gender <gender>. If <gender> is one of the standard genders (e.g., 'male', 'female', 'neuter',...), your various pronouns will also be set appropriately, making exits and certain other objects behave more pleasantly for you.
> The second form tells you the current definition of your player's gender, your current pronouns, and the complete list of standard genders.
> It should be noted that some of the "genders" on the standard gender list need verb conjugation in order to work properly and much of the MOO isn't set up for this (...yet). For example, you should expect to see 'they is' a fair amount if you @gender yourself 'plural'.
> Your gender is currently female.
> Your pronouns: she,her,her,hers,herself,She,Her,Her,Hers,Herself
> Available genders: neuter, male, female, either, Spivak, splat, plural, egotistical, royal, or 2nd[5]

However, as Kolko and others (2000) have noted, the MOO does not allow the user to set a "race" category. Kolko (2000: 214) writes, for instance, "in the case of textual worlds, race tends to be missing as an element of virtual identity".

In her work, Kolko (2000: 213) describes, "how race as a category has been elided in such media through various design choices", while investigating "how the construction of `raceless' interfaces affects the communicative possibilities of virtual worlds". She goes on to describe efforts at reintroducing race as an articulated notion on MOOscape in order to "ask how an explicit marking of race online might affect the social environment". Because of work done by previous researchers on race in cyberspace, we've come to understand that in many online environments, explicit mention of race becomes an anomaly, unless used as a particular kind of identity tourism (Nakamura, 2002), for which it is employed nearly completely stereotypically. In fact, Kali Tal (1996: 1) goes as far as to assert that:

> In cyberspace, it is finally possible to completely and utterly disappear people of color. I have long suspected that the much vaunted "freedom" to shed the "limiting" markers of race and gender on the Internet is illusory, and that in fact it masks a more disturbing phenomenon--the whitinizing of cyberspace. The
>
> 5 This excerpt was taken from Lingua MOO's help menu on gender
>
> invisibility of people of color on the Net has allowed white-controlled and whiteread publications like WIRED to simply elide questions of race.

In employing the MOO pedagogically, our goal was not so much to reintroduce race-as-an-articulated-notion as a textually recognizable label or category, as it seems to have been in Kolko's invaluable experiment, but to engage the apparent invisibility of being raced. Our strategy was to create a racial awareness implicitly and explicitly in our face-to-face class environment. In an effort to refuse to allow race (and other nuances of identity grounded in the body) to remain unremarked, students entering the MOO textual environment had been sensitized to issues of race, sexuality, geography and class within the face-to-face classroom environment, in face-to-face group discussions and through class readings. Thus, when they entered the textual environment the analytical and conceptual lenses they engaged in trying to make meaning of their encounters with the MOO – as their identity and MOO interface were explored – led them to be very aware of racial, sexual and cultural codings in interpersonal and socioeconomic contexts within both their daily lives and in their online activities in class.

Part of the goal of this project was to conduct auto/ethnographic observation and analysis of the ways that the self was produced at the intersection of the face-to-face classroom, MOO classroom, and MOO analysis.

Unsettled White Male Privilege?

The very idea that a mediated form of communication technology could serve to disguise identity and even prevent those of privilege from asserting their identity (particularly white, European-American males) became a center to my engagement with course materials. ... Such technology has shown to have the ability to disguise one's true identity.... The main issue underlying all of this is that there are certain forms of technology within the realm of communication that in some form or another make it difficult for people to assert their physical identity." – "Ray", graduate student in Research Methods Course.

What is interesting to us here is that Ray's experience does not match what theorists such as Kali Tal would suggest about whiteness as the default category of identity in cyberspace. Ray failed to realize that even though the visible physical markers of his identity are not present, the seemingly ubiquitous white maleness in cyberspace marks him with the unmarked default category of white male. According to other research on race in cyberspace, we should expect his privileged race/gender position to be preserved even though HE can't see himself that way—he is still going to be read that way. Our research suggests that the "whiteness of cyberspace" functions as an extension of the whiteness of everyday life. In addition, a closer look at how race was used and functioned in this classroom environment shows that:

- The function and definition of race and privilege is radically dependent on the context and specifics of the interplay of cyber- and real-spaces that are being considered.
- Multiple understandings and experiences of race are employed in cyberspaces and the real spaces with which they intersect.

To understand his experience, we have to look at the real world context in which he engaged the technological interface—as described above, the classroom context was designed specifically to try to counter the insistence that race remain unremarked. First, the visible identity markers of the instructor, which identify her as a third world woman. Next, the context of the course readings were heavily influenced by critical theory and postcolonial feminist theory. Third, we have the makeup of the class room participants— Ray was one of only 2 white males, and the other class members included three international students (two Chinese and one Indian), 1 African American and 1 "out" lesbian, and several straight appearing white women, some of whom were fluent and articulate in the theoretical language of postcolonial feminism and critical theory used in class readings.

We see from the beginning that the MOO was "R's MOO"—most students could not pronounce Professor R's first or last name. Thus, the space became racialized in a very particular way. Students were required to program an object that would illustrate a concept coming out of the readings, and then asked to analyze the effect of the object they programmed. This created a reflexive space.

Because of the context and design of the real life space in which students encountered the MOO, the MOO space was racialized, creating a reflexivity on the production of the students' own racial identities (and other characteristics of identity) in the space.

> I'm sitting in front of this terminal trying to figure out what in the world I'm supposed to be doing for this class. What are these commands? I'm supposed to create a home? I'm supposed to generate artifacts that represent me? I can't figure out the basic functions of this MOO. I hate this assignment. – "Ray"

Ray goes on to describe how he would rather use the Moo at home even though his access is an older, super-slow, dial-up connection, compared to the relatively speedy direct connections he could access at the university computer lab. His anxiety about identity and meaning manifest themselves in this choice, evoking not just the absence of visible physical cues about his everyday self, but also the lack of validation of his identity that he is granted from others in his everyday life.

> Here, I have the smell of home, the taste of my wife's cooking, and the security that she is there for me. She knows who I am—she can see me, she understands me, and she knows all of my quirks – "Ray"

In addition to this idea of the way the MOO was raced/affiliated in this context, we see how critical it is that students were unfamiliar with this technological interface. The technological interface, because of its design, can force us to negotiate cultural cues that function differently in familiar everyday life. This can make the process of producing the self visible.

> A personal encounter with a technology that strips me of much of my everyday privilege. This is a way to sum up my personal encounter with the MOO. Let me explain—I am a white, European-American, male, of middle-class status. These very marks of identification have been taken from me during this encounter.... I noticed my desire to assert some sort of privilege on this technology. Can't they see I'm white? Can't they see that I'm male? Can they see anything about me at all? I couldn't seem to produce the privilege that I seemed to take for granted. –"Ray"

Ray's response is also a kind of racial anxiety. What we observed was how he was more anxious about the presence of his body than someone who was more confident about his ability to communicate wholly through text might have been. After examining some of his responses and articulations, we wondered if his anxiety around the absence of his white body to assert his privilege in a social space may have been linked to his obvious struggle with academic articulation. Thus, while his own analysis of his encounter with the anonymity of cyberspace via the MOO might suggest that he was a white male – privileged in many ways in comparison to other students in class, he may indeed have been slightly more disadvantaged in terms of particular kinds of academic or cyberliteracy when compared to some of the other students who may have appeared more disadvantaged socially based on their race-based, gender-based, sexuality-based and geography-based locations. Lori Kendall (2002: 183) states that:

> [C]lass background may be the single most important factor influencing online participation. Over 60 percent of Internet participants (63-75 percent, depending upon the data source) hold some form of professional, technical, managerial, or other white collar job ...Yet in their depictions of interactive forums such as muds, online researchers rarely discuss class, usually focusing instead on gender. This tendency reflects online culture itself, where gender and sexuality are much more frequent topics of discussion than class or race identity.

If race is expected to be an invisible category, in everyday life and in cyberspaces – class is even more so. Both these categories are often subsumed under discussions of the "digital divide", where the specifics and complexities of race and class in relation to the Internet examine issues of access and literacy in non-problematic ways as purely economic, geographic or a combination of both (as in, "the poorer regions of the world experience the [singular] digital divide"). In actuality, both existing connected populations as well those who are on the unconnected edge of the digital divide are variously raced and classed, and likewise have varying cultural competencies in different online spaces. The particular pedagogic process that was engaged here was designed to reveal the complex interplay of race, class, sexuality, gender and geography in relation to the negotiation of online environments. As is visible in the two examples discussed, issues of literacy, access and class were as much a factor in the production of hierarchies as race and gender. Thus, we used a practice of pedagogy that relies on dislocating students out of privilege, then asking them to reflexively analyze the loss of privilege and the everydayness of the privileges they experience. This practice resulted, as we shall see in the next example, in helping students articulate the different cultural competencies and literacies that impacted their experiences in the virtual learning environment.

But how might this pedagogy of dislocating students out of privilege work with an Asian female student who had come to the U.S. to study only about a year prior to taking this course? What sorts of privilege or lack might this encounter reveal in relationto her? In what ways does her gendered, classed, and raced experience reveal the nuances of techno, academic, language or other literacies that impact virtual learningenvironments?

Y, a female Chinese student in the class, was very silent when the MOO assignment was first introduced as a requirement. Her non-verbals indicated that she wasnot particularly happy. As it turned out, she later went to meet the instructor in an effort to learn to "MOO". During this meeting, she gently questioned the need for the MOOexercise in a course that was supposed to be about "research methods." Upon being asked if she felt angry at being asked to do this assignment and if she was could she please articulate that anger in discussion via the online course discussion space so that we could raise the topic in class discussions, she did so. Below, we reproduce the post that she contributed regarding her response to the MOO.

SUBJECT: POWER AND NEW LITERACY

I have always considered myself to be literate because I can not only read and write in my native language, Chinese, I am also quite proficient in English.

However, my literacy is completely challenged in the MOO world because here I don't know the codes, the commands, and the icons. Suddenly, I realize that I'm illiterate in this world. To be confident, I have to learn the MOO language which takes time. I feel kind of embarrassed for sleeping all the time in MOO. Not only that, I accidentally built my room in auntpearl's room and infringed on her private space. To make things worse, I even didn't know that I was sleeping in somebody else's room right from the first day I had a room in the MOO. Now with the help of the patient professor, I was able to apologize to auntpearl and move my room to my territory. The technological illiteracy (not knowing the MOO language) renders me powerless in this already built and sophisticated world. My impotency makes me suffer from inferiority complex and unnamed anger. Never before have I felt so stupid for a course I've taken. I feel angry with myself and the MOO. I am angry with myself because after several attempts to explore the MOO world, I still feel almost as dumb as the first time and I don't seem to make any progress as far as understanding and mastering another language is concerned. On the other hand, I feel angry with MOO because it is MOO that makes me feel stupid and inadequate.

My frustrating MOO experience leads me to thinking of power structures in terms of entry for the time being. In an already established power structure, the order of entry does matter. The later you come, the more puzzlement you have to experience and the more failure you have to endure. However, there is still some hope. My present situation reminds me of a book Woman/Native/Other. Somewhere in the book, the idea of using the master's language to defeat him is discussed. Whether it is an appropriate analogy, there is the hope for me to know the language and use it for something good. Actually, I did some ethnographic work on my mother's and sister-in-law's life and I'm still working on it. Although they come from different educational background (While my mother is completely illiterate, my sister-in-law can read and write), both of them feel inadequate in articulating their voices. They entrust me with the job of telling their stories, stories of ordinary, everyday Chinese women to the audience in theWest. Thus, I become the agent of their voices in a foreign land where I have to constantly struggle with my place of belonging. The world of academia to them is what the world of MOO to me. But here, I cannot find an agent to do the talking for me and I have to make it out myself.

Through the examples discussed in this chapter, we can understand how the learner herself experienced the socio-cultural space we are studying. Y's reflection on what happened for her in the MOO space reveals nuances we could not have surmised from watching the product of the socio-cultural exchange. In addition, asking students to reflexively consider their experiences in virtual learning environments creates opportunities for the learner herself to better understand the ways that privilege and power are nuanced.

In Y's case, understanding the MOO encounter was about considering "power and new literacy". As a transnational travelling subject, she uses literacy in more than one way in her explanation—and her careful articulation makes it clear that to understand how race, privilege and power interact in online spaces, we must reach for a finely nuanced analysis.

It is obvious both from Y's participation in class and from her carefully written post quoted above that she is highly literate in English as a language. Additionally, we can see her fluency (or literacy) with academic language, the language of theory. In fact, Y's position as a non-native, Chinese woman living in diaspora made her feel comfortable in a classroom steeped in the language of postcolonial feminism, and we saw this proficiency both in classroom discussions and in her written work.

In Y's case, however, she cites two other kinds of literacy that need to be considered in order to fully understand her experience on the MOO. First, she suggests that her lack of comfort with the particular technology, her "technological illiteracy" with the language of the MOO, makes her feel angry and uncomfortable—lost in a world without the right language. Although Ray clearly expresses similar feelings of inadequacy and frustration (and in fact nearly all students first introduced to the MOO in this classroom said the same, including the student co-author of this essay), Y's post articulates this frustration as technological illiteracy.

In later assignments, Y realizes even one more kind of literacy that impacts her experience on the MOO—her literacy with the "soft parts of American culture." A world traveler who is extremely fluent in both Chinese and English, who has studied life in the U.S. and has been teaching students to be prepared to successfully communicate in U.S.

English for several years, pop culture references in the MOO made her feel like an outsider—lost not only in the MOO techno-language but also in the everyday culture references used as students built objects that referred to popular bands, movies, TV shows, and so on.

The ways in which Y nuances literacy can help us build a framework for analyzing what happens in such settings. When we juxtapose Y's varying literacies with Ray's, we see a complex interaction of cultural competencies and/or literacies that allow/produce privilege at the intersection of cyber/real spaces in the classroom.

CONCLUSION

In this chapter, we have described what we would call a methodology of subjectivity and context production based in epistemologies of doing. Through an engagement with the process of building, co-creating and living in online spaces, it is possible for the researcher to understand the production of selves through technospatial praxis. This research suggests not just the need for radical contextualization, but a need to consider closely our methodologies as we study various virtual, digital, and online technologies. While straight textual analysis can yield a particular kind of understanding of what happens in online spaces, considering the processes of meaning making, not just the resulting text, yields another understanding, one that is vital if we are interested in understanding the subjective experience of participants in online spaces. We have shown how this can be done, by using examples from pedagogic situations where exercises for specific kinds of online and offline study and research of such techno-mediated spaces were carefully thought about and developed based on one of the co-author's past experience researching and building online environments (see Gajjala, 2004). The findings from the research described in this chapter also have implications for critical pedagogical use of internet technologies within the classroom.

References

[1] Butler, J. 1990 'Performative Acts and Gender Constitution: An Essay in Phenomenology and Feminist Theory', in S. Case (ed.), *Performing Feminisms:Feminist Critical Theory and Theatre*, pp. 270-282, John Hopkins UP,Baltimore, MD.

[2] Elkins, J., 1996, *The Object Stares Back : On the Nature of Seeing*, Harcourt Brace, San Diego.

[3] Gajjala, R., 2004, *Cyberselves: Feminist Ethnographies of South Asian Women*,Altamira Press, London.

[4] Haynes, C. and Holmevik, J. R., 2000, *Mooniversity: A Student's Guide toOnline Learning Environments*, Allyn and Bacon, Needham Heights MA.

[5] Kendall, L., 2002, *Hanging Out in the Virtual Pub Masculinities and Relationships*, University of California Press, Berkeley.

[6] Kolko, B., 2000, 'Erasing @race', in B. E. Kolko, L. Nakamura, and G. B.

[7] Rodman (eds.), *Race in cyberspace*, pp. 213-232, Routledge, New York.

[8] Kolko, B., Nakamura, L. and Rodman, G. (eds.), 2000, *Race In Cyberspace*,

[9] Routledge, New York and London.

[10] Marvin, C., 1987, When Old Technologies Were New, Oxford University Press,New York.

[11] Munt, S., 2001, *Technospaces: Inside the New Medi*a, Continuum International,London.

[12] Nakamura, L., 2002, *Cybertypes: Race, Ethnicity, and Identity on theInternet*, Routledge, New York and London.

[13] Nelson, A., Hines, A. H. and Tu, T. L. N., 2001, 'Hidden Circuits', in a. Nelson A. and T. L. N. Tu (eds.), *Technicolor: Race, Technology and Everyday Life*, pp. 1-13, New York University Press, New York.

[14] Nelson, A., Tu, T. L. N. and Bald, V., 2001, 'Appropriating Technology', in a. Nelson and T. L. N. Tu (eds.), *Technicolor: Race, Technology and Everyday Life*, pp. 88-99, New York University Press, New York,Slack, J. D., 1989, 'Contextualizing Technology', in B. Dervin, L. Grossberg, B. O'Keefe,and E. Wartella (eds.), *Rethinking Communication Volume 2, Paradigm/Exemplars,* pp. 329–45, Sage, Newbury Park, CA

[15] Sterne, J., 2000, 'Bordieu, Technique and Technology', *Cultural Studies17*,vol. 3, no. 4, pp. 367-389.

[16] Sunden, J., 2003, *Material Virtualities*, Peter Lang Publishing, New York.

[17] Tal, K., 1996, 'The Unbearable Whiteness of Being: African American Critical Theory and Cyberculture'.*<http://www.gse.buffalo.edu/FAS/Bromley/classes/socprac/readings/Kali-Tal-unbearable.htm>*

In: Health Research in Cyberspace
Editor: Pranee Liamputtong, pp. 85-104
ISBN 1-59454-819-6

Chapter 5

Researcher/Woman/Lesbian? Finding a Voice in Creating a Researcher Position, Trust and Credibility as a Participant Researcher in a Mediated Mailing-List Environment for Lesbian and Bisexual Women[1]

Janne Bromseth

> *The researcher is filled with tales of mask for age and race, gender and class; masks for almost all aspects of identity. These are tales that do not always have happy endings. The stories of on-line cross-dressing that abound, for example, often culminate in narratives of betrayal.*
>
> (Kolko and Reid, 1998: 218)

Introduction

In 2001, I started to get familiar with Sapfo, a women-only discussion group for lesbian and bisexual women in Scandinavia, while browsing around to find an interesting group to look into as an in-depth study.[2] I had previously been studying two online groups with professional and political purposes and subjects – however merely as non-participatory observer. Moving on with Sapfo, I wanted to expand my researcher role, being more active and visible inside of the group, to be able to create dialogues with the list members. This chapter reflects some of the challenges I faced during the process of establishing a researcher position, and creating trust and credibility within the mediated context. Both initially when asking the community for permission to do research, but more importantly, in maintaining

[1] I would like to thank Isabelle Dussauge for useful comments on drafts of this chapter.
[2] This article is based on my Ph.D. dissertation. See Bromseth 2006.

trust in a period of severe conflicts in the previously stable group, when four of the female long-term participants were 'revealed' to be written by one man (see later section about this). The changes that took place in the group following what happened forced me to reflect around my research position as participant observer, along with adapting my research strategies to the developing interaction-context.

What will be an appropriate 'voice' and methodological approach is always situated – in relation to context: a group' purpose, its participants and their background, and always implies an ethical perspective (Markham 2005). Using an ethnographic approach studying online groups, research strategic choices are not only relevant when creating a research design, but also as the project is carried out and moves along. In what ways could I participate in a group community where everyone suddenly suspected each other of being 'an-Other (fake and unreal)? What position was possible for me to take as a participant observing researcher in the reflections that followed the revelation, that by many participants were interpreted as a betrayal?

The Net As Arena for Minority Groups: Subcultures 'Coming Out' in The Public

In spite of the utopian beliefs of the internet as more democratic and socially equalizing because of the absence of the body, separating the typist from the text, social and cultural divides are re-produced in internet contexts. Bodies matter in differentiated ways also online, through discursive productions and negotiations of cultural hegemonies. Hierarchical social positions are re-produced, amongst others visible through what makes up the normal and the deviant, the marked/unmarked. This is visible both in participation patterns, values and ideology dominating the content of the net. A range of studies show how hierarchies are created online through social practice. This is visible in productions of cultural stereotypes (Nakamura, 2002), as well as through online harassment towards women, blacks and homosexuals (Hall, 1996; Herring,1996 ; Harcourt, 1999; Ward, 1999; Nakamura, 2002). Another aspect is that there will always be a limit to how liberating it can be to 'escape' identity categories online, as related to life offline. Nobody lives their entire life online. As Kolko et al. (2000: 8) points out: "neither the invisibility nor the mutability of online identity make it possible for you to escape your 'real world' identity completely". Race, gender and sexuality matters no less in cyberspace than it does in other social contexts – also as related to power.

On the other hand, research also report of the positive aspects and new possibilities that the net offers to allow marginalized voices to speak and create supportive minority networks across time and place. Mitra (2001) points out that public media in general has been a restricted access sphere with little room for minority voices. The net represents an arena with fewer gatekeepers and more possibilities of visualizing cultural and subcultural minorities that previously have been culturally marginalized and difficult to access. Many scholars within the field of internet-studies have discussed the possibilities and consequences mediated interaction spaces might have for minority groups to create community, and their meanings as half-hybrid public space (Wakeford, 1997; Mitra, 2001; Brockington, 2003; Gajjala, 2004; see also Chapter 1 in this volume). Or rather, the meanings of creating community on the basis of minority positions that are generally constructed and interpreted as 'the deviant other' – as homosexuality.

SAPFO AS CULTURALLY SITUATED COMMUNITY OF PRACTICE

Sapfo is a half-closed e-mail-distributed listserv without public archives. All women are welcome as list members, but the primary target group was lesbian and bisexual women. It was started in 1999, as part of several mailing lists owned by the Organisation for sexual minorities in a Scandinavian country, which also has the formal responsibility for the list. When I joined the group, it had approximately 350 members, where of 20% were actively writing. A list mistress was responsible for technical issues related to running the group, as well reporting to the board of the Organisation if there were social difficulties within the group. Because of the lack of a participating list mistress, several list members took social responsibilities that a list administrator usually takes care of on mailing lists. This included everything from welcoming new members, encouraging each other to write in periods of low list traffic and collaboratively working themselves out of conflicts. The flat collaborative structure is a common organizing form of feminist groups in general, and the women-only context of Sapfo was also pro-feminism. As compared to many other countries, feminist political perspectives have a relatively strong position in the Scandinavian countries.

TROUBLED SUBJECT POSITIONS: COMMUNITY AS A REPAIRING FORCE

The participants on Sapfo and other groups for queer people create subcultural community on the basis of non-heterosexual subject positions that are 'potentially troublesome' in the heteronormative society (Staunæs 2003: 104, building on Wetherell 1998) "[...] positions that challenge the normativities at stake in certain everyday contexts of lived experience". This is to a large degree related to how taking these positions are perceived and responded to by others. There is, thus, a pattern of what causes the trouble in the first place: others' responses and interpretation of oneself as non-heterosexual. What is at the centre for creating a shared frame of reference for the interaction is related to living a sexual minority position. Lesbian or bisexual can be categorized as minority subject positions that are made more or less relevant throughout most social contexts. If and how the position is made relevant and experienced then, vary between social contexts; and further, a sexual minority position always intersect with other social identity positions (class, ethnicity, gender, place, age, profession and so on) in unpredictable ways. Sexual orientation, in line with gender and race, are not static and essentialized master identities, but identity positions that are socially and culturally constructed on all levels, through discourse and social practice (Staunæs, 2003). They gain meaning through culturally situated processes. Living marginalized minority positions implies to be questioned in relation to a central part of identity, and the processes of dealing with these experiences implies, amongst others, "the psychologies of interaction and negotiations of subject positions/identities when they become inappropriate, destabilized, difficult – when they are challenged and must be repaired"

(Wetherell 1998, in Staunæs, 2003: 104). The challenges non-heterosexuals take place in social situations in everyday life, often related to coming-out-processes, discrimination and harassment. Groups like Sapfo, thus, often have a supportive function, through creating a space where amongst others 'reparations' of identity challenging social experiences can take place – but also as spaces where it is possible to escape feelings of otherness. As long-term list-member Kaisa says:

> To belong to a minority [...] is equal to being questioned and vulnerable and then I do not necessarily mean by the crazy people with shaved head except the feeling of always being special. That is why it is so liberating with a forum where you don't have to be The Lesbian Guru. I can write about recipies and tell about my coughing wife without getting fifty-two follow-up-questions about my existence, but I can also write about feminist work without having to defend men in every and every-other meaning (the ones who have discussed feminist strategies in a mixed group know exactly what I am talking about).

However, creating a sense of community on the basis of a specific position of otherness – whether the subcultural community is mediated or not - does not imply that minority communities are one happy big family without internal struggles of power. As Radhika Gajjala (2004: 19) points out in relation to her study of mediated networks for South Asian women:

> Because this is a 'community' (though in several ways different from a 'real-life' (RL) community, the 'virtual community' is embedded in real-life communities), I expected that there were/are several discourses being marginalized. Thus my project was also to study what kind of discourses/opinions were being marginalized or silenced in this Internet community.

What is quoted above is also true when it comes to lesbian communities. On one level, hierarchies of 'normality' are on Sapfo turned upside down regarding sexuality, where 'non-heterosexuality', usually in a subordinate position in society, is in a superior position. Parallel to creating a 'we' in opposition to the heterosexual 'other', though, they also create and negotiate *internal hegemonies* of what identity positions and practices that should be considered right/wrong, good and bad. In these processes, participants also relate to other social arenas within the lesbian community within this Scandinavian country. In general, non-heterosexuality is marginalized and troubled as identity positions in most societies. In what ways these positions are troublesome, how they are made sense of and what characterize the positions that are available *within the subcultural community* in different countries, vary and are thus culturally situated (Blackwood, 1995; Chao, 1999; Fitzgerald, 1999). The sense of community that is created amongst participants in queer online groups is to a high degree related to the cultural frames participants share and relate to. In a study of The queer sisters' bulletin board for queer women in Hong Kong, initiated by a political group in Hong Kong with the same name, Joyce Nip (2004) found that the fact that the participants related to the physically based local queer/lesbian subculture was important for their sense of 'being part of the community' – both online and offline.

Cultural situatedness is central to the content of what gains validity when performing identity/presentations of selves in the interaction processes: what is talked about, how and with what effect. During the last decade, there have been extensive discussions about identity political issues both in the western and eastern world. This has been caused by the queer critique of essentialzing understandings of gender, sexuality and identity, challenging restricting norms of gender and sexuality for how an individual should live and perform sexuality. Identity politics and the queer influence have also been reported as major topics in other online groups (Nip, 2004; Munt et al, 2002). These conflicts and debates were also central in the discussions on Sapfo, and the list became one of several important arenas in the national subculture where ideas of identity politics was discussed. The Organisation for sexual minorities, who owned the list and who are the main actor in sexual minority policy making in the country, thus came in contact with a more extended group of queer people in the country, something that the board members expressed as very valuable in itself.

For me as a researcher, studying an online community like Sapfo implied studying a vulnerable context, in several senses, that required a cautious interaction with the community. It was clear that the list serv was very important to its participants, amongst others through being an arena for 'repairing' troubled subject positions that were to a high degree related to experiences from participants' offline life. Further, for some of the members who lived in small places, or who were not open about their sexual orientation, the list was the only place where they met other queer women. In order to develop an interactional approach with the list members, I needed to learn about the social frames of the community, both to understand how I would be interpreted within then *and* to actively use them as resources to gain confidence in the community.

An Ethnographic Approach

During my education, I was never trained in doing ethnography. As I did my master thesis though, or maybe more correctly, after doing it, I discovered that this was the name of approach that came closest to what I had actually done in practice: being present and observing the processes of group communication as situated cultural practise, trying to learn about the interactional codes and norms that were constructed over a longer stretch of time.

Many qualitative researchers have written about the particular possibilities of studying cultural processes mediated through the Internet in conducting material in online contexts. Christine Hine, author of Virtual Ethnography (2000), talks about 'a re-birth of ethnography' following the rapidly growing field of studies of net-culture. During the recent years, a few publications have addressed methodological issues in using qualitative approaches to online contexts (see Jones, 1999; Hine, 2000; Mann and Stewart, 2000; Markham 2003, 2005) as a result of the research experience doing internet studies the last decade. Although online contexts are quite diverse when it comes to what characterize them in form and purpose, they have one important thing in common, framing the interaction processes as well as the processes of doing research: the absence of the physical body and co-presence:

> The question ethnographic work online has attempted to answer is how people deal with this very absence [of the body]; how very specific online modes of communication develop and how shared systems are created (Sundén, 2003: 49).

Additionally, a great deal of interaction online takes place through non-vocal modes, mainly through text, as opposed to face-to-face interaction. In the synchronous online environments, like chats and MUDs, this has created new forms of dialogue, or 'textual talk' as Sundén (2003) calls it in her study of online community. These new kinds of social interaction that has features from both oral communication and written texts. Mailing lists and news groups operate through asynchronous modes, even if the rhythm of the exchanges of posts can take place within minutes, getting a feeling of same-time presence.

That participants are not physically present at a common place, and that the communication is taking place in written texts, influence the interaction. These two conditions for group interaction create specific frames for social processes for the people participating in it, as well as for the researcher studying online groups (Markham, 2005). As Annette Markham (2005: 799) points out, even if the Internet on the surface can seem like a more accessible and easy way to conduct studies of culture; the mediated setting adds quite a few challenges as well:

> But in the virtual field, as one interacts with anonymous participants, tracks disjointed, non-linear, multiple participant conversations, and analyzes hundreds of screens worth of cultural texts, one can begin to feel like the Internet might cause more headaches than it cures. Deceptive in its apparent simplicity, qualitative inquiry in this environment requires careful attention to the tradition by which social life is interpreted and the adjustments that must be made to give value to the online experience and internal consistency to one's methods.

These challenges appeared all along the way, and forced me to become very aware of how my position within the group could affect the community I studied – as well as the knowledge I was producing. In this chapter, I want to stress how my need to be "one of us" but with a responsibility and interest as a researcher necessarily created a vulnerable position to be negotiated within the frame of the community.

Defining the Research Context

> To have the option to pick a nice place, as opposed to picking a place out of necessity, might sound like an ethnographer's dream (Sundén, 2003: 31).

Like many other researchers studying mediated culture also have experienced, it is fairly easy to gain access to a diverse universe of groups as compared to doing field work on physically situated groups. However, the work of defining a research context then is, as Annette Markham (2003) points out, not located within and limited by specific physical places, but defined by interaction. The different stages in using an ethnographic approach in studying internet-mediated groups, can be roughly divided into two main phases (Kendall 2002). The first phase is related to 'casing the scene' as Sundén (2003) characterizes it, which in my case implied browsing around the Net to try to figure out what exactly existed of discussion group activity out from certain criteria, and by getting a picture of this, decide on which groups that potentially could be used for an in-depth study. The second phase is related to the process of the in-depth study itself, consisting of many different stages; most importantly getting permission and then, the period I spend in the field collecting material. During the preliminary observation phase, I followed many paths. My main interest was to focus on community building in non-commercial Nordic women-only spaces that had some sorts of counter-discursive aim and target group. In the end, I decided to look closer into discussion groups for lesbian and bisexual women[3]. Both because of their women-only group of participants, and because of thetiies to an established local lesbian subculture outside of its net-mediated context. Personally, I had experienced mediated groups as important arenas in my own sexual identity process, and since very few studies had been conducted on Nordic groups for queer people, I was eager to do the job. I decided to do an in-depth study of Sapfo, that I had been a member of since 2001.[4]

When I discovered Sapfo, I was enthusiastic about the well-functioning community that in spite of not having an active socially responsible list mistress (see later section) managed to work out things on a group level. Compared to many other women-only groups I had come across, it both had a high activity and the participants seemed to be able to discuss and disagree with each other. Simultaneously, list members took collective responsibility for reaching consensus before the disagreements got to a destructive level. New members were warmly welcomed by regulars, proud of their group:

> People,
> In every little cell in my seventeen year-old body I'm looking forward to sharing thoughts and reflections around different topics. I hope that Sapfo will give me plenty.
> Unna, who has been informed about the list by her girlfriend Fia, listmember
> **
> Welcome, Unna!
> You will not be disappointed, Sapfo enriches your life!
> Krista – who has a soar throat today
> **
> Hi Unna
> I hope so too. Welcome to us. Hope we get to
> see a lot of you in the time to come *s*
> Gyda
>
> (List messages)

I started preparing the first step in my research design: getting permission to be present.

---

[2]During my search, I also did some observation in 3 Nordic online GLBT-communities (Gay/Lesbian/Bisexual/Transgender), something that provided a useful broader context for my in-depth-study later on. (See Bromseth, 2003).

[3] During the first pre-liminary phase of the study, observation and field notes were the primary tools that I made use of. In relation to the second phase, I used several additional tools to help me enlighten my research questions from different angles. Qualitatively I chose two extended threads of discussion that I printed and used as a basis for in-depth analysis. I also printed and categorized several other discussions that in one way or another were characteristic for the interaction culture, or important episodes that affected the group in a particular way. During the formal period of doing research in the group, from November 2002 to July 2003, I was actively participating in the group myself, as well as having a few private exchanges of e-mails with some of the participants to enlighten particular issues. I also made five interviews face to face with the Organisation that owned the list, as well as four of Sapfo's members, and conducted one extended e-mail interview with one of the participants.

KNOCKING

Asking for Permission, June 2002 – Nov 2002

Who is the intended audience of an electronic communication – and does it include you as a researcher? (Ferri, 1999, cited in Mann and Stewart, 2000: 46)

The stage of getting permission to take part in the groups as a researcher is an important transition, where the control suddenly is not in your own hands anymore. Even if I at this point had chosen the group that I wanted to study, it all depended on if they wanted me to look at them. The question then, is not so much about what is practically possible in itself, but of what is possible to do within the frames of informed consent as a ground principle for the study – and with what effects. In preparing my research desing, I defined at least four possible effects to consider:

> There are at least four obvious main issues in preparing a functional research design that will be affected by choosing to obtain informed consent or not: 1) How will the research purpose be affected in informing group members? What research strategies would be possible? 3) How and can informants' privacy be protected and 4) What effects on the group as a social unit can occur? (Bromseth, 2002: 53)

In Norway, observation studies can normally be carried out without consent if they take place within public areas, and if they are not recorded digitally (The National Committee for Research Ethics in the Social Sciences, Law and Humanities (NESH) , 2001). Many net-researchers have argued that net-mediated groups are 'like a public town square'; Because they are situated in a half-public space, easily accessible for others it should not be necessary to obtain consent to do research there.[5] In my case, I had decided that no matter how accessible or open the groups I decided to use were, I would ask for consent. Even if online spaces are highly accessible, participants' primary purpose of communication is not necessarily 'speaking in public', but more a secondary consequence of meeting others online (Bromseth, 2002: 38). The lack of visual and audible cues also lowers the awareness of having an audience (Sixsmith and Murray, 2001). Since reading and writing takes place in isolation, it is easy to get a feeling of perceived privacy – not being conscious of the fact that the interaction is potentially accessible to a large silent audience. Considering the topic of the group I wanted to study, sexuality is moreover explicitly characterized as a sensitive issue by NESH, which always requires informed consent.

The main ethical consideration in not informing about the ongoing research is primarily related to potential consequences of harming individuals or groups **after** the study is done, in publishing the results from it. Deciding that obtaining informed consent **is** necessary, the implications are to a larger extent related to the process of collecting the material (Bromseth, 2002: 53).

My argument was, thus, that as a researcher, I have the superior responsibility of taking these issues into consideration. Rather then defining a priori that a context is 'public' because

---

[4] Important debates the latest years have however nuanced this picture, separating different net-spaces based upon how accessible they are on one hand – and the kind of social activity that takes place within it (see Association of Internet Researcher's ethics guidelines, 2004)

of its mediation form, which could be said to be an 'outside-position' of defining the context, I based my definition on an 'inside-position'; on the type of social activity that took place in the group, and by asking the participants themselves of their definitions. This choice was further related to my qualitative approach, wanting to take actively part in the groups, as well as intending to use an extensive amount of context information, and not least, document my findings with verbatim quotes. The process of obtaining consent implied that the owners and members of Sapfo would agree to participate in my project. But how would *I* participate in their community as an observer?

Asking For Permission in a Time of Conflict: Whose Consent? Now or Later?

1/10

> I am really worried now since I haven't heard anything from the list mistress yet. The last e-mail I sent was September 12th, 3 weeks ago. Now I have to send yet another reminder, and that sucks. This time I will try to call, it is obviously not committing enough with e-mails – more difficult to sneak away on the phone.. If I don't get permission, then what??? God forbid!!!!! (From research diary)

The first step in the process of approaching the group for permission was to contact Sapfo's web-master – or, 'list-mistress' as she was called, the person administratively in charge of the list. June 2002, I sent her a description of myself and the project, and what I intended to do in the period I would be present in the group. On the basis of this information, I was asking her if I could ask the participants on Sapfo themselves. When she finally replied after several repeated requests, she said that she needed to discuss it with the board of the Organsation first. November 1st, I called the list-mistress to inform her that I would contact the board myself, if she had not heard anything from them yet, something that really got the snowball rolling. Talking to the leader made me believe that the project finally was about to come to live. After one week the leader had discussed my request with the board, and Nov 8th I finally received green light to send my letter of introduction to Sapfo:

8/11

> What a weird day! Got an e-mail from the leader today, and finally permission to send the letter of introduction to Sapfo – under the condition that it is the board that makes the decision of if I can move forward with the project on the background of the reactions on the list. It was however obvious that they had discussed it thoroughly, and they expressed worries that the research can harm the list. Instead of jumping up and down with joy, I was caught with a horrible anxiety..and lots of 'what-if-fears'... (From research diary)

The most important thing when asking for consent, is of course to ask in a way so that people say 'yes' and to make sure that they know what they say yes to. It is impossible to have control of all aspects influencing these decisions – but one good thing is always to be as clear as possible when describing the project; what will be done? why?, and how?. I took a look at the letter of introduction that I had prepared for the list four months earlier. I thought of other aspects related to the self-presentation, most importantly the tone of voice I chose to use and if it would appeal to the participants in the group. Even if the basic information that should be included in asking for consent, the 'wrapping' that will create credibility and goodwill is dependent on the context and group of people. What would work well in one context will not necessarily work the same way in another one. At this point, I knew the context a lot better than when I started, after having followed the group closely while I waited for my permission to come through. As I reflected in my research diary:

> What is it that sounds weird with the letter as it is now?
> […]
> Because I know more about the group now I feel like looking at the letter critically again […] Maybe in particular when it comes to the conflicts that have dominated recently – will it f ex appeal more to one group of participants than another (the defined queer feminists vs the radical feminists f ex? (From research diary)

While I was waiting for my permission, the group was having a big conflict about identity politics and understandings of gender, sexuality and feminism: were male-to-female transsexuals to be accepted in the woman-only community (see Bromseth 2006)? The conflict that had been going in waves through-out the fall affected my slight over-preparing paranoia, also in relation to picking a good time to post the request to the group. Should I wait for less agitated times, or chance now? The board in the Organisation informed me that they were planning to exclude several members from the list because of this, and advised me to e-mail the group before they went through with it. Having a gender focus myself, I worried that the way I presented my research aim and focus could be understood as supporting one view more than the other in the conflicting views on the list, and thereby influence how my project was perceived.

Since getting all of the participants to agree is close to impossible, I had decided that if no-one had difficulties with my presence and purpose, it would be ethically satisfying to interpret a 'silent agreement' as consent to be present in the group to do research. As for quoting directly, I promised to obtain permission directly from the participants that I wanted to quote, and to get back to them individually about this at a later point. Since the group had a practice of being able to work out solutions on their own, I felt satisfied with leaving it up to them – an interpretation list members also shared with me in the discussion that followed my request:

> Personally I think that it would be really fun if we are used for research purposes, in particular when it is as sympathetic as yours seem to be *s. I have difficulties of seeing any risks for our integrity. The question is if we start to write more seriously because what we write might be part of a dissertation *s – no, I don't think so! So I don't mind – but then there are 349 more of us…You might ask if there are 'anyone against it'..
> (List message, Lina)

Reply, me:

> >Good and important point. This is some of the challenge in research on Internet-mediated
> >groups: who should one ask for permission? The owner, the list mistress or the group itself?
> >And in that case, must every member of the list say yes? As I see it, it depends to a large
> >degree on the group in question – and my impression as a member here is that you are quite
> >good at reaching decisions through common discussion. So that's why I ask you as a group,

>hoping that if there are strong disagreements , it will show during the debate. This counts for
>the part that is about the observation and general descriptions of the group. [..]
(List message, me)

MOVING FROM THE OUTSIDE TO THE INSIDE

Participant Observation, Nov 2002 – July 2003

..online, perception of another's attention is only known by overt response [...] 'I am responded to, therefore I am (Markham, 2005: 795)

One of the challenges of the next phase; well 'inside', was to try to establish an interactive dialogue with the group. I wanted both to encourage reflections about issues that I found interesting in the group itself as well as through writing privately to specific participants. In all my posts, I tried to communicate that I wanted a two-way dialogue, and invited participants to write to me directly if they had questions or thoughts about anything related to the project. As a participant in the group, I had previously only had a 'lurking' position; reading the posts, but had never spoken myself (see also Chapter 1 in this volume). This was a choice I made out of ethical reasons; I wanted to have permission to do research before I started speaking in the group,[6] as I did not want to mix my roles of participant vs researcher. Of course, by this time then, I knew the group – but they did not know me.

Taking the step from looking from the outside to participating on the inside implies a shift in position. Observing interaction without speaking, my gaze was completely focussed on what happened in the group. Starting to participate, the point from where I observed shifted, and it also made me more self-conscious of my role as a researcher (as I now also was looked at). In sharing reflections aloud with participants in the group, they were able to join in, and contest my interpretations. The positive aspect of this, is that they made me aware of other perspectives that I had not thought of, something that I would not have achieved if I continued to let my own pair of eyes be the only ones filtering what I saw. The one-on-one interviews at a later point, and private e-mails, further gave room to develop my interpretations. Getting to the point where I felt comfortable when interacting, and actually was responded to, took time, the text-mode posing specific frames in the process of finding my way in.

---

[6] This choice was not based upon positivist reasons, but out of caution that it could have created more difficulties in getting permission if f ex certain participants did not like my opinions, as I had experienced in my previous study of a political group that I was active in before doing research there. Nancy Baym (1999) experienced it easier to communicate with the group when she announced her research project because she was already a participating member in the group. What is a wise approach is however dependent on the group's purpose and your own relation to it, I would suggest. Radhika Gajjala (2004), who was also 'an insider' when asking for consent to study a South-Asian female network, SAW-net, experienced that her previous posts might have had the opposite effect when changing her position from participant to participant observer.

Creating Relations and a Credible Self in The Mediated Context

Doing research in a text-based mailing-list community like Sapfo, and the work of creating credibility and trust, allocates specific frames of communication and limitations when it comes to the actual tools you have at hand. This poses some very particular challenges in trying to create trust in building relations between researcher and informants, as compared to doing ethnographic studies in physical environments (see Gajjala 2004: 29-40 for a discussion of these issues). All that should be said and done must take the form of explicit text only. During the different parts of the participant observation of the group, I was to most people text – and they to me. I found this fact challenging in many aspects; not being able to be silently present, but still visible as in a physical context, deprived of my smile, lacking the possibility of making encouraging nods to make people talk, to approach the silent observer in the group and invite her to talk to me. Not being able to read other participant's facial expressions to something I said or asked when trying to interpret lack of responses when initiating or inviting to reflections on an issue, also created feelings of insecurity (see also Chapter 1 in this volume). The text-mode is clever, in the sense that it focuses on content and leaves out the important self presenting cues we give off in everyday interaction (Goffman 1959) that might have helped humanize me and lower the threshold a little; that my outfit are jeans, my notebook is full of spots and that I twitch my curls when I am nervous. These little non-content-oriented actions are often unconscious and unintended, as compared to the well-planned posts that I sent to the list. I really twisted my brain as to how I could establish trust and create responses through the texts that I wrote, words carefully weighed in gold, something that is of course advantageous (avoiding embarrassing slips of the tongue), but also restricting. This does not mean that the text mode makes it impossible to show emotions and other sides of the self than the content-focussed researcher. In fact, the communication norms on the list were to a large degree informal. This included using features from the synchronous chat modes; smileys and other emotes (*hug* as a closing greeting to the group for instance; see also Solomon in this volume), as well as situating oneself by relating to what was going on in the off-line surroundings at the time of writing. In striving to find a position and a voice to speak with in the group, I adopted some of these informal ways of writing, as well as chose to share parts of my own private life with the group when participating. For instance as in this closing greeting:

> Thank you so much for letting me be here – I learn so much from it!
>
> (and so engaging that I now will be late for a premade trout-dinner that my 3 beloved flatmates have made…ha, who needs a girl-friend..)
> Have a continued good week-end!
>
> Janne (List message)

Identity Norms and Group Requirements: Researcher, Woman, Lesbian, Feminist

> Our personal characteristics as individuals – our ethnic identity, class, sex, religion and family status – will determine how we interact with and report on the people we are studying. (Dewalt and Dewalt, 2001: 25)

As Donna Haraway (1988) reflects in her writings on and criticisms of scientific objectivity, the researching observer is always situated; the gaze is positioned, and must see from somewhere: 'Location is the always partial, always finite, always fraught play of foreground and background, text and context, that constitutes critical inquiry. Above all. location is not self-evident or transparent. [...] There is no way around this polluting criterion for strong objectivity.' (cited from 2004, 237)

Identifying as lesbian, was an important part of filtering what I observed in the group, as well as a central resource in communicating with the list in the active part of the research.

Using informal communication features to adjust to group norms also included sharing more personal sides of myself other than the 'researcher'. Being a group aiming at women, and a sexual minority-related community, my credibility as a 'researcher' was simultaneously dependent of creating a culturally appropriate image of myself through an intersection of subject positions as woman/lesbian/researcher, both initially when asking for consent, and afterwards, trying to 'get on the inside' and establish a dialogue. In short, I wanted to be perceived as a serious, 'well-intended' researcher, supportive towards the lists aims and its group of users. By doing so, I wanted in particular to avoid a potential scepticism of being interpreted as the heterosexual 'other', which in general can be a more difficult subject-position when establishing trust in research on sexual minority communities (Fitzgerald, 1999).

In the absence of the physical body, embodiment is created actively through text in text-based online environments, and used as resources for participants to interpret and make visualized images of the Other (Sundén, 2003). How do you create a credible image of a gendered body with a same-sex orientation through textual means, in a discussion group environment where content-oriented discussions through asynchronous e-mail exchanges is the main activity? If I had met the group physically, I could have communicated my sexual orientation more implicitly, through subcultural signifiers telling a silent tale for themselves; through the way I dressed, my thumb-ring, or my body language. Instead, I had to make everything explicit in text. For instance, when I introduced myself to the group in my first post, motivating the project with basis in a shared a subject position of being a non-heterosexual woman:

> I am lesbian myself and I have because of this become particularly interested of the Net as arena for discussion and social meeting place for lesbian and bisexual women as a sexual minority in a heteronormative society, and in Scandinavian culture. In line with other international and Norwegian lesbian networks that I have been part of, I have been enthusiastic about Sapfo and the huge activity here on the list, as well as the broad range of the subjects discussed. I would very much like to use Sapfo as part of my project, and after having permission from the board of the Organisation I now write to you.
>
> (From the introductory letter to the list)

Or as later on, communicating it more implicitly in diverse ways; through telling stories of a lesbian holiday place I had been to, mentioning girlfriends and discussing queer-related issues.[7] Using the lesbian identity actively as a resource also made it easier for me to engage in dialogues, by referring to a common ground and a shared frame of reference of living a sexual minority-position. Because of this 'insider' knowledge of the subculture, I was also able to recognize many of the issues discussed as well as to make use of my own experiences when I participated myself.

Speaking from an 'insider'-position, using personal experiences when discussing topics related to sexual identity as part of the research process was also challenging in different ways. On one hand, clarifying my role as a researcher in the group, and not an ordinary participant, was important. On the other, speaking in a tone of voice that was close to the cultural norms was important to be able to both build down the fear of the researcher that is often present, and to 'fit in'. Trying to find a balance between what felt 'too private' or 'too informal' when writing wasn't always easy, and at times it gave me the feeling of having to undress because of the research context:

> March 03
>
> [...] since the norms on the list have been so informal and oriented towards private life, it has been impossible to both be able to keep a distance and at the same time get inside. I have had to make visible more sides of myself as a human being – in particular as a queer woman. It has been a balance project that has been very difficult, to judge where the line goes for informality. On one hand it is important for them to remember that I am a researcher in order to make them aware that what they say and do will be used in research. On the other I would never have been able to break the ice if I had continued to be 'too researchy'. (From research diary)

Finding a Key to Dialogue in the Changing Context: Humour as Ice-Breaker

Many ethnographers can point to the moment when they experienced a breakthrough in trying to establish contact with the group they conduct their studies on, feeling accepted from participants in the group (Dewalt and Dewalt, 2001). This was also the case for me. Paradoxically, it was related to the episode of the revelation of the male cross-dresser on the list, something that changed the context severely. One of the list members revealed, after her own inquiry "off-list", that four of the long-term active women on the list was produced by the same person, who additionally was a man. The list was in shock and many participants did not believe the news at once. However, when it had been accepted as a fact, the climate became highly suspicious towards all members: Are you really the one you say that you are? In the period following the revelation, there was in general a suspicious mood on the list, where list members started suspecting each other for being the product of the cross-dresser:

[7] Gaining acceptance and credibility in subcultural environments is of course tightly connected to the hegemonic cultural norms for what is seen as 'right and relevant' ways of acting; experiences, opinions, positions etc, and is not always and easy task. As Chou reports from her ethnography of a lesbian community in Taiwan, with strict sexual roles and codes, getting inside was not a matter of 'saying ' that she was a lesbian, but rather a

>The list runs a high risk of dying, it seems like, and it isn't at all strange considering
>what has happened. Because everyone now is suspicious towards newcomers, I have to
>write a few rows. I have followed the discussions for a year, but because of the weird
>discussions that took place I didn't feel like participating in the discussion. And I am
>me, it is simple to check because I don't have any need to be anonymous. Maybe I will
>introduce myself more thoroughly when I see how everything develops here.
(Annema, Dec 17th 2002)

Subject: [Sapfo] …what can you say..

It is a rather quiet list right now…or very quiet
I guess nobody want to write anymore. Almost me neither. ☹
Oh well, wish everyone a happy new year at least!

Mette (List message)

At first I experienced this incident as making my efforts of creating credibility and trust in the bodiless context even more difficult than before, having fears that list members would also start suspecting me and my intentions for being there, and how I should move forward:

4/1
Methodology:
I am really uncertain of how I am going to move forward methodologically in the time to come, in particular regarding my own participation on the list. On one hand I am dying to ask the list members to go deeper into certain issues related to the meta-discussion that is now taking place on the list. […] Should I continue to ask the list about the things I wonder about – and how should I obtain credibility? Is it right or wrong of me to express my own opinions and feelings towards what has happened? Is it better to ask each participant directly and with what effect? (From research diary)

I was careful to state explicitly that 'I was me' – amongst others by referring to my home page and offering to answer any question they would have. The use of humour became an important part in the period after the revelation in different ways, something that had always characterized the interaction culture on Sapfo. Both in list messages in general, but also as a strategy to solve conflicts and disagreements and be able to move on (also found by Baym, 1999). Using humour was also my key to 'breaking the ice', I felt, in that it was the first posts that gave many replies and useful reflections, either as just comments or more content-oriented messages. As several of us were trying to figure out who and how many of what I had interpreted as women were in fact written by the same male person, I sent a post where I self-ironically started to make fun of myself and my project, regarding how the revelation ruined my research project:

>Hi Frida!

>It has come up that Flisan, Malin_and_Agira,

process of 'proving' it by performing in accordance with one of the two strictly pre-scribed identity roles within the community (see Chou, 1999).

>Anyone else?? Are made up by one and the same
>man; 'Hansie'

>So, Agira never existed for real…

>Hugs
>Mette

Reply, me 9/1:

From: Janne Bromseth janne.bromseth@hf.ntnu.no
Subject: Re: [Sapfo] Small presentation!
At 10:54 09.01.03 +0100, you wrote:

Hi Mette –

Agira too? I guess I have missed that too..

scratches her head and throws yet another analysis in the paper basket

Janne

**

Reply, Marple 9/1:

Janne: Anna, Agira, Flisan, Nicole, Malin.

(Probably Jenny too, or she was so surprised that her fingers stopped working..)

Marple
**

Reply me, 9/1:

Hi Marple
The other 4 I have registered ;)

In making fun of myself and my own naivety, I also pointed to the fact that I, in line with many of the others, also felt naive and fooled. I tried to reflect openly about the analytical issues on my mind and invite them to reflect around it, either on the list or to write to me in private e-mails. In some ways, it was easier for me to find a position to speak from after the revelation. This was firstly connected to the meta-reflections the episode caused, as the participants explicitly discussed their previously taken-for-granted expectations of the Other on the list – and why they experienced it as upsetting when the image of the gendered body writing did not match with reality. But it was also, I think, related to the fact that - as opposed to previous political conflicts on the list, that made me feel insecure about how to position myself – the betrayal contributed to construct a 'we' on the list again; 'us women' against 'the male cross-dresser'. It made the members gather around a common experience that invoked anger and hurt, but that also created an extended use of humour. In this process, I included myself as part of this 'we' – 'the real lesbian/bisexual women who had been fooled by the multiple male-crossdresser '. I was increasingly included and responded to by the others, they shared their reflections with me, and also, laughed with me about the surprising turn my project had taken.

THE VULNERABLE OBSERVER

At the same time, a strong identification with the researched group also had its problematic sides, in trying to get an analytical distance when interpreting events in the group. As Ruth Behar (1996: 5) discusses, the positions of being both participant and observer at the same time implies a paradox; the participant engaged from the inside, while the observer-position usually requires some sorts of distance. Letting 'the culture enmesh you', as Clifford Geertz (referred in Behar 1996: 5) puts it, is important in the process of trying to understand the culture one wishes to learn something about. Just how far one lets the culture enmesh you differs, Behar argues in her book 'The vulnerable observer – anthropology that breaks your heart' (1996). Taking an empathic stance when doing participant observation of human behaviour involves observing not only with the head but also with the heart. It involves an emotional recognition or a strong identification with the people and culture one interacts with in a research project on a long-term basis. In my case, experiencing both the struggles living a sexual minority position implies, my sexual orientation is something that is a very vulnerable part of my identity. It makes me feel some kind of emotional bond to other queers in a very sensitive way – even if I like them and their opinions or not.[8] After finishing my fieldwork, it took some time before I was able to distance myself from some of the things that happened while I was present in the group, because I experienced as emotionally upsetting as a participant, in line with other long-term participants. I was angry because the organisation owning the list never did anything actively to answer all the questions about safety and regulation that list members were left with after the revelation. Sad because as time went by, I could see the community suffer a slow death before my eyes as a result of the distrust and insecurity that grew in the group, but uncomfortable with the thought of actively doing anything about it myself from my researcher-position. This was in a sharp contrast to the enthusiasm for the lively list community that was a driving force in the beginning of the project: the fairytale turned into a Greek drama. In this phase, I struggled with feelings of shame over having these emotions. Even if I knew better, the 'positivist ghost' whispered to me that being emotionally affected could be a sign that I was 'out of control', biased, and non-objective = non-scientific. Until I started using these emotions actively as resources in my writing, situating my researcher position and point of departure as 'engaged insider', as a wall to discuss the other participants reflections against when doing my analysis, trying to reach "a keen understanding of what

[8] This does not mean that all queers are the same or experience their identity processes in the same way or that they are mostly negative. What I mean is that they are for most people an emotional process, for good and bad, and do for most people involve some struggles in everyday life in a heteronormative society (varying between cultural contexts; from being severely oppressed and deprived from human rights in many countries to mainly consisting of cultural suppression in a few European countries).

aspects of the self are the most important filters through which one perceives the world, and more particularly, the topic being studied" (Behar, 1996:13).

Concluding Remarks

In this chapter, I have wanted to make some reflections around connections between participant observation as a situated process and its relations to research strategies within a mediated context, and show how specific intersected subject positions became central filters and recourses for developing a gaze and an interacting voice in my study.

Ways to approach individuals and the group have to be adjusted and changed during the time of study dependent of what happens within the group, along with changes in research foci that follows from increasing knowledge about the context. Online groups are developing social units in constant processes, where the frames of the interaction can be more or less stable over certain amount of time, both in terms of participants as well as levels of conflict. Finding a voice and position as participant observer then, requires reflexivity and sensitivity towards the dynamic context during the research process, to be able to develop fruitful dialogues on the groups' premises (Markham, 2005).

What is important is to acknowledge are the different points of departure when starting a long term ethnographic study online as compared to off-line, and be aware of the specific frames the online mode create in doing participant observation. As Kolko and Reid (1998: 220) discuss, the text mode seems to restrict flexibility in performing social relations when it comes to sorting out and dealing with conflicts: "online we are what we say in a far more intimate and inflexible way than we are ever purely or merely what we say face to face". This is challenging both when it comes to participants in online communities as well as for the researcher studying them. Building trust textually in a group setting is more of a challenge than face to face – something that also Radhika Gajjala (2004) reflects on in relation to her request of doing research on SAW-net, where a few strong critical voices got to dominate when the group was to decide whether they wanted to be part of her project or not. Building 'quality relations', that is an outspoken ideal in feminist research, is more difficult since the textual mode is very content-oriented. Can ethnography be compared to online studies at all? Gajjala asks in her reflections.

Gaining informed consent as well as getting on the inside of a group as participant observer can thus be harder work than first imagined, in particular in restricted access stable discussion groups where trust and credibility is build upon textual presentations of self as a main source. In doing online ethnography of group communities, there's a lot of fragility and vulnerability under the text-based, seemingly non-personal discursive surface, for participants as well as researcher.

References

[1] Baym, N., 1999, *Tune in, Log on,* Sage Publications, Thousand Oaks, CA

[2] Behar, R., 1996, *The Vulnerable Observer. Anthropology that Breaks Your Heart,* Beacon Press, Boston.

[3] Blackwood, E., 1995, Falling in Love With an-Other Lesbian, in D. Kulick and M. Wilson (eds.), *Taboo. Sex, Identity and Erotic Subjectivity in Anthropological Fieldwork,* pp 29-51, Routledge, London.

[4] Brockington, Wanda Goins, 2003, *Searching the Internet: Black Space in the Public Sphere*, unpublished paper presented at AOIR's *conference Internet research 4.0: Bordening the Band*, Toronto October 16th-19th.

[5] Bromseth, J., 2002, 'Public or Private?', in *Researching ICTs in Context*, A. Morrison (ed.), *InterMedia Report 3/2002*, pp 33 – 63, Unipub Forlag, Oslo.

[6] Bromseth, J., 2003, Nettets 'Private Sfærer' – Arena for Utvikling av Seksuell Identitet, NIKK-magasin, Seksualitet og identitet, vol.1, pp 9-13.

[7] Bromseth, J., 2006, *Genre Trouble and The Body that Mattered. Negotiations of Gender, Sexuality and Identity in a Scandinavian Mailing List Community for Lesbian and Bisexual Women.* Doctoral thesis at Department of Interdisciplinary Studies of Culture, Norwegian University of Technology and Science, Norway.

[8] Chao, Y.A., 1999, 'The Indigenous Lesbian Circle in Taiwan', in F. Markowitz and M. Ashkenazi (eds.), *Sex, Sexuality and The Anthropologist*, pp. 128-145, University of Illinois Press, Urbana and Chicago.

[9] Correll, S., 1995, 'The Ethnography of an Electronic Bar. The Lesbian Café', *Journal of Contemporary Ethnography*, vol. 24, no 3, pp 299-322.

[10] Dewalt, K.M and Dewalt, B.R.,2001. *Participant Observation. A Guide for Fieldworkers*, AltaMira Press, Walnut Creek, CA.

[11] Fitzgerald, T.K., 1999, 'Identity in Ethnography: Limits to Reflective Subjectivity', in F. Markowitz and M. Ashkenazi (eds.), *Sex, Sexuality and the Anthropologist*, pp. 117-128, University of Illinois Press, Urbana and Chicago.

[12] Gajjala, R.,, 2004, *Cyberselves. Feminist Ethnographies of South Asian Women,* Alta Mira Press, Walnut Creek, CA.

[13] Goffman, E, 1959, *The Presentation of Self in Everyday Life,* Penguin Books, Great Britain.

[14] Haraway, D, 1988, 'Situated Knowledges: The Science Question in Feminism and the Privilege of Partial Perspective', *Feminist Studies*, vol. 14, no. 3, pp. 575-99.

[15] Harcourt, W, 1999, *Women @ Internet: Creating New Cultures in Cyberspace*, Zed Books, London.

[16] Hall, K, 1996, 'Cyberfeminism', in S. Herring (ed.), *Computer-Mediated Communication: Linguistic, Social and Cross-cultural perspectives*, pp. 148-170, John Benjamins Publishing, London.

[17] Herring, S., 1996, 'Posting in a Different Voice: Gender and Ethics in Computer-Mediated Communication.', in C. Ess (ed.), *Philosophical Perspectives on Computer-Mediated Communication*, pp. 115-147, State of New York Press, Albany.

[18] Hine, C., 2000, *Virtual Ethnography,* Sage Publications, Thousand Oaks, CA.

[19] Jones, S., 1999, *Doing Internet Research. Critical issues and methods for examining the net,* Sage Publications, London.

[20] Kendall, L., 2002, *Hanging Out in the Virtual Pub*, University of California Press, Berkeley and Los Angeles, CA.

[21] Kolko, B. and Reid, E., 1998, 'Dissolution and Fragmentation. Problems in Online-Communities.', in S. Jones (ed.) , *Cybersociety 2.0*, pp. 212-231, Sage Publications, Thousand Oaks, CA

[22] Kolko, B., Nakamura, L. and Rodman, G. (eds.), 2000, *Race in Cyberspace*, Routledge, New York

[23] Mann, C. and Stewart, F., *Internet Communication and Qualitative Research. A Handbook for Researching Online,* Sage Publications, London.

[24] Markham, A., 2003, 'The Internet as Research Context', in C. Seale, G. Gobo, J.F. Gubrium and D. Silverman (eds.), *Qualitative Research Practice*, pp. 354-375, Sage Publications, London.

[25] Markham, A.H., 2005 'The Methods, Politics, and Ethics of Representation in Online thnography', in N.K. Denzin and Y.S. Lincoln (eds.), *Handbook of Qualitative Research 3rd edition*, pp. 793-820, Sage Publications, Thousand Oaks, CA.

[26] Mitra, A., 2001, 'Marginal Voices in Cyberspace.', *New Media and Society*, vol. 3, no. 1, pp 29-48

[27] Munt, S, Bassett, E.H., O'Riordan, K, 2002, 'Virtually Belonging: Risk, Connectivity and Coming Out On-line', *International Journal of Sexuality and Gender Studies*, Vol. 7, Nos. 2/3, July 2002, pp 125 - 137

[28] Nakamura, L., 2002, *Cybertypes. Race, Ethnicity and Identity on the Internet, Routledge,* London.

[29] Nip, J.Y.M., 2004, 'The Relationship Between Online and Offline Communities: The Case of the Queer Sisters', *Media, Culture & Society*, vol. 26, no. 3, pp 409-428

[30] Sixsmith, J. and Murray, C., 2001, 'Ethical Issues in The Documentary Data Analysis of Internet Posts and Archives', *Qualitative Health Research*, vol. 3, pp 423-432

[31] Staunæs, D, 2003, 'Where Have All The Subjects Gone? Bringing Together The Concepts of Intersectionality and Subjectification', *NORA, no.2 2003*, vol. 11, pp 101-109

[32] Sundén, J., 2003, *Material Virtualities. Approaching Online Textual Embodiment,* Peter Lang, New York.

[33] The National Committee for Research Ethics in the Social Sciences and the Humanities, 2001, *Guidelines for Research Ethics in The Social Sciences, Law and The Humanities,* NESH, Oslo

[34] Ward, K., 1999, The Cyber-Ethnographic (Re)-Construction of Two Feminist Online Communities, *Sociological Research Online,* vol.4, no.1. <http://www.socresonline.org.uk/4/1/ward.html>

[35] Wakeford, N, 1997, 'Cyberqueer', in A. Medhurst and S.R. Munt (eds.), *Lesbian and Gay Studies. A Critical Introduction*, pp 20-39, Cassell, Virginia.

[36] Wetherell, M., 1998, Positioning and Interpretative Repertoires: Conversations Analysis and Poststructuralism in Dialogue', *Discourse & Society*, vol. 9, no. 3, pp 387-412.

In: Health Research in Cyberspace
Editor: Pranee Liamputtong, pp. 105-120

ISBN 1-59454-819-6

Chapter 6

THE METHODOLOGY OF INTERNET RESEARCH: SOME LESSONS LEARNED

Richard M. Hessler

BACKGROUND

The Internet has great potential for data gathering in the social and behavioral sciences. For example, we were able recently to conduct a needs assessment entirely on-line for only $40.00 each month that the survey was in the field. For a total of $80.00, we received a tab-delimited data set of 35 variables, 1500 respondents, and marginal frequencies as well. Our experience is a small part of a rather significant use of the Internet for survey-type quantitative research (Jerome et al., 2000), but less use for qualitative research. In this chapter, I draw on my quantitative and qualitative Internet research experiences that my colleagues and I have carried out in order to discuss the methodological costs and benefits of data gathering on the Internet. One study focused on income and other barriers to child and adult day care among hospital workers. The other study used e-mail to study adolescents' thoughts and behaviors as part of an assessment of teen risk, including drug use, unprotected sex, reckless driving, and violence (Bagnall and Plant, 1991). In this latter study, we adapted from an important British study of adolescent risk (Furlong and Cartmel, 1997) that clearly portrayed a knowledge gap between societal level opportunity structures such as labor markets and the subjective meanings that adolescents use to frame those structures. Given the statistical data, we sought to understand what it all meant to the adolescents.

THE INTERNET RESEARCH PROBLEM

The Internet is a significant force affecting the global marketplace. A testable hypothesis would posit that a country's economic development is hurt by any attempts, either public or private, to censor or otherwise restrict access to or the content of the Internet. On the other hand, community and ethical standards increasingly are perceived as threatened by growing Internet access.

We are concerned particularly about the twin issues of privacy and quality control of data given our research experience and a review of recent literature indicating a relationship between rising privacy risk and the development and dissemination of Internet technology. The same relationship seems to hold for quality control of data gathered over the Internet.

Privacy

U.S. Supreme Court justices Samuel Warren and Louis Brandeis, in the *Harvard Law Review 1890-91*, defined privacy as the right to be left alone. Keeping this basic definition in mind, we see risk to privacy increasing with technological advances in online research. Germany is an interesting case in terms of the perspective that the growth of Internet data threatens privacy. German public policy and law place great value on the right to privacy. Since the early 1960s, Germans have systematically protected privacy over freedom of information. For example, the German national census was dropped in the 80s and in 1983 a constitutional law was passed that gives all German citizens the right to know about any data that exists about them. In 1996, a German research project established computer capability to link Auschwitz prisoner numbers with names. Also in 1996, the German government waged a losing battle against Compuserve over the government's desire to control public access to Internet porn. Had Germany succeeded, the principle of government regulation of the Internet to protect privacy would have been established.

The Internet was introduced to China in 1994. At the time, Chinese officials embraced the new technology for its economic development potential, but did not like the concomitant freedom of information. Two years later, the Chinese government took a very different approach than Germany to privacy and the Internet. First, officials tried to have e-mail users register with the police. That failed. Then the government committed to building an Internet that would be imminently censorable and consequently a perfect threat to privacy. I recall having to scramble e-mail messages to my son who was serving in the Peace Corps in China around that time because local censors were reading and deleting some of our messages. James Chu argued that one could "join the information age while restricting access to information", pointing to firewall software from Sun Microsystems as the technological means to achieve this censorship (Kahn et al., 1996). Unfortunately for Chu's theory, cable and wireless rendered moot this and other subsequent efforts to control the free flow of information on the Internet in China. By 1997, Beijing had over twenty Internet providers and in 1998, a magazine named Tunnel was written in Chinese, in China, and distributed throughout China by e-mail from the United States. According to The Economist (1998), *Tunnel*'s main objective was to "break through the lock on information and controls on expression". Interestingly, the first revolution using the Internet occurred in Indonesia in 1998 as well, all this while cyber-censorship raged in China, Malaysia, Cambodia, Burma, Indonesia, Vietnam, Laos, North Korea, and Singapore.

In 1991, the U.S. Congress formalized into law the technological innovation of massive linked data files that all computer users would have free access to, a concept that one of the Senate sponsors, Albert Gore, Jr., called the "information superhighway" (Business Week, 1991). This was known as "The High Performance Computing Act". Senator Gore's

Information Infrastructure Task Force laid out the guiding principles of the Information Superhighway in 1993. These were: 1. Open public access; 2. Universal service; 3. Security for individual confidentiality; and 4. Authenticity procedures in place. Again, the theory of open public access to enhance economic development clashed with privacy threats, now in the form of national security concerns. However, the fight took a surprising, almost contradictory twist. Growing national security fears prompted the government to restrict access for the general public. Researchers included, while the desire for security (and business profits) led to the growth of centralized data sets, super computers, and more access for security agencies and some large businesses. Federal publications and government data have been harder to come by as a consequence of this policy.

The myriad security and quality flaws inherent in large linked data sets came into public consciousness in the U.S. in 1980. An Arkansas newspaper obtained Representative Tommy Robinson's private medical records electronically and a medical researcher at St. Luc's Hospital in Montreal, Canada, admitted that data in a large multi-hospital linked cancer trial had been falsified. The Children's Online Privacy Protection Act of 1998 has led to mandatory Internet filters for public school and libraries that receive federal funds for Internet access. Legal battles ensued over the possibility of blocking legitimate Internet sites based on political or religious values. Interestingly, a study done in 2001 by Consumer Reports found that the filter software tended to block harmless sites as well as the intended ones. In 2004, a commercial data merchant named Choicepoint sold personal information on 145,000 unsuspecting U.S. residents to a crime ring and an elementary school in Sutter, California, required students to wear electronic ID badges to track students with RFID technology. The program was eventually dropped in the wake of strong citizen protests concerning the children's privacy rights. To summarize, privacy is threatened by Internet filters and other barriers to public access along with corporate violations of confidentiality principles and advances in computer software and hardware have not reduced the problem. We seem to be faced with a technology nemesis.

Quality of Data

Of course, access to falsified data is worse than no access at all. In fact, false data becomes reified when linked to multiple files and the harm to scientific inquiry, privacy, and public perception of the scientific community is greatly magnified. For example, a colleague of mine in another department had a student who did quite well in his course, but basically falsified a course evaluation and pilloried the professor. One can only surmise here, but my colleague, who recognized the student by the handwriting, recalled several conversations and other hints of religious zealotry on the student's part. The best guess is that my colleague somehow conveyed the fact that he is a liberal with no membership in any organized religion and the student took it out on him in the final course evaluation. This would not be much of a problem at all as long as the data remained in the department. But, with linked files, the data is merged into several other files, some that actually can be easily read by anyone with Internet access. At the moment, there are no systematic methods for validating the data. Assuming that this evaluation might occur with similar students over time, researchers using the data would be treated to reliably invalid results.

In our two online studies, we had no way of knowing exactly who was filling out the e-mail diaries or completing the Survey Monkey questionnaires. In graduate school, I was taught to standardize the data collection method as much as possible and to be vigilant and present while respondents were filling out questionnaires. In the case of face-to-face interviews, I always checked a random sample of the respondents to make sure that the interviewer actually showed up and that questions were asked exactly as worded and in the proper order. None of this quality control occurs with online data gathering today.

Lessons from the Adolescent Risk E-Mail Diary Study

A low budget coupled with past experience led us to choose e-mail as the main data-gathering tool for the study of adolescent risk. In an earlier qualitative study of peer mediators (Hessler, 1998), we learned that face-to-face focused interviews between adult researchers and young boys and girls were very difficult to do. In the mediation study, the words we used in asking questions and the presence of researchers themselves seemed to intimidate many of the respondents and rapport always seemed to be a concern. We found that the age gap was eased a bit by letting the respondents spend more time telling us about their world while we listened and occasionally reacted with a request for elaboration or clarification. But, we had poor luck in getting to that stage of rapport and when we did, usually the time for fieldwork had run out.

With this experience in mind, we decided to use e-mail daily diaries as the primary data gathering method for the adolescent risk study. We asked the following research questions:

- What are adolescents' pathways to meaning as they negotiate their everyday lives?
- How do adolescents frame behaviors and attitudes that are defined as defined as risky by adults?
- What future research strategies might we recommend based on what we learned?
- We wanted to explore the ways in which the adolescents viewed or portrayed their everyday lives. We decided that we could do this best with a panel so we followed a small group of adolescents over roughly ten weeks. We expected that sex, drugs, and other sensitive topics would arise so we decided to use daily diaries and e-mail as the main field methods. Anticipating a sizeable data set for each respondent, we used a qualitative electronic data analysis program called HyperQual2.

Field Methods

We found a sizeable scientific literature on technical difficulties associated with e-mail (Rosencrance, 2000), a smaller literature on privacy issues surrounding e-mail (Samoriski, et al.,1996; Fonseca, 2000), but many fewer articles that discussed using e-mail as part of qualitative data gathering in social sciences (Workman, 1992) and medicine (Spielberg, 1998). Security of data or confidentiality was the common theme running through most of the articles and was best summed up by Fonseca (2000: 18) who writes, "at the heart of the problem is the fact that these communication methods were not initially designed to have strong security features because they were not originally intended for mission-critical tasks". Transmitting confidential information was not part of the original e-mail plan, apparently. Similarly, Cho and LaRose (1999) accuse on line surveyors of committing multiple violations of physical, informational, and psychological privacy that the authors conclude are more egregious than those found in conventional surveys. On the positive side, two articles presented finding that suggested that interaction and rapport might be enhanced through Internet communication (Kawaura, et al., 1999; Janney, 1996).

Entry to Respondents

It was asking a lot of adolescents to write a two to four page daily diary for 8 weeks, so we had budgeted $100 dollars for each respondent who completed the job. The money was to be paid directly to the respondent by check at the end of the fieldwork phase of the study. This introduced a potentially serious privacy problem.

We divided the state into five cultural areas. These were the northwest, northeast, Ozark, Bootheel, and central regions. Also, we included the St.Louis and Kansas City areas because of high accidental injury rates there. Counties within the regions were grouped into low, average, or high risk depending on their overall injury rate for adolescents relative to the average for the state as a whole. We did this based on an analysis of a state data set called E-code.

We gained access to respondents at two high schools in the northwest region, both in low injury counties. In one case, one of the researchers had a friend whose sister was the principal of the high school. The researcher contacted the principal after his friend had called her and the principal expressed strong interest in participating as the contact person. The researcher sent a packet along with a reminder that the study was seeking a range of student backgrounds, some college bound, and others on the verge of dropping out. That was all that it took to get 15 students online almost immediately. In the other case, one of the researchers called the school counselor who referred the researcher to the principal. The researcher explained the study to the principal, stressing that participation would be a unique opportunity for students and faculty. The researcher asked the principal to think it over and then called the following day. The principal agreed to participate and gave the researcher back to the counselor who agreed to be the site liaison person. This was all accomplished before any written materials had been sent. A packet was sent to the counselor and she helped select six respondents who all worked from their home computers. These cases proved to be ideal in terms of ease of entry and the quality of the data received. In fact, one of the counselors asked us to be sure to include her school in any other studies that we might do.

We gained respondents from the St. Louis area through a University of Missouri student. This student used an existing network of family members and friends to secure 10 respondents, nine of whom ended up completing the required 8 weeks of journal entries. This was during the summer months which also shed light on adolescent activities outside of the normal school year. In addition to this site, a central Missouri site was developed, again using contacts that one of the researchers had through family and friends. That site yielded four respondents.

Because we needed the names, Social Security Numbers, and addresses of the respondents in order to pay them, we devised a system for getting the consent forms distributed, signed, mailed, and ultimately for paying the respondents. The key was to recruit seemingly trustworthy adults who lived in the same areas as the respondents. These field coordinators were unpaid volunteers, mostly high school teachers, who agreed to recruit respondents, process the informed consent forms, and finally to serve as a conduit for payment. Hence, the field coordinators and the university person authorizing the payments were the only people, other than the respondents, who knew the identity of the respondents. We researchers knew only e-mail pseudonyms.

After exhausting most of the entry strategies that we had used successfully in past qualitative research and with time running out, we ended up with 31 respondents whose daily journal entries formed the data.

Institutional Review Board (IRB) Requirements

Because the target research population was 18 and under, our campus IRB insisted that we obtain signed permission from parents or guardians. The IRB members argued that e-mail created potentially significant enough confidentiality risks for the respondents to warrant signed consent forms from the respondents. Computer files are never completely secure and the university e-mail system was no exception. In this case, the e-mail was backed up and saved on tapes. The back up process was unpredictable, too, making it all the more difficult to protect the anonymity of users. For example, the computer operators told us that e-mail was saved randomly three or four days a week, depending on capacity and use. The messages were stored on tapes by date and were kept from three weeks to six months. Of course, this meant that all e-mail users were vulnerable to invasions of privacy, legal or otherwise. We instructed the respondents to use a fake e-mail name that we then would use to identify and collate the downloaded files. "Flutebud" would send daily letters and one of the research staff would import the text into HyperQual under the same name. All of "Flutebud's" entries were located in one HQ file called "Flutebud." Once the text was imported, then the original e-mail message was deleted from the project account, but it might have been backed up on the mainframe computer.

This potential break in security was compounded by the existence of signed consent forms and the fact that the field coordinators knew all of the respondents' e-mail names, real names, and SSNs. The researchers had to keep the signed consent forms on file in case of an IRB audit. There was no question that a determined investigator would stand a decent chance of being able to line up at least some of the HQ text with real names. We listed all of these potential threats to privacy on the informed consent forms.

The negotiations with the campus IRB uncovered another more interesting privacy issue. If a respondent wrote about any threat to self or others, we would have to try and prevent the harm from occurring. For example, if "Cookie Monster" wrote that her friend was threatening to commit suicide, we would inform the field coordinator about this. We let the respondents know that we would do this and listed this as a warning on the consent form as well.

Interestingly, in spite of all of these caveats, the respondents were remarkably open and candid about behaviors and thoughts that certainly could cause trouble for them in the hands of school authorities, police, or parents. Fortunately, nothing arose to cause us to break the confidence that we had promised to do our best to protect.

Problems in Gaining Entry to Respondents

The original plan called for recruiting 50 adolescents who would keep daily journals for a ten-week period. That plan ran into some knotty unforeseen problems and we had to scrap it.

Dozens of potential respondents declined our offer to participate in the study. The majority who declined seemed to be doing so because they viewed the $100 payment as simply not worth the effort. The most interesting of these cases occurred in a small town located in the Bootheel region of the state. We had enlisted the support of an influential administrator of the county juvenile court. She had agreed to contact 15 adolescents, some of whom were college bound, some not, along with several high school dropouts. The administrator knew the potential respondents through her court work and community leadership activities. As the contact person, she helped devise the confidentiality system that we ended up using at the other research sites. Finally, after several weeks of trying, the administrator threw in the towel and drew a halt to her recruitment efforts. She told us that most of the adolescents whom she contacted were unwilling to write daily journal entries for $100 dollars. The administrator felt that a few of the adolescents were poor enough writers that the prospect of writing something every day frightened them. But, the majority was not attracted particularly by the $100 stipend. Surprisingly, almost all of the adolescents contacted by the administrator came from moderate to low income backgrounds, a fact that would seem to favor participating in the study.

At another site in a northwestern county, we utilized a former MU sociology student to help us gain entry to a large high school that she had attended several years ago. The former student offered to serve as the local contact person since she was home from law school for the summer. Furthermore, she offered to introduce the researchers to a high school guidance counselor with whom the former student had been close. One of the researchers spoke with the guidance counselor on the phone and was in turn referred to the principal. Subsequently, the researcher went to the school and met with the principal who agreed to participate. The principal offered to let the respondents use the school's computers and he allowed the researcher to attend two study hall periods to introduce the study to the students. The researcher met with over 70 students, introduced the study, and answered questions about confidentiality, payment, and the journal. The researcher told the students that if they had a time problem, they could send the journal entries twice a week instead of daily. The researcher reported later that some of the students appeared interested, but the majority was not. The uninterested students stated that the $100 dollar consulting fee was not enough money to entice them to participate. Also, the students admitted that they were not responsible enough to commit to the study over the summer break. They said that if they could have done the project during school time, they would have considered it. However, the students were unwilling to drive either to the public library or to the school campus to send the e-mail. The researcher told the students that if they wanted to do the study, they could contact either the school secretary who had all of the appropriate information, and IRB forms, or they could contact the former student who had offered to be the contact person. Later, one of the high school students called the researcher and expressed interest in participating. However, he had concerns about having to send the journal entries twice a week. Since he was the only potential respondent out of 70 students contacted, the researcher told him to reconsider and to get in touch with the contact person in his hometown. That student never called the contact person. Two other students called the contact person directly and expressed interest in participating. However, both backed out when they got full-time summer jobs.

In summary, the majority of the students who declined our invitation to participate probably did so because they thought that the consulting fee of $100 dollars was insufficient for 10 weeks of daily submissions in a journal. Also, trepidation about having to write down one's thoughts and actions on a daily basis seemed to be a factor. None of the reasons given involved concerns about confidentiality or the informed consent forms.

Thirty-one adolescents between the ages of 14 and 18 wrote daily journals and sent the entries to the researchers through e-mail. Twenty-one respondents participated for 10 weeks during the 1998 academic year while the other 13 respondents sent journal entries over an 8-week period during the summer of 1998.

Public Secondary School Educators

We believed initially that high school teachers and administrators would be interested in helping us do the study. The e-mail approach could be part of computer education for their students, the daily journal writing might be incorporated into writing classes, and the research problem seemed relevant to social science courses, so we thought. We seem to have been wrong. By far, the most troubling barrier to our access to respondents was high school teachers and administrators. We had virtually guaranteed that no school would be liable for any problem stemming from the study, primarily because of our carefully crafted consent forms and procedures for maintaining anonymity. Furthermore, the study seemed to have significant educational value for all concerned and participation required only 15 or so minutes of time at the very end of the study for the contact person. In one notable case that we will describe in more detail below, the study would have given the students real e-mail to use and the experience of participating in a sociological study while they were taking a sociology course. In another case, a horrific automobile accident that involved a couple of potential respondents was the reason cited by administration for pulling out of the study. A letter from the principal investigator to the high school principal reminding him of that our study would shed light on the causes of such accidents went unanswered. In another instance, the high school guidance counselor refused to help because he was not to be paid.

One of the low accident rate counties in the northwestern part of Missouri contained a fairly large high school that we contacted for help in securing nine respondents from the student body. We contacted the high school principal and discussed the study overview, the IRB procedures, the data collection procedures, and the consulting fee. The principal put us in contact with a community/school coordinator and we faxed all of the letters and forms. The coordinator called us and agreed to serve as the local contact person. We put together nine packets of materials consisting of study overviews, consent forms for students and parents, and instructions for respondents and for the contact person. We had asked the contact person to meet with the summer school computer teachers to explain the study and then to recruit nine students. She would have given packets of materials to willing students, collected all the signed consent forms later, and then slip the self addressed stamped envelope in the mail to us at the sociology department. Two weeks later, we received a phone call from the contact person at the school who informed us that the computer coordinator at the school was concerned about liability issues. One of the researchers spoke with the computer coordinator by phone and explained the IRB approval process and the protection that we had in place. The researcher mentioned that the computer lab would need to insure that the respondents would have privacy in typing and sending the e-mail. The researcher reported that the coordinator appeared satisfied and had agreed to set aside 20 minutes a day in two of her computer sections for the respondents to send their journal entries. The contact person informed us that she had secured the participation of 6 students. When we had not heard from her for a couple of weeks, we phoned her. She informed us that she had decided not to participate in the study because several students from the high school, including a couple who had agreed to be in the study, had been in a pile up auto accident. She told us that several students were injured, some seriously, and that she was too busy dealing with distraught parents and students to continue with the study. We offered to give her some time for things to settle before starting the fieldwork, but she declined, offering to take part in our "next project". After two weeks had elapsed, the principal investigator called the principal, left a voice message, and wrote an extensive e-mail letter in which he reiterated the need for the study, particularly given the accident. Neither communication was answered.

We had difficulty recruiting respondents in the northeast part of the state as well. Two counties in this region had been selected based on their low injury rates. We picked high schools and contacted guidance counselors as the starting point for gaining entry. In one school, the counselor stated that students there recently had been involved in an auto accident that resulted in one death. Also, violence and racial tension were concerns at the school. Finally, the guidance counselor stated that the students had poor writing skills and thus he concluded they would be uninterested in participating. The guidance counselor at a different high school in the same county told us that she would seek permission for the study from the superintendent of schools. Permission was granted and packets were sent to the school while the guidance counselor was seeking someone to serve as contact person. Later, the packet was returned with a letter stating that the school would not participate due to time constraints. At another high school in the other county, the guidance counselor agreed to ask the principal. After doing this, she contacted us and told us that the school would not participate because the students were too busy applying to college. This is in spite of the fact that we were seeking non-college bound students for the study. We tried to gain the cooperation of representatives of the FFA and 4-H organizations, but they had a policy against releasing the names of their members and they were unwilling to contact members for us.

In St. Louis County, a high accident site, one of the researchers had a friend who was teaching at a high school that we had decided to try and get involved in the study. The researcher contacted the teacher who in turn talked with the principal. A week later, the principal called the researcher who described the study, its importance, funding source, and so forth. The researcher faxed the packet of materials to the principal. After reading the forms, the principal called the researcher again, expressed interest in participating, but told the researcher that she the principal had to get approval from the school board. After a week, the researcher called the principal and was informed that the school board had rejected the study out of concerns about school liability. According to the principal, the board members were concerned about the students having access to the Internet from the school campus, something that had not been allowed up to that point. In this case, the school administration refused to recruit students who might have had home computers and thereby could have avoided the problem of Internet access from the school.

An attempt within the City of St. Louis ended in failure, too. We had a contact person in the St. Louis Public Schools who had worked with an administrator of a state agency that had contracted with the public schools in the past. We telephoned this person who put us in contact with a school administrator who was involved in the drop out problem. This person transferred us to the evaluation research office and we filled out a formal application to do the study. We had chosen a high school that was struggling with a high drop out rate and it was located in a high injury area. The principal of this high school suggested that we contact a computer science teacher at the school which we did. The teacher offered to contact students in her class and a packet of consent forms was sent to the teacher for distribution to respondents and their parents. The teacher requested that the researcher visit the school to help the respondents start their e-mail. Upon arriving at the designated time, the researcher discovered that the students had been dismissed from class and had left for the day. The researcher returned to Columbia and sent an e-mail letter to the teacher who wrote back and explained that she was unable to get the students to remain after class because they had to work. Then the teacher attempted to arrange an evening meeting time, but that failed, too.

The following school refusal was the most troubling. We had located a high school in a low accident county in the Ozark region of the state. The situation seemed perfect as we sought the participation of 15 students. It just so happened that a sociology teacher had exactly 15 students in class. The students were representative of the qualities we needed, such as some college bound, others on the verge of dropping out, and so on. Furthermore, the students were in the process of learning about the Internet and e-mail. Fortunately for us, at least I thought so at the time, the students needed real e-mail contacts as they had been sending messages to each other in class. The principal investigator contacted the principal who put him in contact with the guidance counselor. The counselor in turn got him in touch with the sociology teacher, a young man who had been teaching at the high school for a couple of years. The principal investigator explained the study, and then he offered to travel to the high school to talk with the students about qualitative research and careers in sociology. The teacher seemed to be very interested and the researcher offered to bring his lap top computer and a Proxima projector to demonstrate the qualitative data analysis program that the research was using. The researcher sent 15 packets to the teacher. After a couple of weeks had elapsed with nothing in the return mail, the researcher called the teacher only to learn that the teacher had decided that he was too busy to participate. The researcher called the guidance counselor and asked her to distribute the material to any 15 students she thought might want to participate, but she declined, again citing a busy schedule.

At another high school in the same region, a guidance counselor at first agreed to participate and then refused when he learned, upon his inquiring, that he would not be paid for serving as the local contact person.

The last "failure" in the Ozark region was based on parental concerns about access to the Internet. In this case, one of the researchers utilized her own social network that she had established growing up in the area. Because the local high school had very limited resources and could not afford to let the respondents use the computers, we loaned a computer with e-mail access to a parent who was willing to serve as the local contact person. After some thought on the matter with the computer in place and ready to go, the parent decided that he did not want his children to have access to the Internet.

These several reasons why we failed to gain the cooperation of these high school administrators and teachers can be viewed as risks to the subjects. We felt that the benefits of the research outweighed these risks and we remain puzzled by the problems we had gaining access to respondents. The results of the study would have shed light on aspects of the everyday lives of adolescents that might have helped the school staffs design policies and programs to lessen the myriad risks to this age group. Furthermore, the teachers and administrators would have been privy to qualitative information not contained in the currently available survey data and the students would have been given the opportunity to reflect on their lives and to contribute to something positive. Being too busy, for example, to help students take part in research that could affect the opportunities available to them seemed almost capricious from our perspective at the time.

Data Gathering: The Electronic Journal

We decided to put the burden of measurement on the shoulders of the respondents by asking them to write a daily journal. Generally, we asked the respondents to write each day about what they did and why they did it. In this way we avoided direct contact with the respondents who sent their journal entries via e-mail. This approach was anonymous enough to override the usual adolescent self-consciousness about sharing sensitive thoughts and actions with adult researchers. It was free and very efficient in the sense of being able to gather quickly a large amount of descriptive and attitudinal information. It would have been impossible to achieve the same degree of depth and coverage of the lives of the respondents using the interview and/or questionnaire methods. Aside from the few times that we wrote to the respondents, the researchers were basically an e-mail address. The entire data-gathering phase of the study was a one-way flow of information from respondent to researcher, which is exactly what one wants if the goal is to understand the thoughts, and actions that occur in the every day lives of adolescents.

Each respondent used a pseudonym, but was asked to begin each of his/her entries with the name of the county in which he/she lived. Also, respondents were sent a single sheet that discussed how to write journal entries and which questions or issues the respondents might consider. Only one respondent made the mistake of sending his/her real name with the first journal entry. Because Whitley Vale, a co-researcher on the project, was receiving the journal entries, he alone saw the name and replied immediately instructing the respondent to use a pseudonym. Otherwise, there were no breaches of confidence that we know about during the entire one -year study period.

E-Mail Technology

Internet providers included AOL and particular high school systems. Respondents used a variety of e-mail programs, including Netscape, Yahoo, and Eudora. Once the e-mail connections were established, one member of the research team was responsible for receiving the entries and distributing them to the other research team members on the University Pine Mail system. Research team members were assigned responsibility for particular respondents. Each of the researchers had their individualized Pine Mail folders into which appropriate journal entries were saved. The research team members would read their assigned entries and would respond to respondent requests or for clarification. In this sense, turnaround time was minutes as opposed to days using regular mail.

However, the University of Missouri-Columbia's e-mail system presented the researchers with a particularly knotty problem. All University e-mail was backed up and saved every couple of days. This meant that persons other than the researchers could have retrieved the respondents' journal entries for those days at any time. All of the respondents used code names, but the messages were saved in folders according to the counties that they were sent from. This was done for record keeping purposes. Ultimately, if someone got their hands on the back up tapes and wanted badly enough to find a particular respondent, probably it could have been done. We refused to compromise the confidentiality of the respondents, so we warned them and their parents in the consent forms to be careful about what went in to the journal entries. Most probably this had somewhat of a dampening effect on the willingness of respondents to divulge sensitive material. Still, several respondents wrote about highly personal matters that would have caused conflict with their parents had the information leaked out. Generally, the problem was not as bad as it might have been, probably because we were able to reassure several concerned respondents that we would protect their confidence. The words of an 18-year-old male are instructive: "Don't get me wrong. I really want to be open about everything and I want to talk to you. But I need to be assured, just one more time, that this is just between me and you and my real name, if you ever find out, will not be released in any way. I really hope that I can continue to talk to you about my life because you always need someone to talk to and get things off your chest so everything is not a big secret". Again, e-mail seemed to break down the inhibitions normally associated with interviewing or keeping a physical journal to be mailed to the researchers.

Another advantage to using an electronic journal was that the researcher could read entries daily and react to them while they were still fresh. For example, a couple of respondents began their participation in the study by sending very superficial and terse journal entries. Immediately, the researchers keeping track of those respondents replied and reminded the respondents that they had agreed to send detailed descriptions of their daily lives. In all but one case, this produced excellent results. The temptation was always there to respond to the respondents, but we avoided doing this as much as possible. We did not want the respondents to become dependent on us for ideas to write about nor did we want to influence unduly the emergence of what the respondents found interesting and relevant. The less input from the researchers, the more likely that the study would capture how the respondents thought and what they thought about. In the absence of direct questioning from the researchers, the respondents would write what was on their minds. Theoretically, the behaviors and issues that got the most attention would be the most salient parts of the respondents' every day lives.

Particularly in the beginning of the study, many of the respondents asked us to reply to their e-mail messages. Mostly, they wanted to be reassured that what they were writing was of value to the study. A few were concerned that their e-mail messages were not getting through, and others just seemed to need the stimulation of a researcher's question in order to write journal entries. We wrote each respondent within the first week of them sending entries to acknowledge receiving their mail. Occasionally during the 10 weeks, we wrote some of the respondents to ask for clarification on journal entries that we thought perhaps were incomplete or tantalizingly close to discussing a decision that led to risk taking. Also, occasionally we presented each respondent with the same case study derived from a current news event. These cases involved moral dilemmas surrounding acts that the media considered "risky". We asked the respondents a series of questions about the event. The response to our queries was uniformly positive. In the words of a 17-year-old female, "I didn't really have much to tell you today. I told you so much yesterday. I like when you write back and ask questions though because I have more to write about".

Qualitative Data Processing and Analysis

This study used HyperQual2 software to record and analyze the hundreds of textual journal entries received. HyperQual2 is a Macintosh HyperCard-based program that enables the analyst to categorize and retrieve sentences and paragraphs.

All of the journal entries were downloaded from the mainframe and converted into HyperQual2 data files. Thus, each respondent's journal entries became a single HyperQual data file for that respondent. Each HQ2 file was named using a combination of the pseudonym, county, age, and sex of the respondent. This name and date of entry followed the data through the categorization process.

HyperQual2 data files were printed and three more researchers were brought on board, one graduate student and two undergraduate social science majors. Copies of the raw journal texts were distributed to the researchers who then began the difficult task of establishing broad categories into which journal entries could be placed. These categories, called "exemplars", eventually emerged to form the backbone of the analysis. For several weeks the research team members followed this pattern. All would read the same portions of the journal entries, code the text, and then meet to discuss the results. Whether the researchers agreed or disagreed, the reasons for choosing a particular exemplar for a given segment of text led eventually to three important outcomes: 1.Inter coder consistency; 2. An exhaustive and mutually exclusive set of exemplars; 3. Clear definitions for the exemplars. Coder consistency meant that other researchers coding the journal entries would place entries in exemplars similarly. The fact that any given sentence appeared in only one exemplar meant that the categories were exclusive and being able to find a category for every sentence meant that the exemplars were exhaustive.

With the final exemplar list in hand, researchers coded journal entries and created exemplar files. Each coder read all of the journal entries for a limited number of respondents and coded every sentence of every journal entry. This resulted in two data sets, one the HQ raw journal entries that contained all of the journal entries in chronological order exactly as written by each respondent, and the other the exemplar files. Each exemplar file was made up of pieces of journal entries from any respondents who wrote about the exemplar. A quote or sentence was "tagged" as belonging to the exemplar and so on until the exemplar file was complete, that is, until we could no longer find information that fit the category. These exemplar files were made up of the raw data found in the HQ2 data files and each journal entry "tagged" as a particular exemplar constituted an individual card. This is different from the HQ2 raw data where all of the journal entries for a given respondent were on just one card. The number of cards for a given exemplar reflected the attention paid to that exemplar by the respondents in the form of the number of journal entries about that exemplar. For example, the exemplar "sex" had 11 cards compared to 148 cards in "family relationships". That meant that the respondents wrote approximately 17 times more about family relationships than they did about sex. This gave the researchers a rough picture of the relative attention that respondents paid to those two aspects of their everyday lives, for example.

Essentially, the data files were a collection of diary entries organized according to the particular topic or exemplar. For example, friend relationships had 93 entries that 20 or more respondents wrote. Each entry had identifiers that contained the respondent's e-mail name, the date it was written, and the exemplar name. Sorts by name within an exemplar file would have produced a list of everything that a given respondent wrote about that exemplar. Also, we had kept the raw data HQ files for each respondent as a permanent record. While not as easily accessible as field notes on paper, nevertheless the HQ files posed a significant privacy risk given a determined investigator in possession of the respondents' real names and addresses.

Conclusion

The e-mail approach had its advantages and weaknesses. On the plus side, e-mail worked well to transmit large text files quickly and accurately to the research team members. It seemed to facilitate writing every day, possibly in part by eliminating the usual hassles associated with "real" mail. We were able to "motivate" respondents quickly when we felt that entries were inadequate or lagging. Also, we noticed that the quality of the writing improved week by week. By writing every day, respondents seemed to reflect better on their experiences and thoughts with each passing e-mail.

HyperQual2 served us well as a type of electronic filing system for storing and retrieving the diary entries. We gained most, however, from its "exemplar" system. Tagging quotes as belonging to specific exemplars or topics, such as family relationships, forced the researchers to define each topic clearly and code behind one another until we reached agreement about the appropriate home for the quotes (inter-coder reliability). Patterns among the exemplars emerged as the number of diary entries grew. We obtained a picture of everyday life framed by the topics and meanings deemed salient by the adolescents. By counting the number of entries in each exemplar file, we got some idea of the relative importance of those issues for the respondents. By sorting respondents into exemplars, we were able to think in a Weberian fashion about types of adolescents and patterns of meaning associated with risk. We were able to download the e-mail text into the HQ2 data editor on a daily basis and could add to each respondent's text data file consistently and easily this way.

A few of the respondents mentioned feeling pleased about being asked to contribute to real social science research, adding that they thought it was unusual for adults to listen to them so carefully. Generally, the anonymity of e-mail appeared to break down some of the almost innate age gap associated with face-to-face interviews and observations between adults and adolescents. Respondents discussed very private thoughts and behaviors pretty early on in the data-gathering phase of the study and seemed to do this easily and without hesitation. Remember that the IRB worked with us to produce informed consent forms that left no risk unturned, so the fact that the respondents were so open with us was quite impressive.

Finally, getting daily data entries from so many respondents was relatively inexpensive and it kept us focused on analysis and interpretation, too. We read new data daily, assessed the theoretical framework, and regularly revised our thinking about how the adolescents negotiated their everyday lives. If something emerged that we wanted clarification on, we instantly sent a query out to every respondent and usually we had dozens of responses by the end of the workday.

A significant negative aspect of our e-mail methodology stemmed from the inherent security problems all e-mail systems have at present. Interaction with the campus IRB helped us anticipate and address in writing the key ethical issues. In spite of the safeguards discussed earlier, we knew that a truly committed and knowledgeable sleuth could probably match e-mail diary entries with the actual respondents. For example, if one of the field contact persons had decided to make trouble for the respondents or researchers, it would have been relatively easy to do so given the technology. Several respondents had put themselves on the line, so to speak, and if their teachers, parents, or friends found out what they had written, it might have been very difficult for all concerned. At the moment this problem appears to be miles from any solution and in fact may have just gotten worse. Recently, the Pentagon admitted that it had designed and was using an e-mail tracking system appropriately called "Carnivore". An investigator can use this program to eavesdrop systematically on e-mail sent and received anywhere on Earth.

Another less technical problem had to do with what Rosalie Wax (1975) called "immersion". In her wonderful book on field work, Wax discussed the explanatory power that a researcher gets from delving into the field setting and participating as widely as possible in the life of the community. Probably the problems we had with educators in the field would have been better handled by us if we had spent some time on site and therefore had a better sense of the best entry strategies to use. No shortcuts exist for time spent gaining entry to the field, and we paid a rather stiff price in time and lost opportunities by not showing our faces and negotiating directly with adolescents. We lacked the funding to do much of this on-site work plus we thought it best at the time to avoid face-to-face interaction with respondents because we felt that it might counteract the anonymity of e-mail. Of course, one can go overboard and "go native" by getting too emotionally involved in the research setting, but there is no good substitute for first-hand experience of the research setting. E-mail used alone as the data gathering technique precluded researcher mastery over the research setting that Wax so correctly urged us to strive for.

Again, we had no good way to insure that the "right" respondents filled out the diary entries. Nor did we have any way of checking on the substantive accuracy of the entries, in short, the validity of the data.

Clearly, e-mail and adolescents are a good fit for qualitative researchers. Technical problems and their attendant ethical consequences need to be attended to before we can begin to systematize methodological principles and techniques in using the Internet for research. Privacy risk and the quality of data remain as unsolved methodological problems for Internet research.

REFERENCES

[1] Bagnall, G. and Plant, M.A., 1991, 'Aids Risks, Alcohol and Illicit Drug Use Amongst Young Adults in Areas of High and Low Rates of HIV Infection', *AIDS Care,* vol. 3, pp. 355-361.

[2] *Business Week.*, February 11, 1991, #3199, p.28

[3] Cho, H. and LaRose, R., 1999, 'Privacy Issues in Internet Surveys', *Social Science Computer Review*, vol. 17, no. 4, , pp. 421-434.

[4] *The Economist*, February 7, 1998,. 346, # 8054, p. 43

[5] Fonseca, B., 2000, 'Ensuring Secure Transmission', *Infoworld*, vol. 22, no. 14, , p. 18.

[6] Furlong, A. and Cartmel, F., 1997, *Young People and Social Change: Individualism and Risk in Late Modernity*, Philadelphia, Open University Press.

[7] Goffman, E., 1974, *Frame Analysis: An Essay on the Organization of Experience*.

[8] New York, Harper Colophon.

[9] Hessler, R.M.,1998, 'Peer Mediation: A Qualitative Study of Youthful Frames of Power and Influence'. *Mediation Quarterly*, vol. 15, no. 3, pp. 187-198.

[10] Janney, R.W., 1996, 'E-mail and Intimacy', in B. Gorayska (Ed.), *Cognitive Technology: In Search of a Humane Interface. Advances in Psychology*, pp. 201-211, Amsterdam, Netherlands, Elsevier Science Publishing Company.

[11] Jerome, L.W., Deleon, P.H., James, L.C., Folen, R., Earles, J. and Gedney, J.J., 2000, 'The Coming Age of Telecommunications in Psychological Research and Practice', *American Psychologist*, vol. 55, no. 4, pp. 407-421.

[12] Kahn, J., Chen, K. and Brauchli, M., 1996, 'Fences in Cyberspace: Governments' Move to Limit Free Flow of the Internet', *The Boston Globe*, January 2, p. 15.

[13] Kawaura, Y., Yamashita, K. and Kawakami, Y.,1999, 'What Makes People Keep Writing Web Diaries?', *Japanese Journal of Social Psychology*, vol. 14, no. 3, pp. 133-143.

[14] Rosencrance, L., 2000, 'Netscape Users Lose E-Mail', *Computerworld*, vol. 34, no. 16, p. 67.

[15] Samoriski, J.H., Huffman, J.L. and Trauth, D.M., 1996, 'Electronic Mail Privacy and the Electronic Communications Act of 1986: Technology in Search of Law', *Journal of Broadcasting and Electronic Media*, vol. 40, p. 1.

[16] Spielberg, A., 1998, 'On Call and Online: Sociohistorical, Legal, and Ethical Implications of E-Mail for the Patient-Physician Relationship', *JAMA*, vol. 280, no. 15, , pp. 1353-1359.

[17] Wax, R., 1975, *Doing Fieldwork: Warnings and Advice*, Chicago, The University of Chicago Press.

[18] Workman, J.P., Jr., 1992, Use of Electronic Media in a Participant Observation Study', *Qualitative Sociology*, vol. 15, no. 4, pp. 419-425.

In: Health Research in Cyberspace
Editor: Pranee Liamputtong, pp. 121-132
ISBN 1-59454-819-6

Chapter 7

METHODOLOGICAL ISSUES IN ONLINE SEXUAL HEALTH RESEARCH

Brian S. Mustanski

INTRODUCTION

The use of the Internet for sexual health research represents an exciting new frontier. The anonymity and accessibility of the Internet allow data collection from populations that may otherwise go understudied (such as geographic isolates and young HIV seropositive individuals), especially for research in the sexuality arena. The ease of recruitment and data collection allow extensive samples to be readily achieved. Although benefits are numerous, several potential problems must be prevented to assure the collection of valid data. Many of these potential problems are issues that must be faced with any data collection from human subjects, such as lying and sabotage. Other issues are more particular to online research, such as repeated submission of data from the same individual and greater loss of control over stimulus presentation. The purpose of this chapter is to discuss issues of reliability, validity, and ethics in online sexual health research. Special attention is given to the use of the Internet to collect data from traditionally underrepresented groups (gay, transgender, and so on.). The chapter ends with a look at non-survey sexual health research over the Internet, such as health interventions, experimental designs, and event-level assessments.

To help clarify many of the issues and recommendations presented in this chapter, each is explained in the context of an online daily diary study. The purpose of this Internet-based research project was to explore the within- and between-person relationships between mood and sexual interest, behavior, and risk-taking (Mustanski, 2004). Participants were recruited through U.S. gay and lesbian university student organizations, websites designed to help gay men find sexual partners, and websites targeted to individuals who identify as "sex addicts." This recruitment strategy resulted in a sample of 3,260 gay and bisexual men who completed a set of initial questionnaires. These questionnaires assessed sexual history, sexual inhibition and excitation proneness, and several personality constructs. I designed and programmed this website using Microsoft FrontPage and it was hosted by the university server. The daily diary portion of the study was programmed by The Center for Survey Research at Indiana

University using Cold Fusion technology. It was completed by 155 participants randomly selected from the initial questionnaires. Participants logged on each night and completed diaries for up to 30 days. The quantitative diaries assessed mood and sexual interest and behavior, with a quantitative HIV/AIDS risk score based on response to the behavioral items. The major finding of this study was that daily Positive Affect and Sexual Interest showed significant within-person relationships with fluctuations in HIV/AIDS risk behaviors. More information about this study, such as specific problems that were encountered and how they were overcome, is provided as examples in the following sections when relevant.

Cost

Some Internet-based research projects can be conducted with few, if any, related expenses. Because most universities provide web hosting for affiliated individuals, the server used for data collection may be cost-free. With the advent of easy-to-use website design software, researchers can create websites for most survey studies themselves, without having to hire a computer programmer. Outflows related to printing, mailing, or coding can be eliminated by recruiting participants via e-mails or web-postings and by having data automatically entered into a database.

The majority of Internet-based studies so far have been conducted without offering participant incentives, instead relying on participant altruism (Musch and Reipis, 2000). Research on the degree to which this introduces participation bias is just now emerging. For example, an online experiment randomly assigning participants to an incentive or incentive-free condition suggests that incentives do influence drop out, but not initial interest in participation (Frick et al., 2001). Other Internet-focused studies have similarly found that subject payment influences participation rates (O'Neil et al., 2003; Ross et al., 2004). The effects of incentives on participation will likely increase as the Internet becomes more saturated with online studies and polls.

If providing incentives is preferable as a means of reducing drop-out and thereby decreasing participation bias, the obvious question is how to provide such incentives in the context of Internet-based research? Direct payment to the participant is one option, but it requires the potentially non-optimal loss of participant anonymity. Researchers have begun to develop innovative alternatives, like payment to third party accounts (such as paypal.com) that do not require the participant to reveal identifying information (Konstan et al., 2005). Others have offered compensation to a charitable organization (Ross et al., 2004), although maintaining anonymity here may have the unintended consequence of encouraging multiple submission from the same participant in order to increase the size of the donation. Another alternative is to provide feedback based on the participant's results, which may be considered rewarding for subjects who chose to participate out of curiosity. This option may not be relevant or ethical for all designs, however, because some may have no feedback to offer while other cannot ethically provide the information in such a context (Naglieri et al., 2004). Another option, and the one I used in my on-line daily diary study (Mustanski, 2004), is to conduct Internet-based research with a population with intrinsic motivation for participation, thus potentially ameliorating the importance of providing extrinsic incentives. In this study, participants were not compensated for completing the initial questionnaires, but were paid for the more labor intensive daily diaries. Nevertheless, many participants completed the screening questionnaires without compensation and submitted comments that they enjoyed participating and looked forward to inviting their peers to participate because they found the study to be stimulating and interesting. Many expressed satisfaction about the fact that efforts were being made to include the bisexual and gay population in health research. Fortunately, sex is a subject that many Americans are interested in discussing, especially on the Internet (Mills, 1998), thus making it a topic likely to encourage participation. If no incentives are being offered, the length of the study becomes critical since participation declines as a study becomes more aversive (Korn and Hogan, 1992), possibly explaining why the majority of Internet-based studies require less than 15 minutes for participation (Musch and Reipis, 2000). Incentives or not, of course all research must be discussed in the context of the limitations imposed by the recruitment method utilized.

Ease of Use and Lack of Experimental Control

Another attractive feature of conducting research via the Internet is the extent to which data collection can be automated. For example, in an online quantitative survey participants can complete the study on their own computer whenever they desire, thus eliminating the need for scheduling participants and hiring interviewers and coders. Once the study is set up, participants can participate any time, if allowed, without any further effort by the researchers. For other types of research this automation allows for more advanced designs. Some Internet-based studies have utilized "branching," which means that the questions or stimuli presented to participants are conditional on previously entered information. For example, if a participant positively endorses a question about alcohol use they will then be asked to answer more questions in this area, whereas someone who responds negatively would be taken to the next section. Researchers can build on this method in treatment-outcome or prevention research, with participants automatically and immediately assigned to various arms based on their answers to screening questions. Web-based studies can also be set up to provide real time validity checks and query respondents when they provide illogical responses. In my own online daily diary research (Mustanski, 2004), the diary program was set up to list each participant's diary completion record (without linkage to the participants data) on a password protected website, which allowed research assistants easy assess to the data they needed to ensure participation compliance. The program was also configured to automatically e-mail participants reminders when they forgot to complete a diary. Future developments in Internet technology will allow for even greater automation and therefore innovative ways to take advantage of the Internet for research.

As with any research that takes place outside of a laboratory, the drawback is that it is difficult for the researcher to control the environment in which the individual is completing the study. If the design of the study requires standardized stimulus presentation, such as visual or auditory stimuli, using the Internet to collect data becomes much more complex. Variability in monitor specification, Internet connection speeds, and pop-up advertisements are just some of the possible factors that could confound standard stimulus presentation. Even for research that does not require participants to perceive highly specific stimuli, the quality of the data are potentially decreased because Internet-based research does not take place in a controlled environment, such as a laboratory. Some people may participate in a distracting environment—late at night when they are not fully alert, while visiting erotic web pages or chat rooms, or while intoxicated—thus threatening the validity of the data. Researchers can get around this by using "cookies", which are files placed on users' computers to both collect information and improve site navigation, to collect data about monitor specifications, operating system, and so on. It is also possible to inquire about the environment in which the study took place or request that participants fulfill certain requirements, although there is no guarantee that they will be adopted or accurately reported. It is important to keep in mind that many of these problems have an equal probability of occurring with other off-line survey methodologies.

Sample Size

With over a billion people connected to the Internet around the world the potential sample size far exceeds that of the university classroom often used in social science research. Sample sizes in the thousands are not uncommon in Internet-based research (Musch and Reipis, 2000). Sexual health researchers should be particularly interested in becoming active in on-line data collection efforts because of the large interest in sexual materials and communication via the Internet, so much so that the Internet has been labeled an "erotic oasis" (Ross et al., 2000). Sex related searches predominate the list of most common search terms on the web and sex related chat rooms are extremely popular (Mustanski, 2001; see also Couch and Liamputtong in this volume).

One issue that has yet to be clearly resolved is how to report participation rates in online studies. While the numerator (how many subjects participated) is clear, the denominator (out of how many invited) is less clear. For example, if participants are recruited through banner advertisements on sexuality-related website it is possible to record the number of times the banner was shown and the number of times it was clicked. It is also possible to use cookies to estimate the number of visits and the number of unique visitors that come to the research webpage. I propose that Internet-based research investigators should report all of these relevant statistics, including: number of banner impressions or recruitment e-mails sent, number of unique participants who visit the research page, number of participants who initiate the study, and number of participants who provide usable data. Some researchers may be hesitant about this approach because they fear reporting these numbers may lead to questioning of the validity of their study; It can be expected that only 0.05% of the times a banner is shown it will be clicked (see for example Bull et al., 2004; Ross et al., 2005) and dropout rates can range widely. Nevertheless, this is the reality of Internet-based research and researchers should provide all of this information to allow for evaluation of the relative validity of the study. Similarly, editors and reviewers should realize that the parameters of Internet-based research differ from traditional research.

External Validity

External validity refers to the extent to which conclusions derived from a particular study will hold for people in other places and times. There is no such thing as a study that has perfect external validity; instead the goal is to be able to generalize the conclusions based on a particular sample to the population of interest. In Internet-based research the population of interest may be a subset of Internet users (such as rural gay men who use the Internet to meet sexual partners), all Internet users, or even a population that includes those who do not have access to the Internet. For the first two populations, external validity will largely depend on the recruitment methodology, for the last it will also depend on the degree to which Internet-users are representative of the larger population.

Just as in traditional research, two main recruitment approaches exist for Internet-based research: probability and convenience sampling. Couper (2000) provides an authoritative review of the various types of sampling methods currently available on the Internet, ranging from polls for entertainment purposes to population-based panels. He points out that these approaches vary in their degree of error associated with sampling, coverage, nonresponse, and measurement error, all relative to financial costs. In past Internet-based sexual health research, a variety of different recruitment methods have been used, including banner advertisements on sexuality or mainstream websites, postings in newsgroups or bulletin boards, sending targeted e-mails to members of various organizations or websites, inviting participants in chatrooms either individually or collectively, advertisements in print media, and recruitment in person at STD clinics. There are sexual health studies currently under development that will be population-based, but because of the prohibitive financial costs involved, these studies will continue to be rare.

Demographic data is critical to assess the extent to which the study's results are generalizability. This data will also allow an analysis of possible response correlations with demographic information and whether any significant effects remain after adjusting for demographic differences. Beyond simply asking participants to report demographic data, a number of innovative techniques are available in Internet-based research to collect this information. Cookies allow the researcher to collect a variety of demographic data. Commonly used "web tracker" programs collect the visitor's IP address, an estimate of the city, state, and country of the visitor, how long they visited the website, their computer's Internet browser and operating system software, as well as the URL of the websites visited before and after the study website. If recruiting across multiple domains, using different URLs for each recruitment effort will help to determine if there are any group differences. Reips (2000) refers to this as the *multiple site entry technique*. To do this, set up a number of different entry pages with different URLs, all of which can have the same content, and make sure to track from which URL the data was submitted. Then, when recruiting from different media, make sure to give each a different URL. For example, if recruiting from both chat rooms and banner advertisements, give different URLs to each. It is then possible to determine how participants ultimately found out about the study and then compare results across recruitment methods.

The reach of the Internet into the population is ever increasing. Because of the constant increases in Internet connectivity around the word, any review is inevitably a snapshot that immediately becomes out-of-date. For that reason, instead of reviewing current coverage data, readers are encouraged to visit one of these websites that provides current Internet demographics:

- Nielsen//Netratings: http://www.nielsen-netratings.com/
- Pew Internet and American Life Project: http://www.pewinternet.org/
- Internet World Stats: http://www.internetworldstats.com

In my daily diary study of the relationship between mood and sexuality, the population of interest was gay and bisexual men residing in the U.S. The sample was recruited by e-mailing every GLB student organization in the U.S. and by posting recruitment messages on sexuality websites. The demographics of this sample were more varied than found in a comparison sample of Psychology Subject Pool participants and the sample size was much large than would have been possible to achieve using conventional methods.

Utilizing Virtual Communities to Recruit Underrepresented Populations

The validity of survey research often suffers from the lack of inclusion of some minority populations (Birnbaum and Mellers, 1989). This issue becomes increasingly important for stigmatized groups such as homosexuals, individuals who engage in high-risk sexual behaviors, or individuals who are HIV positive. The anonymity of the Internet may help to solve this problem by allowing subjects to participate without being identified (see also Chapter one in this volume).

The Internet may make sexual minorities easier to recruit because many of these individuals have formed "virtual communities" (Rheingold, 1993) for discussion, support, networking, and entertainment purposes. Many sexuality-based groups maintain web pages, listserves, and chatrooms for their members to exchange information. For example, the PlanetOut network (which includes Gay.com a website catering to GLBT individuals), reports over 6 million registered members world-wide and 6 thousand new members each day (PlanetOut, 2005). Bowen and colleagues (2004) reported some success in using this website to recruit rural men who have sex with men (MSM) for a study on HIV risk behaviors. Other web communities exist that represent a plethora of populations of interest to sexual health researchers. Many of these web communities have online bulletin boards and e-mail lists that may be used to recruit participants. The website may also be willing to post a recruitment message on their website. I can report substantial anecdotal evidence for the willingness of such organizations to help spread the word about on-line research relevant to their organizations. The vast majority of the organizations that replied to my request to help recruit participants were positive. In approaching these organizations for help in recruiting participants, I have found it important to be brief but informative, explain the nature and importance of the study, and make it clear that these organizations are very important in the research process. Offering them access to aggregated results and approaching them with the attitude that they are collaborators in a very important research project also seemed to be advantageous.

Internal Validity

Just as in research on other sensitive topics, sexual health researchers must be vigilant about the accuracy and honesty with which their subjects respond to study questions. In his review of the literature regarding self-presentation bias in sexual health research, Catania (1999) reports that a participant's degree of discomfort is positively correlated with nonresponsiveness and negatively correlated with honesty. Furthermore, assurances of anonymity reduce discomfort and attempts to manage impression (Agnew and Loving, 1998). Internet-based research then has the potential to decrease self-presentation bias to the extent that participants feel that they are anonymous. In fact, studies have supported the fact that participants may feel less social desirability in Internet-based studies (Joinson, 1999). This is an exciting area, where much additional research is needed.

Despite the potential for greater honesty with self-reports via the Internet, researchers should still take steps to identify self-presentation biases, purposeful lying, and careless responding. One possibility is to include a social desirability questionnaire such as the Marlowe-Crowne Social Desirability Scale (Crowne and Marlowe, 1960) or the Balanced Inventory of Desirable Responding (Paulhus, 1988). Another possibility is the inclusion of similar questions with the affirmative response switched to identify participants who are responding to the questions randomly. Finally, it may be wise to include items that everyone would endorse, and check to see that the participant did, in fact, respond appropriately.

When studies are conducted anonymously on-line, it is possible for the same individual to participate multiple times, thereby confounding the results. The probability of this occurring varies with the population under study, the method used to recruit and encourage participation, and prevention methods taken. Several solutions to this problem have been suggested, such as asking participants not to participate more than once, asking them about the seriousness of their answers or if they have already participated, or collecting their e-mail or IP-address (Reips, 2000). In my previous writing (Mustanski, 2001), I have discussed in detail the many problems that accompany the use of any of these techniques, like confounding multiple distinct responders from the same computer. Konstan and colleagues (2005) offer a validation protocol to identify multiple responders. This protocol involved checking for duplicate IP address, e-mail address, and birthdates/ages, monitoring completion time, comparing start/end times across surveys, and reviewing payment records. Using this protocol, 11% of responses were judged invalid, with most of these cases detected using one of the last three suggested checks. The authors also noted the importance of only using these checks to "flag" suspicious entries; because of poor sensitivity and specificity the final decision to exclude should be made by a human. It is important to point out that the 11% rate of repeat responders in this study is higher than has been reported in some other studies (Reips, 2000; Gosling et al., 2004).

Violating the rules of on-line etiquette, also called "netiquette" (see also Chapter one in this volume), can also increase the probability of sabotage occurring. McMurdo (1995) provides a digest of general netiquette advice. Binik and colleagues (1999) discuss the importance of solicitation advertisements telling participants about compensation, timing, recruitment criteria, identifying researchers and their affiliations, and being in good taste. Along these same lines, it is important to note that e-mails soliciting participation in sexual health research may be problematic, depending on the nature of the study, because many people may read their e-mail at work where it could be monitored by employers. Additionally, new "spam" filters may block e-mails that use words related to the topic of a sexual health-focused study. Researchers should be aware of this and consider alternative language, or using a solicitation e-mail that invites the reader to visit a website to find out more about the study.

Because it is difficult to ascertain a subject's motivation for participating in an on-line study, researchers should be cautious about informing potential participants that they are ineligible because of particular characteristics. If the prospective subject is particularly curious about the contents of the study, or has little interest in following the rules set out as criteria for participation, they may falsify characteristics that would exclude them. This is especially the case if enticing participation incentives are being offered. To get around this problem it is preferable to simply ask participants about all relevant characteristics and then exclude those who do not meet the study requirements from analyses or invitation for further participation.

Comparing Internet and Traditional Research Samples

There has been much interest in research attempting to compare results from studies conducted online to those using more traditional research methods. These studies have focused on demonstrating the internal and external validity of Internet-based research. In regards to internal validity, researchers have found generally equivalent or superior results using the Internet. Gosling et al. (2004) reviewed this literature and found evidence for cross-method consistencies for constructs as diverse as reaction-time and personality. They also reported that when differences were found, the evidence supported less socially desirable responding via the Internet.

Sexual health studies have focused on the generalizability of Internet data by comparing demographic and behavioral reports to those found using traditional recruitment means. Some studies have reported demographic differences (Rhodes et al., 2002; Ross et al., 2000; Ross et al., 2005), while others have not (Bowen et al., 2004). What is to be made of these findings? Do they reflect true demographic and behavioral differences or do they reflect a lack of comparability of the two samples (that is third variable problem)? Do they reflect putative differences in internal or external validity? All of these questions will need to be answered as Internet-based sexual health research evolves.

Ethical Issues

Researchers must remember that depending on the methodology used, materials placed on the Internet are potentially accessible to anyone, including minors. In the sexual health arena, there is the potential that some guardians would object to minors observing research materials. The prevailing attitude seems to be that it is the responsibility of guardians to shield minors from accessing materials they deem offensive as long as the website's owners have made a reasonable attempt to prevent them from reaching the site. Researchers and their Human Subject Review Boards must evaluate what constitutes such reasonable attempt.

It is important to recognize that obtaining informed consent and receiving Human Subjects Committee approval is an important part of any research project, and collecting Internet-based data is no exception. How to go about this within the confines of current technology is still a matter under debate (see also Chapter one in this volume). In my online daily dairy study (Mustanski, 2004), two informed consent forms were used. The first one, for the initial questionnaires, was the first page participants accessed after viewing a short description of the study. Following the informed consent information was the statement, "By clicking the AGREE button you are indicating that you have read the statement, printed a copy for your files, agree to participate in the study, and that you are over 18 years of age." Following this was a button, which took the participants to the study questions. For the online daily diary portion of the study, participants were taken to the appropriate consent form after logging in with their unique user ID for the first time. The website recorded the fact that they had viewed the informed consent form, and on subsequent visits participants were not required to again provide consent, instead a link was provided in case they wished to view the consent form again.

Web Page Design

The aesthetic of the web page is important for convincing participants that the research is legitimate and important. Hosting the survey on a university or departmental server will add legitimacy over hosting it on a commercial server. Adding a departmental logo to the site will likely provide additional confidence (see also Couch and Liamputtong and Merkes in this volume). A well-laid-out site that is easy to follow and formal in appearance will inspire confidence in potential participants. Couper and colleagues (2001) review the literature and report on a study testing the effects of various web designs. They discuss the importance of considering issues like the number of items included on each page. One long page may seem confusing or overwhelming, while multiple pages may increase the download time and not allow participants to evaluate their commitment at the start, thus potentially increasing dropout rates. On the other hand, using multiple pages allows the collection of data from participants who do not complete the entire study; partial data cannot always be collected from single-page forms. Reviewing other studies currently being conducted on the Internet will provide some assistance in addressing this and other similar design issues.

In my daily diary study (Mustanski, 2004) a lot of attention was paid to the aesthetic and usability of all of the pages. All webpages were testing on different computer platforms (Macintosh and PC) and with different software (Internet Explorer and Mozilla Firefox), as well as on different screen resolutions and monitor sizes to make sure that the page layout was robust across all of these variables. Extensive testing was also done to assure the accurate submission of data. Researchers would be well advised to try everything they can to derail the data collection program before "going live." At minimum consider: the effects of using the "back" and "forward" buttons, all possible characters that might be entered into all fields (what happens if your delimiter character is entered into a field by a participant?), that ID numbers consistently are linked with participants across multiple pages, and that new submissions do not unintentionally overwrite existing data. Ask your colleagues to help you try and sabotage the webpage. Repeatedly, I have heard stories of woe from colleagues who had to write off data from hundreds or thousands of carefully recruited participants because of a programming problem. You cannot be too careful with this step.

Innovative Designs and Future Directions

The majority of research conducted on the Internet so far has consisted of surveys based on convenience samples (Musch and Reipis, 2000). Experimental studies taking advantage of the ability to provide real-time random assignment to condition are now being routinely conducted online. For example, experimental studies have been conducted in the areas of perception (Hecht et al., 1999), decision making (Birnbaum, 1999), personality (Buchana and Smith, 1999), psychoacoustics (Welch and Krantz, 1996), and cognitive tests requiring the collection of reaction time data (McGraw et al., 2000). My own online daily diary study (Mustanski, 2004) took advantage of several aspects of web-based research. The web diary automatically sent participants reminders when they forgot to complete a diary, assuring very high completion rates. The program also automatically asked participants a set of questions when they logged in after failing to complete a diary entry the previous day. This methodological innovation helped to prevent important confounding of dairy completion with reportable events (in this case mood or sexual behavior). Researchers are now designing sexual health interventions online (note that 80% of MSMs in one study (Bolding et al., 2004) reported they would participate in an online HIV prevention intervention). Several commercial companies now allow true probability sampling to be achieved on the Internet, and sexual health research using these methods is now underway. The best and most cutting-edge research will involve designs that take advantage of the benefits of Internet-based research to overcome methodological limitations inherent in more traditional research designs.

As technology becomes more advanced, bandwidth increases, and connectivity increase, the use of the Internet to conduct sexual health research will surely proliferate. It is important to remember, however, that although the use of the Internet to collect sexual health research has many potential benefits, risks to experimental validity must also be combated to insure the collection of quality data. Many of these risks also need to be put in the perspective of current limitations inherent in traditional research methodology. Further methodological research is clearly needed to assure the collection of valid data as sexual health researchers continue to explore this new frontier.

References

[1] Agnew, C.R. and Loving, T.J., 1998, 'The Role of Social Desirability in Self-Reported Condom Use Attitude and Intentions', *AIDS and Behavior*, vol. 2, pp. 229-239.

[2] Binik, Y.M., Mah, K. and Kiesler, S., 1999, 'Ethical Issues in Conducting Sex Research on the Internet', *The Journal of Sex Research*, vol. 36, pp. 82-90.

[3] Birnbaum, M.H., 1999, 'Testing Critical Properties of Decision Making on the Internet', *Psychological Science*, vol. 10, pp. 399-407.

[4] Birnbaum, M.H. and Mellers, B.A., 1989, 'Mediated Models for the Analysis of Confounded Variables and Self-Selection Samples', *Journal of Educational Statistics*, vol. 14, pp. 146-158.

[5] Bolding, G., Davis, M., Sherr, L., Hart, G. and Elford, J., 2004, 'Use of Gay Internet Sites and Views about Online Health Promotion among Men who Have Sex with Men', *AIDS Care*, vol. 16,no. 8, pp. 993-1001.

[6] Bowen, A., Williams, M. and Horvath, K., 2004, 'Using the Internet to Recruit Rural MSM for HIV Risk Assessment: Sampling issues', *AIDS Behavior*, vol. 8, no. 3, pp. 311-9.

[7] Buchana, T. and Smith, J., 1999, 'Research on the Internet: Validation of a World-Wide Web Mediated Personality Scale', *Behavior Research Methods, Instruments, and Computers*, vol. 31, pp. 565-571.

[8] Bull, S.S., Lloyd, L., Rietmeijer, C. and McFarlane, M., 2004, 'Recruitment and Retention of an Online Sample for an HIV Prevention Intervention Targeting Men who Have Sex with Men: The Smart Sex Quest Project', *AIDS Care*, vol. 16, no. 8, pp. 931-43.

[9] Catania, J., 1999, 'A Comment on Advancing the Frontiers of Sexological Methods', *The Journal of Sex Research*, vol. 36, pp. 1-2.

[10] Crowne, D.P. and Marlowe, D., 1960, 'A New Scale of Social Desirability Independent of Psychopathology', Journal of Counseling Psychology, vol 47, no. pp. 155-164.

[11] Couper, M.P., 2000, 'Web Surveys: A Review of Issues and Approaches', Public Opinion Quarterly, vol 64, no. pp. 464-494.

[12] Couper, M.P., Traugott, M.W. and Lamais, M.J., 2001, 'Web Survey Design and Administration', *Public Opinion Quarterly*, vol. 65, no. 2, pp. 231-253.

[13] Frick, A., Bächtiger, M.T. and Reips, U.-D. 2001. 'Financial Incentives, Personal Information and Drop-out Rate in Online Studies', in Reips, U.-D. and Bosnjak, M. (eds.) Dimensions of Internet Science, pp. 209-220, Pabst Science Publishers, Lengerich, Germany.

[14] Gosling, S.D., Vazire, S., Srivastava, S. and John, O.P., 2004, 'Should We Trust Web-Based Studies? A Comparative Analysis of Six Preconceptions about Internet Questionnaires', *American Psychologist*, vol. 59, no. 2, pp. 93-104.

[15] Hecht, H., Oesker, M., Kaiser, A., Civelek, H. and Stecker, T., 1999, 'A Perception Experiment with Time-Critical Graphics Animation on the World-Wide Web', *Behavior Research Methods, Instruments, and Computers*, vol. 31, pp. 439-445.

[16] Joinson, A., 1999, 'Social Desirability, Anonymity, and Internet-Based Questionnaires', *Behavioral Research Methods, Instruments, and computers*, vol. 31, pp. 433-438.

[17] Konstan, J.A., Rosser, B.R.S., Ross, M.W., Stanton, J. and Edwards, W.M., 2005, 'The Story of Subject Naught: A Cautionary but Optimistic Tale of Internet Survey Research', *Journal of Computer-Mediated Communication*, in press.

[18] Korn, J.H. and Hogan, K., 1992, 'Effect of Incentives and Aversiveness of Treatment on Willingness to Participate in Research', *Teaching of Psychology*, vol. 19, pp. 21-24.

[19] McGraw, K.O., Tew, M.D. and Williams, J.E., 2000, 'The Integrity of Web-Delivered Experiments: Can you Trust the Data?' *Psychological Science*, vol. 11, pp. 508-512.

[20] McMurdo, G., 1995, 'Netiquettes for Networkers', *Journal of Information Science*, vol. 21, pp. 305-319.

[21] Mills, R., 1998, 'Cyber: Sexual Chat on the Internet', *Journal of Popular Culture*, vol. 32, pp. 31-47.

[22] Musch, J. and Reipis, U.D. 2000. 'A Brief History of Web Experiments', in M.H. Birnbaum (ed), Psychological Experiments on the Internet, pp. 61 - 87, Academic Press, San Diego..

[23] Mustanski, B.S., 2001, 'Getting Wired: Exploiting the Internet for the collection of Valid Sexuality Data', *Journal of Sex Research*, vol. 38, pp. 292-301.

[24] Mustanski, B. S., 2004, 'The relationship between mood and sexual interest, behavior, and risk-taking', *Dissertation Abstracts International: Section B: The Sciences and Engineering, 65*(5-B), 2640.

[25] Naglieri, J.A., Drasgow, F., Schmit, M., Handler, L., Prifitera, A., Margolis, A. and Velasquez, R., 2004, 'Psychological Testing on the Internet: New Problems, Old Issues', *American Psychologist,* vol. 59, no. 3, pp. 150-62.

[26] O'Neil, K.M., Penrod, S.D. and Bornstein, B.H., 2003, 'Web-Based Research: Methodological Variables' Effects on Dropout and Sample Characteristics', *Behavioral Research, Methods, Instruments, and Computers*, vol. 35, no. 2, pp. 217-26.

[27] PlanetOut, 2005, 'Sales Kit'. <http://www.planetoutinc.com/sales/>

[28] PlanetOutPartnersSalesKit.pdf

[29] Paulhus, D.L., 1988, Assessing Self-deception and Impression Management in Self-reports: The Balanced Inventory of Desirable Responding. Manual available from the author at the Department of Psychology, University of British Columbia, Vancouver, B.C., Canada V6T 1YT.).

[30] Reips, U.D., 2000, 'The Web Experiment Method: Advantages, Disadvantages, and Solutions.' in M.H. Birnbaum (ed), Psychological Experiments on the Internet, pp. 89-114,Academic Press, San Diego.

[31] Rheingold, H., 1993, *The Virtual Community: Homesteading at the Electronic Frontier*, Addison-Wesley, Reading, MA.

[32] Rhodes, S.D., DiClemente, R.J., Cecil, H., Hergenrather, K.C. and Yee, L.J., 2002, 'Risk Among Men who Have Sex with Men in the United States: A Comparison of an Internet Sample and a Conventional Outreach Sample', *AIDS Education and Prevtion*, vol. 14, no. 1, pp. 41-50.

[33] Ross, M.W., Månsson, S.-A., Daneback, K., Cooper, A. and Tikkanen, R., 2005, 'Biases in Internet Sexual Health Samples: Comparison of an Internet Sexuality Survey and a National Sexual Health Survey in Sweden', *Social Science and Medicine*, vol. 61, pp. 245-252.

[34] Ross, M.W., Rosser, B.R., Stanton, J., and Konstan, J., 2004, 'Characteristics of Latino Men who Have Sex with Men on the internet who Complete and Drop Out of an Internet-Based Sexual Behavior Survey', *AIDS Education and Prevention*, vol. 16, no. 6, pp. 526-37.

[35] Ross, M.W., Tikkanen, R. and Mansson, S.A., 2000, 'Differences Between Internet Samples and Conventional Samples of Men who Have Sex with Men: Implications for Research and HIV Interventions', *Social Science and Medicine*, vol. 51, pp. 749-758.

[36] Welch, N. and Krantz, J.H., 1996, 'The World-Wide Web as a Medium for Psychoacoustical Demonstrations and Experiments: Experience and Results', *Behavioral Research Methods, Instruments, and Computers*, vol.28, no. pp. 192-196.

In: Health Research in Cyberspace
Editor: Pranee Liamputtong, pp. 133-146

ISBN 1-59454-819-6

Chapter 8

Online HIV Research: Assessing Three Case Study Methodologies

Anthony P. Lombardo and James Gillett

Introduction

In her recent discussion on virtual ethnography, Hine (2004: 4.5) notes that "for each social group that might be the focus of sociological attention, the appropriateness of Internet technology as a research medium may need to be evaluated afresh." The utility of Internet research, in other words, should be justified for each research question at hand (Illingworth, 2001). Hine's words hold true for the suitability of the Internet for the purposes of HIV/AIDS research. In this chapter, we use three of our research studies (Gillett, 2003; Lombardo, 2003, 2004) to examine the strengths and weaknesses of the Internet for conducting HIV-related qualitative social research. We begin by outlining the focus and findings of our case studies researching HIV/AIDS-related topics online, and specify here why Internet methodologies were appropriate for each study. The case studies are then used as the basis for a discussion of the strengths and weaknesses of online HIV studies and the process of negotiating the ethical consideration involved in this type of research. We conclude with our personal reflections on using the Internet as a "research medium" and suggest directions for future areas of study.

Media Activism Study

The first case study, Gillett (2003)—herein the media activism study—examines the Internet as a forum for self-representation among people living with HIV/AIDS. In this research, prominent themes regarding the underlying purpose or rationale for Internet sites by people with HIV/AIDS were identified and examined. The majority of sites emphasized the first theme, the autobiographical, which referred to individuals using the Internet to tell their own story of living with HIV/AIDS. A second theme was the lay expertise of people with HIV/AIDS and the importance of sharing this knowledge via the Internet. Less prominent were the themes of self promotion, or people with HIV/AIDS using the Internet as a means of sharing personal projects that they were involved in (writing, music), and dissent, which were those who used their site to question conventional theories regarding the origin and existence of HIV and AIDS. It was found that there is a connection between Internet use among people with HIV/AIDS and the use of media by AIDS activists generally as a component of the AIDS movement. The use of media to create cultural spaces as a forum for those with marginalized or stigmatized identities has become a common feature of contemporary social movements. The Internet has been taken up as a strategy for activists to speak out about social problems and public issues. This use of Internet for such purposes is not limited to activists; there are numerous people with HIV/AIDS who have created their own sites for the purposes of self expression and mutual education, support, and advocacy. To varying degrees, the Internet sites in the study were created in order to challenge or transform conventional understandings of what it means to be a person living with HIV/AIDS.

The methodology for the media activism study followed the approach developed by Hine (2000) in her book *Virtual Ethnography*. Hine makes the case that Internet research does not necessarily require the development of an entirely new set of methodologies. Online social spaces are distinctive, particularly in that they created and experienced through media technologies (Kendall, 1999; Mann and Stewart, 2000). Established qualitative methods may need to be modified or augmented to take into consideration the nature of virtual realities; however, this does not mean that they cannot adequately guide research on virtual or online social life. The data collection and analysis occurred in three stages: field work, semiotic analysis, and e-interviews. The fieldwork involved identifying and visiting a wide range of Internet sites (N=165) by people with HIV/AIDS in order to obtain an initial understanding of prominent themes. From this broad sample of Internet sites, twenty three sites were selected for the purposes of conducting a semiotic analysis of the meanings encoded in the sites following the themes of autobiography, expertise, self promotion and dissent. In the final phase, authors of the Internet sites were invited to participate in an online interview about the themes that emerged from the semiotic analysis.

Governmentality Study

The second case study, Lombardo (2003)—herein the "governmentality" study—is a study of the interactions between "posters" and experts in a "Safe Sex and Transmission" forum of an HIV/AIDS information website. In this forum, users submit questions about safe sex and HIV transmission to the forum's experts, and the questions and responses are posted publicly. The paper situates this case of online HIV/AIDS information within the larger socio-political context of neoliberalism, governmentality (Foucault, 1991) and the "new public health" (Lupton, 1995; Petersen and Lupton, 1996) characteristic of Western societies. It argues that the poster-expert exchanges in the forum can be considered the enactment and reinforcement of central tenets of new public health discourses, such as expertise-seeking and self-governance. Such forums can function as "technologies of the self" (Foucault, 1988: 18) for its users, allowing them to take responsibility for their health through accessing expert advice, learning about sexual activities and their risk factors, and questioning health behaviour they should undertake; thus, the forum offers it users "tools through which they can learn techniques and procedures to transform their conduct for better health" (Lombardo, 2003: 22). The forum, in this fashion, also functions as a "governmental apparatus" (Lupton,

1995: 10) to disseminate expert knowledges and concomitantly make those knowledges easier to access.

The governmentality study is based on the analysis of 79 postings from the "Safe Sex, Prevention and Transmission" forum in the "Ask the Experts" section of the HIV/AIDS information website, collected in March 2003. Online research was particularly justified for this study as it focused specifically on how an online forum can be considered, in one respect at least, as a tool of governmentality. The online forum offered data which would otherwise have been extremely difficult, if not impossible, to obtain in any other more "traditional" research fashion.

Worried Well Study

Lombardo (2004)—herein the "worried well" study—is the final case study we discuss. This study is a sociological analysis of the HIV/AIDS "worried well" experience. Briefly, an HIV/AIDS worried well is "someone who is excessively worried about AIDS or HIV infection despite being uninfected or being objectively at little or no risk" (Green and Kentish, 1996: 147). While the HIV/AIDS worried well are rather well documented in the psychological literature, there has been little sociological analysis of the experience. This study analyzed narratives of prior "worried well" persons posted onto another forum of the same HIV/AIDS information website. The analysis delineates a framework of common worried well experiences, and uses George Herbert Mead's theory of the past (Mead [1929], 1970) to conceptualize the experience in its entirety. Empirically, this study lent credence to the existence of the HIV/AIDS worried well. Theoretically, it illustrated that, as Mead contended, pasts are not concrete entities, but are rather elastic and configured to fit present realities, and that notions of "self" and "biography" are "emergent phenomena, intricately bound up with the meanings they [respondents] gave in the present to past experiences" (Lombardo, 2004: 545). The study also suggested that notions of "biographical disruption" (Bury, 1982) and "narrative reconstruction" (Williams, 1984), experiences commonly associated with those with a chronic illness, should be expanded to include those who merely *believe* themselves ill, in the absence of any confirming proof of illness.

The worried well study is based on the analysis of 25 narratives written by individuals who posted their experiences as worried well onto the "Messages to the 'Worried Well'" forum of the same website. Here, the shortest posting was 146 words in length; the longest, 651 words. Postings averaged about 331 words. The sample included one posting from 1998; five from 1999; two from 2000; eight from 2001; six from 2002; and three from 2003. Like the governmentality study, Internet research here, again, offered data which would otherwise have been difficult to collect.

The governmentality and worried well studies used similar methodologies. Both studies approached the postings collected from the online forums from an inductive analysis method (Glaser and Strauss, 1967; Patton, 2002; Strauss and Corbin, 1998) to allow the data to "speak for themselves" and capture the themes important to the respondents as they related them. In both studies, the Internet forums were used, following Bordia (1996), as a passive source of data. By this, we mean that participants were not actively recruited or interviewed, nor was participant observation carried out; instead, the analysis relied upon the archived postings in the forums on the Internet website. The postings were treated like interview transcripts, or field notes, and imported into the qualitative data analysis software package, *NVivo 2.0,* for analysis. Following the inductive method, the postings were coded for common and prevalent themes.

ASSESSING INTERNET METHODOLOGIES

There is a growing literature on Internet methodologies, largely for quantitative work, but also for work on qualitative research in cyberspace (Jones, 1999; Mann and Stewart, 2000). In either case, there are certain areas of agreement about the strengths and weaknesses of Internet research that transcend methodological boundaries. In this section, through an examination of the existing literature, we highlight the relevant strengths and weaknesses of the Internet research approaches we took in our respective case studies.

Strengths

The Internet offers researchers access to large numbers of diverse potential respondents for their studies, even across geographical barriers (Hewson et al., 1996; Coomber, 1997; Schmidt, 1997; Buchanan and Smith, 1999; Chen and Hinton, 1999; Illingworth, 2001; Fox et al., 2003; Rhodes et al., 2003; Sade-Beck, 2004; see also Chapter 1 in this volume). With the media activism study the Internet provided access to the perspectives of people with HIV/AIDS from diverse geographical locations and social backgrounds. The Internet has enabled citizens to link and communicate with one another across traditional barriers of time and space (Jordan, 1999). The fluid and virtual qualities of the Internet provide researchers with vast and increasing opportunities to participate in online cultures created by people with their own interconnected sites. The media activism study relied on several webrings – a group of Internet sites that are linked by subject and monitored by moderator – of HIV/AIDS Internet sites. The recent rise of web-logs and group web-logs (also known as blogs) has increased the ease by which individuals can created their own site and share with others with similar interests.

In addition to overcoming geographic barriers, the Internet also makes available to researchers "specialized" populations, which might otherwise be unavailable (Hewson et al., 1996; Coomber, 1997; Schmidt, 1997; Smith and Leigh, 1997; Chen and Hinton, 1999; Mann and Stewart, 2000; Koch and Emrey, 2001; Mustanski, 2001; O'Connor and Madge, 2001; Fox et al., 2003; Rhodes et al., 2003; Bowker and Tuffin, 2004; see also Mustanski and Couch and Liamputtong in this volume). This latter point is a particularly important one, especially with respect to the governmentality and worried well studies. While, as above, the data collection for these studies was more passive than active, the Internet forums made available data on very specific topics which would have otherwise been unavailable. For example, the poster-expert exchanges in the governmentality study would have been nearly impossible to obtain elsewhere, save for attempting to navigate the murky ethical and practical difficulties of, for instance, observing client-physician interactions in a public health clinic. In this way, the Internet forum allowed access to what would be an otherwise "closed site" (Mann and Stewart, 2000: 18). Internet research was also useful in the worried well study, as it may have been difficult to locate and recruit people in person to discuss their worried well experiences, both with respect to numbers of potential respondents and their interest in participating in the study. Indeed, as Smith and Leigh (1997: 497) note, the Internet makes available specialized populations to researchers who might otherwise have "difficulty establishing an adequate subject population." As we discuss next, however, Internet research also has significant implications for the validity of the data obtained.

HIV/AIDS, and its related concerns, are particularly difficult and sensitive issues to discuss. The Internet is notably helpful in researching these areas as it offers an arena where potential research participants can engage in studies in a largely anonymous fashion. For this reason, the Internet is a particularly well-suited venue for conducting research on sensitive topics (Coomber, 1997; Mann and Stewart, 2000; Illingworth, 2001; Mustanski, 2001; Hessler et al., 2003; Rhodes et al., 2003; Liamputtong and Ezzy, 2005), such as sexual health and HIV/AIDS. Studies have shown, for example, that the anonymous nature of the Internet may play a role in encouraging "self-disclosive" and/or "disinhibitive" behaviour among participants, leading them to disclose more intimate details about themselves online than they would in person (see for example, Salem et al., 1997; Joinson, 1998, 1999, 2001; Illingworth, 2001; Shields, 2003). Indeed, Griest (1973) suggested that computer interviews freed patients to reveal concealed information about psychiatric symptoms, while clients at an STD clinic reported more sexual partners, number of previous visits and more symptoms to a computer than to a physician (Robinson and West, 1992).

It has also been suggested that Internet research methods reduce the "demand characteristics" present in traditional, face-to-face data gathering, which can also increase the validity of the data (Hewson et al., 1996; Smith and Leigh, 1997; Hessler et al., 2003; Shields, 2003). Importantly, for example, Internet data collection can remove the interviewer effects which are acutely problematic in sexuality research (see for example, Catania, Binson, van der Straten and Stone, 1995). Internet research further differs from traditional face-to-face research in that it allows participants time to reflect on their responses (Shields, 2003; Sade-Beck, 2004), unlike face-to-face interviews, where respondents must provide answers relatively quickly.

All of these points have special significance for data validity in the governmentality and worried well studies. First, as participants submitted their questions to the forums' experts anonymously, it is reasonable to assume that they were more comfortable in detailing their sexual activities and expressing their concerns honestly, without fear of how they might be perceived by a researcher, physician or nurse. They were also able to make their inquiries using "street vernacular," or non-medical terms, to express their questions and stories. In fact, with the governmentality study in particular, posters gave very detailed descriptions of their past sex acts, ostensibly with the purpose of making sure the expert had the "full story," to make the answer as accurate as possible. For example, some posters submitted questions which had been answered elsewhere, but the poster assumed they had experienced a "unique" case of transmission, different than the others already addressed. To differentiate their case, they provided extremely rich descriptions. The Internet forum made this sort of data available in two respects: first, as earlier, the online forum made the poster-expert exchanges available for study, and second, it allowed posters to discuss their sexual health questions in more detail than they might have face-to-face with a physician. Indeed, Hardey (1999: 830) suggests this very fact of seeking health information online:

> The participants in [Hardey's] study took advantage of their computers to find health material....They did this in the familiar space of the home, largely with only self-imposed limits on time. *This is a very different venue from the consulting room.* Embarrassing or difficult questions they wanted to ask were shared only with the computer or anonymous others. (emphasis added)

Second, with respect to both case studies, the nature of the forum allowed posters to craft their questions or tell their worried well stories "in the moment." In other words, in the governmentality study, the posters wrote their submissions largely when they were experiencing the concern of having contracted HIV, and, in the worried well study, when they had, for the most part, concluded their worried well experience. This process made the data collected more naturalistic, as opposed to interviews after the fact, when posters would have recalled their experiences with experts, or the events of their worried well experience. The Internet data, in this sense, were "live." Furthermore, the submitted "worried well" stories in the Internet forum allowed posters to write that which was salient to them in the manner they wished, again without the need to "please" a researcher or being guided by a researcher. Siegel et al. (1989: 370) noted that unstructured interviews which do not utilize probing "captured the respondent's subjective perceptions and definition of the situation and insight into what factors were personally most salient," and a similar statement can be made about these data: they are untouched by a researcher. Again, such rich data would not have been obtainable without the Internet medium and its effects on research subjects.

The media activism study also benefited from the "naturalistic" quality of the Internet as a source of data for research. The perspectives of people with HIV/AIDS who had created their own sites were expressed without the guidance or direction of a preset research agenda or methodology. In addition, the format of the Internet itself provides for a broader range of information than conventional qualitative methods. On an Internet site, a person with HIV/AIDS can use text, images, sound and video to represent their experiences. Medical charts and scanned articles from medical journals or newspapers can be added to their interpretation of HIV/AIDS. In many cases authors of Internet sites made use of providing linkages from their site to other sites which could be a link to another site by a person with HIV or a link to the latest medical journal article on opportunistic infections. In a similar vein, the content of Internet sites as data can be valuable in its historical significance. The medium has been in existence for long enough that Internet sites can potentially contain over ten years of information about HIV from the perspective of those living with the disease.

On a more purely practical level, Internet research makes conducting research somewhat easier and more cost effective. Certainly, conducting research online incurs fewer costs than more traditional methods, as there is generally little need for travel, transcription, data entry or even multiple interviewer payroll. Further, data collected in electronic form can increase data accuracy, as data entry and transcription errors and biases are circumvented, and the data can easily be managed in statistical or qualitative analysis software (Schmidt, 1997; Buchanan and Smith, 1999; Chen and Hinton, 1999; Mann and Stewart, 2000; Mustanski, 2001; Hessler et al., 2003; Shields, 2003; Hine, 2004; Bowker and Tuffin, 2004). Indeed, for the governmentality and worried well studies, the data were collected and analyzed by only one person, and they were imported into the *NVivo* software with minimal effort. Similarly, the media activism study was completed by one person using relevantly few resources compared with most qualitative research projects. The ongoing challenge, which software programs like *NVivo* have helped to address, is the difficulty of downloading and analyzing data from the Internet. *NVivo* is useful when examining texts and to a certain extent audio and video. However, there is need for software programs that can assist in capturing and analyzing information that is provided through the Internet.

Weaknesses

Social scientists would "agree that it is preferable to conduct research with admitted limitations rather than to ignore certain topics altogether because of methodological difficulties" (Koch and Emrey, 2001: 132). While Internet research can offer many benefits, it also brings certain disadvantages (see also Chapter 1 in this volume). One central problem, especially in qualitative studies, is the generalizability of the research results to other populations (cf. Chapter 7 in this volume). Indeed, this becomes an especially acute problem when conducting research online. There is, for example, the inherent problem that respondents recruited and/or responding through the Internet, by definition, have Internet access, which generally means they possess certain characteristics which may not represent the population at large, such as a higher socio-economic status and higher educational level (Coomber, 1997; Schmidt, 1997; Mann and Stewart, 2000). This issue is not particularly problematic with the governmentality study, as it takes as its unit of analysis the interactions between posters and experts as they exist in an Internet forum: that the posters have Internet access is implicitly understood, and the results are not meant to be generalized beyond such a population. For the worried well study, however, generalizability is limited, since the results apply, in the end, only to HIV/AIDS worried well *with* Internet access and the characteristics that bestows. Since, in some cases, the Internet played a role in a worried well's experience (for example, using the Internet to seek health information on HIV/AIDS and its symptoms), the experiences of those without Internet access might have been different. This is, in fact, a very interesting research area in itself: to what extent does online health information contribute to fostering "worried well" persons? For this precise reason, the study included a proviso that this was an exploratory study to generate hypotheses for further study, perhaps using other methodologies.

The "passivity" of the data collection for the governmentality and worried well studies is also somewhat problematic for generalizability. First, because the postings were anonymous and there was no actual contact with their authors, there was no opportunity to gather demographic information. Instead, the studies relied on the largely sparse demographic information included in the individual postings. For example, in the governmentality study, demographics in the postings indicated that 27 of the posters were male and six were female; forty-six were unknown. Only four postings indicated a poster's age, which ranged from under 20 to mid-30s. Two postings came from persons in Europe and four from persons in North America; the rest were unidentified. The only solid statistic available was an almost even split in numbers of responses from each of the forum's two experts. Similarly, in the worried well study, only fourteen informants identified their sex in their posting—eleven males and three females—and only two males identified their ages as twenty-three and thirty.

Further, Internet research presents a unique problem of repeated submissions of responses. While this may seem to be a problem related only to quantitative work, such as online surveys (see Mustanski in this volume), it can be an issue in passive data collection as well. For example, in dealing with forums where posters submit questions, it is entirely possible, if not likely, that the same person might make multiple submissions on the same topic in the hopes of receiving a response. For the "forum" studies, however, two safeguards were in place. First, not all submitted questions are answered and posted; instead, there is an editorial process which filters out questions, especially repeated ones. Second, a watch was kept during data analysis of the postings for similarities between postings which would suggest a repeated submission, such as postings written in ALL CAPS, similar or same "unique" transmission factors, phrasing, terminology, spelling errors, and so on.

While earlier we argued that Internet research can enhance the richness of qualitative data, there are a number of drawbacks which can affect that richness. With the media activism study, the transitory nature of Internet use proved to be a drawback in obtaining consistent data on the perspectives of people with HIV/AIDS. Often it is difficult to know whether an Internet site is "live" or not simply by viewing it. The site may have been created years ago and not updated with few indications from the viewer that this is the case. There may also be significant gaps in the information that is provided by a person on their Internet site and unless the researcher is able to make contact with the author of the site the gaps can take away from the quality of the data that can be collected. Lastly, without access to a dependable means of downloading and archiving the information from an Internet site, the availability of information from Internet sites can be unpredictable. There are few resources available to help host or archive sites that have been created by people with HIV/AIDS, or people in general, who can no longer able to sustain their projects because of financial or health reasons. There were numerous very interesting sites by people with HIV/AIDS which are no longer available and have disappeared from the Internet without a trace.

Anonymity, also, for all of its benefits brings certain drawbacks. First, due to the "passive" nature of the data collection in the governmentality and worried well studies, there was no opportunity to ask respondents to clarify or elaborate on their statements in the postings, as a researcher might probe during a traditional face-to-face interview or in the field. Further, because the posters were anonymous, there was no opportunity, as there was in the media activism study, to conduct follow-up interviews. This was particularly problematic for the governmentality study: without offline follow-up interviews, how posters used—or did not use—the information from the posters could not be determined (see for example, Pleace et al., 2000), thus, only speculations could be made about the effect of online health information on the posters.

For this reason, the governmentality study included a recognition of the fact that for the forum to act as a complete tool of governmentality, the posters must internalize and act upon the information they received, not just simply seek the information out. As Lupton (1995: 110) importantly points out, "once health communicators and promoters have discharged their responsibility in disseminating information and promoting awareness, the emphasis is upon the individual to act upon this knowledge to prevent illness." Thus, the governmentality study was limited since there was no data available to indicate whether or not posters actually adhered to the expertise they were given, and, if they did, how long the adherence lasted. Although the posters took steps towards self-governance by seeking expertise on the website, without follow-up interviews, there was no evidence of whether posters actually applied that expert knowledge to their lifestyles.

Internet interviewing and data collection further removes the ability to note and study verbal and visual cues present during a traditional face-to-face interview (Chen and Hinton,

1999; Illingworth, 2001; O'Connor and Madge, 2001; Bowker and Tuffin, 2004; Sade-Beck, 2004). In this respect, then, no data was available for any of the studies with respect to body language and the like, which might have had some impact on the analysis. Finally, the gate-keeping practices also limited the data available for the governmentality and worried well studies: when submitting a question to an expert forum, posters are warned that "Due to volume considerations, not all questions will be answered and [the forums'] experts will try to group together similar questions" and, in the "fine print," "While neither [the website or its governing organization] regularly reviews posted content, we reserve the right to delete, move, or edit postings if we deem it appropriate under the circumstances".

With the media activism study, there were difficulties in the response rate of authors to requests for online interviews. A number of authors felt that they had already said everything that they had to say on their Internet site and discussing it further via e-mail seemed redundant. In such situations another medium of communication other than e-mail might have proved more effective in obtaining information. Telephone conversations with authors of Internet sites, or even real time instant messaging, proved to be a more effective means of conducting interview than using e-mail. It is safe to assume that data collection through electronic means is not an effective replacement for face to face interviewing; rather, they provide access to another form of a data which has both benefits and limitations.

Negotiating Ethical Issues in Online Research

The ethics of Internet research are somewhat unclear. Nowhere is this more evident than in studying (so-called) "public" information on the Internet. While the ethics of consent, anonymity and confidentiality might be more clear cut among data collection through e-mail or online real-time interviewing (and where the identity of the respondent is known), the ethics surrounding "passive" data collection in newsgroups and the like is still ambiguous. It is in these areas that questions of consent, data ownership, anonymity and confidentiality become very tenuous (for a sense of this debate, see Frankel and Siang, 1999: 6-10; Mann and Stewart, 2000: 46-47; Eysenbach and Till, 2001; and Chapter 1 in this volume). It is far beyond the scope of this article to discuss the ethical issues involved in Internet research in any great detail; however, we make some statements here about how ethical issues were managed in our case studies.

For the governmentality and worried well studies, the data were collected, analyzed and published without gaining permission from the posters, for a number of reasons. The most obvious reason was, again, the "double-edged sword" nature of anonymity—it prohibited attempts to seek posters' permission to use their postings as data. More to the point, however, is that the forum was considered public domain, where posters (and experts) submitted their questions and responses with the explicit understanding that they would be posted publicly on the Internet forum. This fact is made clear on the form to submit a question to the forum, where a statement reads: "Since your question may be posted publicly, if you wish to remain anonymous, please omit any identifying information" and later, "Visitors submitting questions remain solely responsible for the content of their messages". Following Pleace (2000: 2.4), then, these public postings and exchanges were considered "distinct from the *private discourse* that would be found in a letter, telephone call or e-mail" (emphasis added).

Similarly, Denzin (1999: 123, note 3), in his study of a co-dependency recovery newsgroup, remarks that his role as a researcher was as "a passive, lurking observer. I never identified myself to the group, nor did I obtain permission to quote from postings..." Bordia (1996: 150) likewise notes that in his study of rumour transmission in an Internet public discussion forum, he "was not snooping on private conversations, such as e-mail between two people, but was one of several people...studying the proceedings of a discussion (in case of archived discussions)". Furthermore, unlike research involving specific newsgroups, chatrooms or mailing lists, the posters in these forums did not constitute any sort of "community" or "group," which might want privacy from others (such as addiction-recovery groups, for example). Nor was any sort of membership necessary to access the forums. In any case, the postings themselves did not include any personally-identifying material, presumably by virtue of the editing process.

For the media activism study, the central ethical consideration was over the ownership and use of information that is published on the Internet. The assumption by many researchers and authors of Internet sites is that the information published is open to public scrutiny similar to that of a newspaper or magazine. Obtaining consent or permission to use information from Internet sites for the purposes of research can be problematic. As mentioned earlier, contacting an author seeking permission can prove to be difficult because the site may not be active or live. It is difficult to ascertain whether or not to use information from an Internet site without the permission of the author. There was one author of an Internet site involved in the media activism study who had concerns about the use of his Internet site. The issue was eventually resolved between the respondent and the researcher; yet, it was evident that the boundaries regarding what from the Internet can and cannot be used in research are unclear.

CONCLUSION

The Internet until recently was seen more as a fringe activity among many social sciences researchers. Increasingly, research using the Internet is moving into the mainstream. As this process occurs, it is important to critically examine the methodologies that are being used to raise research question and gather and analyze data from the Internet. In this chapter, we have presented three case studies that highlight different ways of conducting HIV research using the Internet. There are clear advantages to the Internet as a "medium for research" in the case of HIV – the richness of the data, being able access marginal individuals and groups, and the availability of data through online sources. There are many interesting future directions for online HIV research. Like the governmentality and worried well studies, more research is needed on the way individuals use the Internet and the social implications of this information seeking. People living with HIV/AIDS (those infected, along with their friends, family, partners and lovers, and caregivers) have a history of using media for the purposes of self representation and, as a result, have a strong presence on the Internet. Consequently, there are many opportunities for future research on stories and portrayals of HIV/AIDS through the Internet along similar lines as was described with the media activism study. Use of the Internet whether in the form of accessing information or creating information is not a static process; the technology continues to evolve and is being taken up in interesting and unpredictable directions. Yet, there are also many limitations to researching HIV online: access to the Internet on a local and global scale continues to be a limitation; the extent to which it is possible to generalize from online to offline social worlds is uncertain. As researchers, we need to work toward evaluating the strengths and weakness of online research. This work will contribute to the development of new approaches to research that can respond to dynamic quality of new media technologies.

ACKNOWLEDGEMENT

Anthony Lombardo is grateful to the Social Sciences and Humanities Research Council of Canada for the Canada Graduate Scholarships – Doctoral Scholarship which helped fund his studies at University of Toronto during which this article was researched and written.

REFERENCES

[1] Bordia, P., 1996, 'Studying Verbal Interaction on the Internet: The Case of Rumor Transmission Research', *Behavior Research Methods, Instruments, and Computers*, vol. 28, no. 2, pp. 149-151.

[2] Bowker, N. and Tuffin, K., 2004, 'Using the Online Medium for Discursive Research About People with Disabilities', *Social Science Computer Review*, vol. 22, no. 2, pp. 228-241.

[3] Buchanan, T. and Smith, J. L., 1999, 'Using the Internet for Psychological Research: Personality Testing on the World Wide Web', *British Journal of Psychology*, vol. 90, pp. 125-144.

[4] Bury, M., 1982, 'Chronic Illness as Biographical Disruption', *Sociology of Health and Illness*, vol. 4, no. 2, pp. 167-182.

[5] Catania, J. A., Binson, D., van der Straten, A. and Stone, V., 1995, 'Methodological Research on Sexual Behavior in the AIDS Era', *Annual Review of Sex Research*, vol. 6, pp. 77-119.

[6] Chen, P. and Hinton, S. M., 1999, 'Realtime Interviewing Using the World Wide Web', *Sociological Research Online*, vol. 4, no. 3. *<http://www.socresonline.org.uk/socresonline/4/3/chen.html>*

[7] Coomber, R., 1997, 'Using the Internet for Survey Research', *Sociological Research Online*, vol. 2, no. 2. *<http://www.socresonline.org.uk/socresonline/2/2/2.html>*

[8] Denzin, N. K., 1999, 'Cybertalk and the Method of Instances', in S. G. Jones (ed.), *Doing Internet Research: Critical Issues and Methods for Examining the Net*, pp. 107-125, Sage Publications, Thousand Oaks, CA.

[9] Eysenbach, G. and Till, J. E., 2001, 'Ethical Issues in Qualitative Research on Internet Communities', *British Medical Journal*, vol. 323, pp. 1103-1105.

[10] Foucault, M., 1988, 'Technologies of the Self', in L. H. Martin, H. Gutman and P. H. Hutton (eds.), *Technologies of the Self: A Seminar with Michel Foucault*, pp. 16-49, The University of Massachusetts Press, Amherst, MA.

[11] Foucault, M., 1991, 'Governmentality', in G. Burchell, C. Gordon and P. Miller (eds.), *The Foucault Effect: Studies in Governmentality*, pp. 87-104, The University of Chicago Press, Chicago.

[12] Fox, J., Murray, C. and Warm, A., 2003, 'Conducting Research Using Web-Based Questionnaires: Practical, Methodological, and Ethical Considerations', *International Journal of Social Research Methodology*, vol. 6, no. 2, pp. 167-180.

[13] Frankel, M. S. and Siang, S., 1999 (November), *Ethical and Legal Aspects of Human Subjects Research on the Internet*, American Association for the Advancement of Science, Washington, DC.

[14] Gillett, J., 2003, 'Media Activism and Internet Use by People with HIV/AIDS', *Sociology of Health and Illness*, vol. 25, no. 6, pp. 608-624.

[15] Glaser, B. G. and Strauss, A. L., 1967, *The Discovery of Grounded Theory: Strategies for Qualitative Research*, Aldine de Gruyter, Hawthorne, NY.

[16] Green, J. and Kentish, J., 1996, 'The Worried Well', in J. Green and A. McCreaner (eds.), *Counselling in HIV Infection and AIDS, 2nd edition*, pp. 147-153, Blackwell Science, Cambridge, MA.

[17] Greist, J. H., Klein, M. H. and Van Cura, L. J., 1973, 'A Computer Interview for Psychiatric Patient Target Symptoms', *Archives of General Psychiatry*, vol. 29, pp. 247-253.

[18] Hardey, M., 1999, 'Doctor in the House: The Internet as a Source of Lay Health Knowledge and the Challenge to Expertise', *Sociology of Health and Illness*, vol. 21, no. 6, pp. 820-835.

[19] Hessler, R. M., Downing, J., Beltz, C., Pelliccio, A., Powell, M. and Vale, W., 2003, 'Qualitative Research on Adolescent Risk Using E-Mail: A Methodological Assessment', *Qualitative Sociology*, vol. 26, no. 1, pp. 111-124.

[20] Hewson, C. M., Laurent, D. and Vogel, C. M., 1996, 'Proper Methodologies for Psychological and Sociological Studies Conducted Via the Internet', *Behavior Research Methods, Instruments, and Computers*, vol. 28, no. 2, pp. 186-191.

[21] Hine, C., 2000, *Virtual Ethnography*, Sage, London.

[22] Hine, C., 2004, 'Social Research Methods and the Internet: A Thematic Review', *Sociological Research Online*, vol. 9, no. 2. *<http://www.socresonline.org.uk/9/2/hine.html>*

[23] Illingworth, N., 2001, 'The Internet Matters: Exploring the Use of the Internet as a Research Tool', *Sociological Research Online*, vol. 6, no. 2. *<http://www.socresonline.org.uk/6/2/illingworth.html>*

[24] Joinson, A., 1998, 'Causes and Implications of Disinhibited Behavior on the Internet', in J. Gackenbach (ed), *Psychology and the Internet: Intrapersonal, Interpersonal, and Transpersonal Implications*, pp. 43-60, Academic Press, San Diego, CA.

[25] Joinson, A., 1999, 'Social Desirability, Anonymity, and Internet-Based Questionnaires', *Behavior Research Methods, Instruments, and Computers*, vol. 31, no. 3, pp. 433-438.

[26] Joinson, A. N., 2001, 'Self-Disclosure in Computer-Mediated Communication: The Role of Self-Awareness and Visual Anonymity', *European Journal of Social Psychology*, vol. 31, pp. 177-192.

[27] Jones, S., 1999, *Doing Internet Research: Critical Issues and Methods for Examining the Net*, Sage Publications, London.

[28] Jordan, T., 1999, *Cyberpower*, Routledge, New York..

[29] Kendall, L., 1999, 'Recontextualizing 'Cyberspace': Methodological Considerations for On-line Research', in S. Jones (ed), in *Doing Internet Research*, pp. 57-74, Sage Publications, London.

[30] Koch, N. S. and Emrey, J. A., 2001, 'The Internet and Opinion Measurement: Surveying Marginalized Populations', *Social Science Quarterly*, vol. 82, no. 1, pp. 131-138.

[31] Liamputtong, P. and Ezzy, D. 2005, *Qualitative Research Methods, 2nd edition*, Oxford University Press, Melbourne.

[32] Lombardo, A. P., 2003, *(Web)Sites of Governmentality: Neo-Liberalism, the Internet and HIV/AIDS*, unpublished manuscript.

[33] Lombardo, A. P., 2004, 'Anatomy of Fear: Mead's Theory of the Past and the Experience of the HIV/AIDS "Worried Well"', *Symbolic Interaction*, vol. 27, no. 4, pp. 531-548.

[34] Lupton, D., 1995, *The Imperative of Health: Public Health and the Regulated Body*, Sage Publications, Thousand Oaks, CA.

[35] Mann, C. and Stewart, F., 2000, *Internet Communication and Qualitative Research: A Handbook for Researching Online*, Sage Publications, Thousand Oaks, CA.

[36] Mead, G. H., [1929] 1970, 'The Nature of the Past', in *Essays in Honor of John Dewey*, pp. 235-242, Octagon Books, New York.

[37] Mustanski, B. S., 2001, 'Getting Wired: Exploiting the Internet for the Collection of Valid Sexuality Data', *Journal of Sex Research*, vol. 38, no. 4, pp. 292-301.

[38] O'Connor, H. and Madge, C., 2001, 'Cyber-Mothers: Online Synchronous Interviewing Using Conferencing Software', *Sociological Research Online*, vol. 5, no. 4. *<http://www.socresonline.org.uk/5/4/o'connor.html>*

[39] Patton, M. Q., 2002, *Qualitative Research and Evaluation Methods*, 3rd edition, Sage Publications, Thousand Oaks, CA.

[40] Petersen, A. and Lupton, D., 1996, *The New Public Health: Health and Self in the Age of Risk*. Sage Publications, Thousand Oaks, CA.

[41] Pleace, N., Burrows, R., Loader, B., Muncer, S. and Nettleton, S., 2000, 'On-Line with the Friends of Bill W: Social Support and the Net', *Sociological Research Online*, vol. 5, no. 2. *<http://www.socresonline.org.uk/5/2/pleace.html>*

[42] Rhodes, S. D., Bowie, D. A. and Hergenrather, K. C., 2003, 'Collecting Behavioural Data Using the World Wide Web: Considerations for Researchers', *Journal of Epidemiology and Community Health*, vol. 57, pp. 68-73.

[43] Robinson, R. and West, R., 1992, 'A Comparison of Computer and Questionnaire Methods of History-Taking in a Genito-Urinary Clinic', *Psychology and Health*, vol. 6, pp. 77-84.

[44] Sade-Beck, L., 2004, 'Internet Ethnography: Online and Offline', *International Journal of Qualitative Methods*, vol. 3, no. 2. *<http://www.ualberta.ca/~iiqm/backissues/3_2/pdf/sadebeck.pdf>*

[45] Salem, D. A., Bogat, G. A. and Reid, C., 1997, 'Mutual Help Goes On-Line', *Journal of Community Psychology*, vol. 25, no. 2, pp. 189-207.

[46] Schmidt, W. C., 1997, 'World-Wide Web Survey Research: Benefits, Potential Problems, and Solutions', *Behavior Research Methods, Instruments, and Computers*, vol. 29, no. 2, pp. 274-279.

[47] Shields, C. M., 2003, ''Giving Voice' to Students: Using the Internet for Data Collection', *Qualitative Research*, vol. 3, no. 3, pp. 397-414.

[48] Siegel, K., Levine, M. P., Brooks, C. and Kern, R., 1989, 'The Motives of Gay Men for Taking or Not Taking the HIV Antibody Test', *Social Problems*, vol. 36, no. 4, pp. 368-383.

[49] Smith, M. A. and Leigh, B., 1997, 'Virtual Subjects: Using the Internet as an Alternative Source of Subjects and Research Environment', *Behavior Research Methods, Instruments, and Computers*, vol. 29, no. 4, pp. 496-505.

[50] Strauss, A. and Corbin, J., 1998, *Basics of Qualitative Research: Techniques and Procedures for Developing Grounded Theory*, Sage Publications, Thousand Oaks, CA.

[51] Williams, G., 1984, 'The Genesis of Chronic Illness: Narrative Re-Construction', *Sociology of Health and Illness*, vol. 6, no. 2, pp. 175-200.

In: Health Research in Cyberspace
Editor: Pranee Liamputtong, pp. 147-157

ISBN 1-59454-819-6

Chapter 9

EMAIL GROUP DISCUSSION AMONG CANCER PATIENTS: FEMINIST ISSUES

Eun-Ok Im and Wonshik Chee

BACKGROUND

Women are reported to be frequently marginalized in research (McCormick and Leonard, 1996). Even on the Internet, women tend to be marginalized, and even online harassment toward women is reported (Finn, 2004). When research is used to support the predominant androcentric views and interests, those who are not part of this dominant group are marginalized, and their issues and/or health care needs are either not considered relevant to study or not reflected accurately in research (Duffy, 1985; Ford-Gilboe and Campbell, 1996). When health research is uncritically conducted and supporting the predominant androcentric views and interests, health care knowledge that will be developed based on the research will definitely mislead health care practices.

In recent years, the number of health care researchers who are using electronic data collection methods as a data collection method has increased dramatically. One of the most frequently used electronic data collection methods is electronic mails (e-mails). Among currently available electronic data collection methods, email is the oldest and most popular (Fawcett and Buhle, 1995; Frandsen, 1997; Mavis and Brocato, 1998; Kollock and Smith, 1999). Emails have been used for Delphi survey among health care providers (Marsden et al., 2003), continuing education for health care providers (Davies and Cleave-Hogg, 2004), interventions (such as electronic mail reminders to improve oral contraceptive compliance, email triage, or email communication between physicians and patients) (Fox et al., 2003; Hobbs et al., 2003; Patterson et al., 2004), and information delivery sources (Baker et al., 2003). Despite its popularity in health-related research, issues in using email group discussion as a data collection method among a specific group of research participants have rarely been explored. Furthermore, email group discussion has rarely been analyzed and/or critiqued from a feminist perspective. At this beginning era of Internet research, it is imperative to critically explore issues in e-mail group discussions from a feminist perspective and provide future directions for email group discussion as a gender sensitive data collection method. In this chapter, from a feminist perspective, issues in using e-mail group discussion among a group of Internet population—online cancer patients—are explored and discussed based on practical issues raised in a study among cancer patients.

METHODOLOGY OF THE STUDY

The study aimed at exploring gender and ethnic differences in cancer pain experiences among cancer patients who were members of the Internet Cancer Support Groups (ICSGs). As data collection methods, Internet survey and e-mail group discussion were used, and the feasibility of electronic data collection methods among cancer patients online was also determined. The study had both quantitative and qualitative phases. As the quantitative phase, Internet survey was conducted, and the research participants were asked to directly enter their answers through the Internet. As the qualitative phase, e-mail group discussion was conducted with nine topics on cancer pain experience of the patients. In this chapter, only the issues raised in the e-mail group discussion are discussed with a feminist perspective for the convenience of discussion. Issues in the Internet survey can be found elsewhere (Im and Chee, 2004).

To recruit research participants, the first 100 ICSGs that were identified through Internet search using Yahoo! and Alta Vista were initially contacted and asked to announce the study through their e-mail lists. Among them, only seven responded to the initial e-mails, and only four agreed to announce the study without fee. To recruit more participants, an additional 150 ICSGs in the Internet communities of Yahoo.com and MSN.com were contacted, and 2,000 e-mails were sent to potential participants whose e-mail addresses were available to the public. Among those who visited the project website, 46 agreed to participate in the study, and 40 completed the Internet survey. Thirty three (72%) among the 40 participants agreed to participate in the e-mail group discussion. By the end of the email group discussion, only nine (27%) actively participated in the discussions, two (6%) withdrew their participation during the first week of discussions, and the rest never responded (67%).

The participants were cancer patients who were members of the ICSGs and who did not report severe fatigue at the beginning of the study. The fatigue level of each potential participant was checked using a Likert scale question ranging from 0 (not at all) to 4 (severe). When he/she reported the score 4, he/she was excluded. The reason for the exclusion criteria was that patients with severe fatigue from the beginning were unlikely to participate in 4 weeks of e-mail group discussion.

The mean age of the participants was 49.45 years (SD=10.84). 22 participants (67%) were males and 11 participants (33%) were females. 26 participants (79%) reported them as Whites; 4 participants (12%) perceived them as just Americans (not ethnic specific); and 2 participants (6%) reported them as others (one Jewish and one Hispanic). 84% of them were U.S. born. About 55% of them reported their education preparation as partial college, college graduates, or graduate degrees. 67% of the participants were married or partnered. 42% of them were employed. About 67% perceived their income as sufficient. 30% of them were Protestant, 27% were Catholic, and 15% had no religion. Nine participants (27%) had breast cancer; 8 (24%) had lung cancer; 4 (12%) had combined cancer; 3 (9%) had colon cancer; 3 (9%) had leukemia; 2 (6%) had lymphoma; and 4 (12%) had other types of cancer including tong cancer, esophageal cancer, and vulva cancer. 49% reported that they were healthy or very healthy; 36% reported that they were unhealthy or very unhealthy; and 15% reported that they did not know about their health status.

For the study, a project website was developed and maintained while conforming to the policy of the institution where the researchers were affiliated. The information sheet was loaded on the project website so that potential participants could download a copy of the information sheet if they wanted. To participate in the study, potential participants were asked to click the button of 'yes, I agree to participate' to indicate their agreement to participate in the study. When they clicked the button, they were asked if they were cancer patients over 18 years old and how much fatigue they were currently experiencing. When they did not report the score 4 of the fatigue scale explained above, they were asked to enter their answers through the website (see also Chapter 2 and Couch and Liamputtong in this volume). Then, they were asked about their intention to participate in the e-mail group discussion, and they were asked to provide their e-mail addresses when they indicated to participate in the email group discussion. A group e-mail list including the participants' e-mail addresses was made, and e-mail group discussion was initiated using the group e-mail list.

The topics discussed through the email group discussion included: languages (terms) used to describe cancer pain and their linguistic meanings, verbal and nonverbal communication styles used to relate cancer pain, culturally universal and specific descriptions of cancer pain, gender differences in pain descriptions, and patient's responses to cancer pain. All the topics were posted on the project website, and one of the researchers sent 2-3 topics per week (9 topics for 4 weeks) through e-mail to the participants. Then, the participants were asked to discuss the topics through e-mail. All participants received all the e-mails that were sent by other participants and one of the researchers. Based on a feminist perspective, the researcher who was in charge of the actual email group discussion process gently drew group members into the discussion, reviewed the e-mails carefully, encouraged the discussion to flow naturally with a minimum of interruptions, subtly guided the proceedings when necessary, welcomed diversity of opinion, and remained nonauthoritarian and nonjudgmental. The participants were encouraged to use their own words and talk about what was important to them. Open-ended questions were used, and the group members were encouraged to direct the flow of discussion. At the end of the 4th week, the participants were asked to add topics that they wanted to discuss with other participants. Only one additional topic was added and discussed during the following week. Procedures adhered to the Internet Review Board (IRB) guidelines of the institution where the researchers were affiliated. The collected data were confidentially dealt with, and no individual identities were used throughout the analysis process. A serial number that the researchers randomly assigned was attached to the data with the state of residence.

Using the content analysis by Weber (1990), the data from the e-mail group discussion were analyzed. Immediately after the first week of data collection, the data analysis process was initiated, and it was simultaneously conducted with the e-mail group discussion. Data from the e-mail group discussion were directly saved in ASC II format and printed out directly from the saved ASC II files as transcripts. Then, the words in the e-mail messages were classified into idea categories such as ethnic (cultural) difference, gender difference, and patents' evaluation of cancer pain assessment and management. Then, the words considered representative of the categories were selected and counted. Relationships among idea categories were looked for to search for latent meanings within the text.

Main Results of the Study

The feasibility of e-mail group discussion among cancer patients was supported in the study presented in this chapter. E-mail group discussion was found to be an excellent research method for group discussion among cancer patients. E-mail group discussion could provide close relationships between researchers and research participants and among research participants themselves despite its inherent characteristics as non-face-to-face interactions. E-mail group discussion also could bring in-depth discussions on research participants' experience with cancer pain assessment and management. At the beginning of the study, the responses of the participants tended to be very short and concise. As time passed, the participants' responses to the topics were getting longer and more in-depth. Most of the participants responded within 3-5 hours, and some participants were responding within only 5-10 minutes. The researchers could find some patterns of responses according to gender: women participants tended to share their feelings and emotions involved in cancer experience and cancer pain management process while men participants tended to share information resources related to their diseases and treatment processes.

Gender and ethic differences in specific cancer pain experiences were found: there were significant gender differences in sharp pain, hot burn pain, and punishing pain and significant ethnic differences in the least pain in 24 hours. The participants reported ethnic and gender specific descriptions of cancer pain, and most of the participants were satisfied with current pain assessment and management provided by their health-care providers. Only three participants including one white man, one white woman, and one Hispanic man complained about inadequate cancer pain management. Most of the participants preferred oral pain medication to injection, and wanted to know more about the pain medication that they were taking. Three participants wanted to get more information on their diseases and treatment processes including side effects of chemotherapy, treatment measures for the side effects, radiation therapy, and so on. Some participants wanted professional consultation on their diseases from the researchers. A few of them wanted to check on the hospitals where they were currently receiving medical care for cancer treatment.

Feminist Issues in the Study

To explore feminist issues in the email group discussion, research staff recorded issues raised during the data collection process, and wrote memos regarding the issues and possible reasons for the issues. The research staff had weekly group discussions, and a series of email group discussion was conducted as well. The written records of these discussions and emails were kept, saved in asc ii format, and reviewed and analyzed using the content analysis suggested by weber (1990). The words in the data were classified into codes: the unit of analysis was individual words.

Based on the codes, categorization was done while considering the evaluation criteria for rigor in feminist research as suggested by hall and stevens (1991). One of the criteria was sufficient reflexivity to uncover what might be deep-seated but poorly recognized views on issues central to the research and a full account of the researcher's views, thinking, and conduct (hall and stevens, 1991). Dependability was another criterion, which could be ascertained by examining the methodologic and analytic decision trails created by the investigators during the course of the study itself (hall and stevens, 1991). They also emphasized credibility and adequacy of the whole process of inquiry, relative to the purposes of the study, rather than by standards that might focus only on the accuracy of measurements within the study (hall and stevens, 1991). Finally, intersubjectivity between researcher and participant and the mutual creation of data were suggested as one of the criteria (hall and stevens, 1991).

Through the categorization, the following issues were found: (a) a low response rate; (b) white male dominance; (c) confidentiality and privacy issues; (d) security issues; (e) a lack of guidelines for human subject protection; (f) relevance issues; and (g) difficulties in using general topics.

A Low Response Rate

Using electronic data collection methods including email group discussion in health research is innovative in terms of facilitating research participants in different geographical areas to communicate and exchange their experiences and opinions without long distance travel (Fawcett and Buhle, 1995). The existing study findings support richness of electronically-collected data, and informative and prompt responses of research participants (Fawcett and Buhle, 1995; Lakeman, 1998). The use of the Internet was reported to decrease human errors that are associated with the traditional research methods (Ford-Gilboe and Campbell, 1996). A major advantage of electronic data collection strategies was reported to be both speed and cost of data collection (high speed and less expense) (McCormick and Leonard, 1996). Furthermore, a similar response rate and quality (such as item omission, response error, and completeness of answer) between email survey and postal survey were reported, and significantly higher levels of response completeness (that is any answer to the question) were obtained for the e-mail survey compared with the postal survey. In addition, the Pew Research Center (2001) compared online and telephone surveys, and indicated nearly identical results.

Despite the positive views and findings on electronic data collection methods, a low response rate was noticeable in several recent studies (Jones and Pitts, 1990; Mavis and Brocato, 1998; Paolo et al., 2000), and the findings of the study presented here agree with the previous findings on the low response rate. As mentioned above, among the 40 participants, 32 agreed to participate in e-mail group discussions. Yet, as explained above, among the 32 participants, only nine (28%) actively participated in the discussions, two (6%) sent e-mail requesting withdrawal of their participation during the first week of discussions, and the rest (66%) never responded. Because of the low response rate, it was practically difficult for the researchers to administer four weeks of discussions. Even some of the participants (20%) complained the group's low response rate.

Several possible reasons for the low response rate were indicated. First of all, there was a time gap between the Internet survey and e-mail group discussions. Therefore, during the time, the potential participants could possibly change their mind. Indeed, two (6%) who originally agreed to participate in e-mail group discussions by providing their e-mail addresses after completing the Internet survey simply changed their mind and sent an e-mail requesting the cancellation of their participation. Emotional fluctuation was noticeable: the two participants who wanted to withdraw their participation changed their mind at several times. Once, they said that they wanted to participate. Then, they sent another e-mail message just after one minute, and said that they did not want to participate because they did not like the project website or slow responses from other participants. Another possible reason would be that the patients' health status could be changed dramatically during the time gap. Four (13%) experienced changes in their health status (e.g., no more pain, another cycle of chemotherapy, radiation therapy, relapse of cancer, surgery) during the time. A third possible reason is that people are frequently making free e-mail accounts, then cancel the e-mail accounts when the providers of the e-mail accounts begin to request a fee. Among the potential participants who never responded, three (14%) changed their e-mail addresses, and the e-mails sent by the researchers were bounced.

White Male Dominance

With the low response rate, another important issue to consider was white male dominance. Kendall (2000) reported white male dominance in online interactions, and posited the importance of consideration on gender and ethnic issues embedded in online interactions. Han and Belcher (2001) reported that most of the research participants were Caucasian, well educated, and reported annual incomes of more than 50,000 dollars in their Internet study. Klemm et al. (1999) also reported difficulties in recruiting underserved populations through the Internet and gender differences in Internet interactions among Internet cancer support groups: Men were more likely to give information and women were more likely to give encouragement and support. In the study presented here, women participants rarely participated in the discussion, and none of the active participants (nine participants) of the e-mail group discussions were ethnic minority persons. The dominance of White males certainly raised an issue in online research. See also Chapter one in this volume.

Confidentiality and Privacy Issues

In the study presented here, the researchers had difficulties in ensuring anonymity in e-mail group discussions even though real names and any other information connected to identities of the research participants were not disclosed. As mentioned above, a group e-mail list including the participants' e-mail addresses was made, and e-mail group discussions were initiated through the group e-mail list. Yet, when the participants responded to the researchers and other participants, some participants used their real names in the messages that they sent to other participants (such as from Jane Doe in California). They seemed to want to disclose themselves to make contributions to the discussions, get connected to other cancer patients, and have some supports and information from other cancer patients. Therefore, instead of anonymity, the researchers tried to ensure confidentiality and privacy of the discussions. The e-mail messages were saved in floppy diskettes and the messages were eliminated from the project server. Then, the e-mail messages were printed out for data analysis. Only research staff had access to the printed data and saved floppy diskettes. The floppy diskettes were saved in a locked cabinet in the researcher's office.

Security Issues

Security of the e-mail group discussions was a continuing issue to deal with. Technically, several measures to ensure security of the e-mail interactions and the collected data were enacted. The project server was always through the gateway server of the institution. The server was installed with Debian 2.0 Linux; this version of Linux (for more information, visit at *www.debian.org*) has been more stable and more difficult to be hacked than others. The security of the stored data in the server was enforced by SSH (Secure Shell), which restricted the telnet and ftp accesses using 128-bit encryption. Apache server software, the number one web server software in the world (60% of web servers in the world are installed with Apache server), was used. Yet, because of the technical limitations of the current server computer, the Secure Server Layer could not be installed for the study. Despite these technical efforts, 100 percent security could not be ensured because no system is 100 percent hacking-proof, nor is data ever completely safe from intrusion (Frankel and Siang, 1999).

Lack of Guidelines for Human Subject Protection

Many local and national laws to protect privacy of patients and/or research participants are available, but there are no special guidelines for human subjects protection in Internet research (Carney et al., 2000). Health Insurance Portability and Accountability Act (HIPAA) was recently enacted to streamline health care transactions and reduce costs (Saba and McCormick, 2001). This legislation mandates that standards be implemented for the electronic collection and transmission of all federally required data. HIPAA mandates that a concerted effort be employed at the local level to evaluate security measures for the protection of data in the electronic transmission of transactions. In the presented study, the HIPAA requirements were conformed to maintain privacy and security of participants' information. Yet, since very few standardized guidelines for Internet research are currently available at the level of institutions or professional organizations (Frankel and Siang, 2001), the researchers had difficulties in planning specific activities to protect human subjects and ensure confidentiality and privacy.

Recently, in addition to the HIPAA, the U. S. Government has enacted the CAN-Spam Act of 2003 that requires e-mailers to be truthful in their subject lines (Stone and Weil, 2003). Research-related emails cannot be considered as spam as defined by the CAN-Spam Act of 2003, but each institution in different states has their own policies that defined spam (*http://www.spamlaws.com/state/summary.html*). Since the study reported in this paper had been conducted just before the CAN-Spam Act was issued, this act could not impact the study. However, future researchers who consider email group discussion as a data collection method, they need to consider this new change in the federal and state laws related to electronic communication.

Relevance Issues

One of the main issues raised through the e-mail discussions was a relevance issue. Relevance was defined as whether research questions can serve research participants' own issues and interests in improving their lives (Hall and Stevens, 1991). Some of the participants wanted to participate in the study because they expected to know more about cancer through their participation. Others wanted to discuss about practical issues related to chemotherapy, radiation therapy, and surgery that they were currently experiencing. However, since this study focused on issues related to cancer pain, the participants were asked to hold other issues that they wanted to discuss until the end of the study. Yet, at the end of the study, when they were asked to add other issues to discuss, only one added a topic to discuss (which was about experiences with chemotherapy). Also, during the study, for some participants who wanted to know more about specific types of cancer that they were experiencing, website addresses of some professional organizations providing information on the subjects that they were interested in were provided. However, there was no way to check if they had adequate information that they wanted to know about. Since cancer patients were dealing with their imminent health needs such as nausea, hair loss, and osteoporosis, those issues needed to be given a higher priority throughout the research process.

Difficulties in Using General Topics

Some of the participants had difficulties in understanding the discussion topics because they did not expect such general topics. When specific questions such as "what is the language that you are using to describe pain' were asked, the participants did not have any problems in responding to the topics. However, when general topics, such as 'how do you describe your pain' and 'what do you think would be specific for your ethnicity,' were asked, they had difficulties in answering the topics. Some of them sent inquiry e-mails regarding what the topics exactly meant, and the researchers needed to assure that the topics were intentionally broad and general, and that the participants could provide any responses, opinions, and views related to the topics.

CONCLUSION AND IMPLICATIONS

The study presented here indicated several issues in conducting e-mail group discussions among a group of Internet population—online cancer patients—which included a low response rate, white male dominance, confidentiality and privacy issues, security issues, lack of guidelines for human subject protection, relevance issues, and difficulties in using general topics. Based on the discussions on these issues, we want to conclude this paper with the following implications for future research using electronic data collection methods.

First of all, to increase the response rate and to recruit underrepresented groups of participants through the Internet, we strongly suggest future researchers use diverse motivation strategies and ethnic and gender specific approaches. Since very little is known about specific gender and ethnic groups' use of computer networks, it is difficult to predict which motivation method would work better. Yet, in general, reimbursement for participation, free on-line education programs, on-line information sharing, or online counseling can be used to motivate potential participants to participate in e-mail group discussions. Also, one of good approaches would be to provide electronic money and/or gift certificate that usually do not require real name and any other information that can be connected to identities of participants except e-mail addresses. In addition, to recruit African American female participants, researchers could contact online communities that are specific for African American women, which include 'To My Sisters... A Gift for Life' (*http://www.biotechnical.com/*) and Sisters Network (*http://www.sistersnetworkinc.org*). To recruit Asian women, researchers may contact 'National Asian Women's Health Organization (NAWHO)' *(http://www.nawho.org/*).

Second, to ensure confidentiality, privacy, and security of email interactions and to follow the current policies and regulations related to Internet research, we suggest researchers regularly update their skills and knowledge related to Internet research and the regulations and policies related to Internet. As Carney et al. (2000) posit, researchers should be in the front line to develop rules or guidelines to ensure appropriate collection, use, and sharing of data collected through electronic data collection methods.

Finally, to increase the relevance of the studies and to make the studies easy and friendly to the participants, participants' own interests need to be identified before data collection. As indicated in the study presented in this paper, participants may have different interests than researchers. For example, when participants want to have some information about specific aspects of their health/illness, researchers need to provide information or provide external links to other resources that are available to the participants. Or, researchers could develop a section for information sharing on their project website so that participants can use the project website to get some information about their interests while participating in the study. In addition, researchers need to consider the possible changes in status and/or situations of the research participants. As in the study presented in this chapter, the drop-outs of the research participants may mean changes in their health/illness status, especially when the research participants are patients.

NOTE

This paper is a revised version of our paper:

Eun-Ok Im and Wonshik Chee, 2003, Feminist Issues in E-Mail Group Discussion among Cancer Patients, *Advances in Nursing Science*, vol. 26, no. 4, pp. 287-298. Reproduced with permission from Lippincott Williams and Wilkins.

REFERENCES

[1] Baker, L., Wagner, T. H., Singer, S. and Bundorf, K., 2003, 'Use of the Internet and email for health care information', *The Journal of the American Medical Association*, vol. 289, no. 18, pp. 2400-2406.

[2] Carney, P.A., Geller, B.M., Moffett, H., Ganger, M., Sewell, M., Barlow, W.E., Stalnaker. N., Taplin, S.H., Sisk, C. and Ernster, V.L., 2000, 'Current Medicolegal and Confidentiality Issues in Large, Multicenter Research Programs', *American Journal of Epidemiology* vol.152, no. 4, pp. 371-378.

[3] Davies, S. and Cleave-Hogg, D., 2004, 'Continuing Medical Education Should be Offered by Both E-Mail and Regular Mail: A Survey of Ontario Anesthesiologists', *Canadian Journal of Anesthesia,* vol. 51, no. 5, pp. 444-448.

[4] Duffy, M. E., 1985, 'A Critique of Research: A Feminist Perspective', *Health Care for Women International*, vol. 6, pp. 341-352.

[5] Fawcett, J. and Buhle, E. L. Jr., 1995, 'Using the Internet for Data Collection. An Innovative Electronic Strategy', *Computers in Nursing*, vol. 3, 273-279.

[6] Finn, J., 2004, A Survey of Online Harassment at a University Campus', *Journal of Interpersonal Violence*, vol. 19, no. 4, pp. 468-483.

[7] Ford-Gilboe, M. and Campbell, J., 1996, 'The Mother-Headed Single-Parent Family: A Feminist Critique of the Nursing Literature', *Nursing Outlook*, vol. 44, pp. 173-183.

[8] Fox, M. C., Creinin, M. D., Murthy, A. S., Harwood, B. and Reid, L. M., 2003, 'Feasibility Study of the Use of a Daily Electronic Mail Reminder to Improve Oral Contraceptive Compliance', *Contraception*, vol. 68, no. 5, 365-371.

[9] Frandsen, J. L., 1997, 'The Use of Computers in Cancer Pain Management', *Seminars in Oncology Nursing*, vol. 13, pp. 49-56.

[10] Frankel, M. S. and Siang, S., 1999, 'Ethical and Legal Aspects of Human Subjects Research on the Internet'.*<http://www.aaas.org/spp/dspp/sfrl/projects/intres/report.pdf>*

[11] Hall, J. M. and Stevens, P. E., 1991, 'Rigor in Feminist Research', *Advances in Nursing Science*, vol. 13, pp. 16-29.

[12] Han, H. R. and Belcher, A. E., 2001, 'Computer-Mediated Support Group Use Among Parents of Children with Cancer - An Exploratory Study', *Computers in Nursing*, vol. 19, pp. 27-33.

[13] Hobbs, J., Wald, J., jagannath, Y. S., Kittler, A., Pizziferri, L., Volk, L. A., Middleton, B. and Bates, D. W., 2003, 'Opportunities to Enhace Patient and Physician Email Contact', *International Journal of Medical Informatics*, vol. 70, no. 1, pp.1-9.

[14] Im, E. O. and Chee, W., 2004, 'Issues in Internet Survey Among Cancer Patient', *Cancer Nursing*, vol. 27, no. 1, pp. 34-42.

[15] Jones, R. and Pitt, N., 1990, 'Health Surveys in the Workplace: Comparison of Postal, Email, and World Wide Web Methods', *Occupational Medicine* (London), vol. 49, pp. 556-558.

[16] Kendall, L., 2000, '"Oh No! I'm a Nerd!": Hegemonic Masculinity on an Online Forum', *Gender and Society*, vol. 14, pp. 256-274.

[17] Klemm, P., Hurst, M., Dearholt, S. L. and Trone, S. R., 1999, 'Gender Differences on Internet Cancer Support Groups', *Computers in Nursing,* vol. 17, no. 2, pp. 65-72.

[18] Kollock, P. and Smith, M. A., 1999, *Communities in cyberspace*, Routledge, London.

[19] Lakeman, R., 1998, 'The Internet: Facilitating an International Nursing Culture for Psychiatric Nurses', *Computers in Nursing*, vol. 16, 87-89.

[20] Marsden, J., Dolan, B. and Holt, L., 2003, 'Nurse Practitioner Practice and Deployment: Electronic Mail Delphi Study', *Journal of Advanced Nursing*, vol. 43, no. 6, pp. 595-605.

[21] Mavis, B. E. and Brocato, J. J., 1998, 'Postal Surveys Versus Electronic Mail Surveys. The Tortoise and the Hare Tevisited', *Evaluation and the Health Professions*, vol. 21, pp. 395-408.

[22] McCormick, N. and Leonard, J., 1996, 'Gender and Sexuality in the Cyberspace Frontier', *Women and Therapy*, vol. 19, pp. 109-119.

[23] Paolo, A. M., Bonaminio, G. A., Gibson, C., Partridge, T. and Kallail, K., 2000, 'Response Rate Comparisons of E-Mail and Mail-Distributed Student Evaluations', *Teaching and Learning in Medicine*, vol. 12, pp. 281-284.

[24] Patterson, V., Humphreys, J. and Chua, R., 2004, 'Email Triage of New Neurological Outpatient Referrals from General Practice', *Journal of Neurology, Neurosurgery, and Psychiatry*, vol. 75, no. 4, pp. 617-620.

[25] Pew Research Center for the People and the Press, 2001, *Poll analysis: January 27, 1999: A Survey Methods Comparison.* *<http://www.people-press.org/onlinerpt.htm>*

[26] Saba, V.K. and McCormick, K.A., 2001, *Essentials of computers for nurses: Informatics for the new millennium* (3rd edition, McGraw-Hill, New York.

[27] Stone, B. and Weil, D., 2003, Soaking in Spam, *Newsweek*, vol. 42, November 24, p. 66.

[28] Weber, R. P., 1990, *Basic Content Analysis*, Sage Publications, Newbury Park, CA.

In: Health Research in Cyberspace
Editor: Pranee Liamputtong, pp. 159-170
ISBN 1-59454-819-6

Chapter 10

YOUTH AND CHRONIC ILLNESS: DEVELOPING INSIGHT INTO THE LIVES OF YOUNG PEOPLE WITH DIABETES BY USING INTERNET BASED INTERVIEWS

Bibi Holge-Hazelton

INTRODUCTION

In this chapter, I discuss my experience of undertaking a research project on young people and chronic illness in Denmark. In the study, a group of young people with newly diagnosed diabetes was studied for two years using participant observation and qualitative face-to-face interviews inspired by the free association narrative approach (Holge-Hazelton, 2002; Holge-Hazelton, 2003; Hollway and Jefferson, 2000). The study was based upon a phenomenological (Van Manen 1997) and constructionist (Schütz, 1973;Giddens, 1991) approach and the aim was to understand how a chronic illness like diabetes is integrated in the every day life of youth. The original intention was to follow the young people at a local diabetes school and onwards in their private homes for a two-year period.

If anyone had suggested that the Internet was going to play a significant role in the construction of data at the time I planned the project (in 1998), I would probably have backed out due to my lack of interest in and knowledge of this medium. My attention was drawn towards the Internet during a field study at a weekend seminar for youths with diabetes. Here, the Internet was mentioned several times by the participants as a place to find the latest information about products as well as about biomedical research and development. This fits well with observations I made at a local diabetes school. It was also apparent in several of the interviews that I conducted with young people with diabetes. One of the first things they would do after they had been diagnosed would be to search the Internet for information regarding their new life situation. Eventually, I realized that I had to turn to the Internet if I wanted to connect to these young people.

WHY THIS PROJECT IN THE FIRST PLACE?

The background for this project is, among other things, the fact that despite intense research in the medical sciences, many illnesses are still lifelong. This has generated an increased interest in ways that healthcare professionals can optimise the chronically ill individual daily control of the various activities which traditionally belonged to the healthcare staff, such as medication, observation, adjustments and control.

Solutions to this issue are often sought in terms of patient education– which have become progressively more dominant in teaching and educating the staff. The ideology behind this is approach is that the failing of certain patients to respond to or deal with their problem in optimal ways (comply) is due to a lack of sufficient knowledge; a knowledge the patients can obtain by being taught by professionals in the health-care sector.

Diabetes is spreading rapidly all over the world. In Denmark alone, the number of diabetes patients is expected to rise from the present level of some 175.000 (type 1 and 2 combined) to some 250.000 in the course of the next decade. Among numerous causes for this is the fact that only about 10% of the approximately DKK 2.5 billion spend on diabetes annually in Denmark are actually used for prevention. Another cause is that people suffering from diabetes have a tendency to ignore the advice they receive from doctors, concerning examinations, treatment and lifestyle changes. The World Health Organisation (WHO) has projected that the number of late diabetic complications could be cut in half within a period of eight to ten years, but this calls for a concerted effort on several fronts, including systematic education. This is in line with other recommendations (National Board of Health, 1994; Danish Diabetes Association, 1998).

In spite of an increasingly focused teaching, it is recognised worldwide that particular youths have a hard time adjusting to diabetes (Robinson et al., 1995). At a diabetes conference in Mexico (IDF), many of the presentations dealt with education and the term *empowerment*, which connotes helping people in such a way that they can cope with their diabetes as well as prevent late complications. One key learning from the numerous presentations was that this is a very tough issue. We can observe the same trend in Denmark: Too many youth fail to show up for scheduled consultations and have trouble adjusting their blood sugar levels in such a way as to prevent potential future complications.

THE ACTUAL RESEARCH PROJECT

The main theme of the project was, therefore, to come to an understanding of what it is like to be young and think that the future is bright and open and then suddenly face the fact that you now have an illness that you will have to deal with every day for the rest of your life. The intention was to examine the needs and experiences of a youth individually from his or her own perspective, and to discuss whether these correspond to the various offers of help from professionals that the youths met.

In order to gain an insight into the experiences of the youths, I observed and interviewed a small group of young people for a period of two years. However, when I began to participate in the youths´ social activities, I realized that I might learn much more about them through the Internet.

Inspired by this, I placed a small advertisement on a diabetes website, encouraging young people to share their experiences of living with diabetes on-line. This quickly led to contacts with a small group of youths with diabetes. Through these connections, other young people were recommended by their peers to participate in the study. Others read about the study and contacted me directly.

When I started on this, I was only able to locate a very small amount of literature on the subject, and by attending the first Association of Internet Researchers´ Conference in Kansas, USA 2000 (AiOR), I was confirmed in my conviction that qualitative work in this field had been sparse. In a sense, I was venturing out into uncharted territories, and as with anything else, I had to go along by trial and error while drawing upon my general experiences with research.

Among other things, I developed a method inspired by psychoanalysis (Hollway and Jefferson, 2000), in which I posed very few questions, but instead tried to make the individual youth pose key questions and then answer them. According to Hollway and Jefferson (2000), much of the "traditional" qualitative work, done by ethnographers, participant observers and interviewers alike, is based on the widespread assumption that the research participants are "telling it like it is", leading to the "transparent self problem". In their view, the subject refers to the person and how s/he is theorised, but the subject is more than that. In Hollway and Jefferson's work with fear of crime, they develop the notion of an anxious, defended psychosocial subject, for which they argue the need of positioning. Threats to the self, like a chronic illness diagnosis, create anxiety.

> This is a fundamental proposition in psychoanalytic theory, where anxiety is viewed as being inherent in the human condition. For psychoanalysis, anxiety precipitates defences against the threats, which it poses to the self and these operate at a largely unconscious level. The shared starting-point of all the different schools of psychoanalytic thought is this idea of a dynamic unconscious self, which defends against anxiety and significantly influences people's actions, lives and relations (Hollway and Jefferson, 2000: 19).

The approach of Hollway and Jefferson aims at transcending the distinction between the subject being rational or irrational, and they offer a theoretical account of defences against anxiety by which both rationality and irrationality can be explained. This notion of erasing the dichotomy between the rational and the irrational subject is very important in the understanding of my particular research subjects, because these characteristics seem to operate side-by-side, and are not necessarily in conflict.

In this context, anxiety is not treated only as a psychological characteristic. I agree with Hollway and Jefferson, but would like to add that I regard these young people with diabetes, as "bio-psycho-social subjects", because the biological factors of diabetes have a massive influence on their every day lives. The biological aspect of the other participants (mostly the healthcare professionals) has a low profile in the study, but that does not mean that it is not there.

I developed on-line relations with more than 20 young people with diabetes, contributing to a rich, *bottom up* picture of their lived experiences with diabetes. According to Mann and Steward (2000), a shared research agenda can give people a feeling of an opportunity of being heard. Moreover, Mann and Steward (2000) argue that the relationship developed on-line can become strong and personal in a very short time, thus, some participants can become very involved in online interviews if they are committed to the subject of the research for personal or social reasons. These observations are supported by this study where I exchanged e-mails with some of the online participants more than 100 times over an 18-month period.

I developed a practice of answering mails within 24 hours, which meant that sometimes I was unable to provide an exhaustive answer. I could always send my thanks for the mail, and, if unable to report properly, I explained when I would do so. I only failed to follow this routine once, when a young girl had sent me several letters explaining very personal matters. When I read what I thought was the last of her e-mail, I erroneously mistook it for a farewell e-mail, and did not reply. After a while she wrote to me again, asking whether I was on vacation since she had not heard from me for so long. This made me realize the need for a kind of contract with the dual purpose of clarification in terms of what people can expect from the researcher and to protect the researcher from being pushed onto a role that creates dependency between the involved parties.

PERSONAL EXPERIENCES IN DOING MY RESEARCH ON-LINE

Meeting these young people in this way has been a very special experience for me. I had the impression that the contact we made was very much on their terms – they could freely ignore me or abstain from answering my mail, they were free to be anonymous, and they had no obligations towards me. Yet it turned into a more private experience than I had imagined. This was probably due to the fact that I would often reply to e-mails sitting in the comfort of my own living room, with a cup of tea close by and my feet on the couch. I would sit and write e-mails late at night, on weekends and during vacations - definitely unorthodox office hours.

When I received a brief e-mail, and I often did, I would write back something along the lines of “Thank you for your reply, I look forward to hear from you again”, or “I hope that you get well soon, and that you will feel like writing to me again”. They would typically respond with things like “I’ll write more once the fever is broken”, or “I am very busy right now, but you are one of my top priorities”, or simply “Very busy, may write back another time”.

Reading their stories in this way allowed me to quickly respond if I wanted them to elaborate further on certain issues. Hence, this allowed me to ask for more information. I found that this type of communication was very “here and now”, more spontaneous and informative than many face-to-face interviews.

ON-LINE INTERVIEWS

The following is a demonstration of how the method unfolded in practice. The case is an e-mail correspondence with a young girl, Camilla who was sixteen at the time. Camilla’s e-mail address was given to me by one of her acquaintances, and so I wrote to her:

> 27 aug 2000: 20:47
> Topic Diabetes Experiences

Hello Camilla! I got your mail address from Tina who told me you might like to share some of your experiences about being a newly diagnosed youth with diabetes. I am, as she may have told you, conducting a research project, with the goal of examining what it really means to a young person to get such an illness. If you would like to participate, I would very much like to hear what it means to you and to your life. There is no "right" way to tell it, just start where it seems natural, I can always ask more indepth questions later on. I can tell you that I have contact with approximately twenty youths via e-mail. If you have something you would like to ask me, you can do that also- I answer my e-mails as quickly as possible, usually within a day.

Lots of greetings: Bibi

Wed, 30 aug 2000 11:32

Regarding Re:Diabetes experiences

Hello Bibi!

I would very much like to help you, but I am not completely sure what it is you would like me to write about.

I have had diabetes for almost a year now.

I remember, I was really surprised about how little I knew about it before I got it. It is not only I who is like that. I have just begun in 10th grade at a new school. I have, of course, told widely about it, but it still surprises me how little my teachers and schoolmates know about it. As a matter of fact, I have several times experienced that people don't want to drink of the same bottle as I, because they think it's contagious!!! I just laugh about it, but in some way it does affect me, because I have started feeling different and left out.

That is one of the things that is of great importance to me - not to be different from my "ordinary" friends. I have also talked to other diabetics about this, and I have the impression that it is a big problem to many of them.

However, there are also some very good things about having diabetes, for instance I have met a lot of amazingly sweet diabetics this summer, I was on the camp in Germany that Tina also attended. It was the first time I observed other young people who also had to sit and take an injection with a needle!!!!!!! (if one has to use the phrase one so often hears from "normal" youths)

What it means to me and my life to have diabetes! That is really hard to answer, because I don't think it has meant as much as I thought it would.

I have decided;

I control my diabetes and that it isn't controlling me.

I don't gain anything from feeling sorry for myself, and therefore I must not.

That dosen´t answer your questions, but it is the way I have decided to ensure that my illness isn't going to mean anything to me and my life.

It does mean something. It means, for instance, that I have to think more about what it is I am doing and think further ahead than I used to do before I had diabetes. I have to plan more, always to bring a bag with me, and when I am doing things with others , I always feel that I am being a nuisance. Then I have to check my fucking blood sugar and take insulin or having to eat something in the middle of it all, which sometimes can be irritating to the other people I am with and not least to myself.

I hope it was a little help. I would really like to write some more, but I have a feeling that it isn't what I have been writing about that you are interested in, but you are very welcome to ask about some more specific things, and I will do my best to answer you as good as I can.

Love from:

Camilla

31/8 2000 8:18

Topic Thanks Camilla!

Hello Camilla! You are mistaken- what you have written is exactly the kind of things I would like to hear and learn about- namely what it is that occupies the mind of a young person who have had diabetes. What did you think I was interested in? What gave you the hunch that it wasn't the "right" thing? Something I wrote? I am VERY happy that you are sharing this with me. If you can, I would like you to write something about how you made the decisions you mention. Is it something you think about at night, or have you reached these decisions together with others? Can you elaborate more about how you came to that? I was also thinking about how you learned to laugh when your friends think diabetes is contagious…maybe it would help if you tell me a little about what kind of person you are?

Best wishes: Bibi

Sat, 9 Sep 2000 14:00

Regarding: Another bunch of crap from me !!!

Hello Bibi!

I do apologize that I haven't answered before now, but I have so much homework right now, that I almost haven't had time for anything else.

How I am as a person!

The first thing that comes into my mind is that I am very naïve.

I am much too credulous, I can't say no when someone ask me for something. I guess that is also the reason why I am some times taken advantage of. If my friends don't treat me right I quickly forget it. I forgive them, and let them do it again.

I am not particularly bright at school, but on the other hand not extremely stupid. I have been doing all right recently, but I do spend a lot of time on my homework. One thing I really hate is to show up unprepared to class. I am also in the group of people who do our homework every time, and whose work the others can copy. Not that I am wildly " nerdy", but I like to have my things done. I have also been taking a lot of extra lessons, first of all Danish, because as you probably have noted I am not very good at writing.

I am very sensitive, it dosn´t take much to make me cry all night. I just don't think I make people aware of how much they hurt me.

I really think you have come up with some good questions !!! They are difficult to answer, but I really am doing my best.

I have speculated about the decisions I have made the whole winter (and yes there has been many sleepless nights), but when I, little by little, came to the conclusion that my diabetes shouldn't run my whole life, things became much better. I don't think I had organized them like that before I wrote to you. Taking trips this summer with older and more experienzed people with diabetes made me come to terms with my situation. I really had a lot of small talks with different people about different things, not just about diabetes, but everything from heartaches to what we had for breakfast. I was told so many things, that it would be impossible to refer to them all, even though I would like to. I heard about other peoples opinions and experiences with having diabetes. They told me that life doesn't have to end just because some stupid man in a white coat tell you that you have something called "diabetes" that you cant even pronounce (at least I couldn't when I got it ☺).

They showed me that it is possible to have fun even when you have to "inject yourself with a needle!!!" But most important I saw that I was not the only person who has experienced all that, that I am not the only one who's got bad days and really bad times. I haven't really been in contact with them after I came home, but I know that if I really need some advice, someone who understands or someone who is just willing to listen, they will always be there.

People often say that they understand, but they don't. Nobody understands the same way as someone who has been there themselves and who has tried it.

This summer I also learned to laugh about my friends who think diabetes is contagious. Taking turns, we told funny stories, things we had experienced with our diabetes. These were the best times. There were so many funny stories, and some more serious, but we roared with laughter about how stupid some people are and how much we had made fools of ourselves. Stories we could all relate to. The problem of standing in a store with a low blood sugar, not understanding a thing about what it is that one needs.

Or when you are out dining, and have asked for a diet coke, and you watch the waiter take a ordinary coke, and you have to stand up and cause a stir while the whole restaurant is thinking "She cant even tell the difference".

That is bloody irritating!

But you have to learn to laugh of it, if you don't, life becomes too serious or too dull.

My eyelids are drooping, it also got late last night, so I better get to bed at a decent time today.

I hope you find it exciting to listen to, if not write to me about it.

Many friendly greetings Camilla

P.S: I have written 815 words, that's more than a whole essay!!!

10/9 2000 9:52

Hi Camilla! Two things comes into my mind when I read your lovely e-mail: 1. I don't understand why you write that you cant write. You are super! And 2. It is e-mails like the one you have written here that really gives a researcher like me, who hasn't got diabetes, a valuable insight into what it can mean to be young and have diabetes. You might think I am good at asking questions, but I can't come up with more right now. Perhaps I can contact you another time, if I need an experts opinion regarding youth and diabetes?

If you feel like writing to me again, or if you happen to think of something you feel I should know, you are very welcome to do so.

My best wishes and have a nice Sunday! Bibi

11/9, 15:41

Hi Bibi!

I am pleased that you can use some of what I wrote. I would be more than happy to help another time, so just keep my address and write if you think of something I could help you with.

Take care of yourself until I hear from you again

Kind regards from Camilla.

Is the Absence of the Physical Body, the Same as the Absence of Truth?

The e-mail exchange between Camilla and myself, the researcher, contained a goldmine of valuable knowledge about what it means to be a young girl learning to deal with a chronic illness. This particular material, along with the other e-mail based interviews and the face-to-face interviews formed a shared knowledge base. For some, the absence of the physical in cyberspace means the same as the absence of truth. According to Gotved (2000), statements that overlook the potentials of a type of truth on the Internet stem from the missing presence of a disturbing stigma. In this study, I often found the absence of the body and the possibility of anonymity in cyberspace to be short lived. Many of the young people presented themselves in great personal and demographic details; sometimes even including pictures.

Like Gotved, I believe that representations of self are constructions of a retrospective story. It is never "Telling it like it is". Hollway and Jefferson (2000) believe that although it is far from transparent, there is a relationship between people's ambiguous representations and their experiences. In this respect, I see no difference between the authenticity of the stories I was told in the face-to-face interview situations and in the on-line narratives. All the young people I have been in contact with via e-mail have, at their own initiative, given their full name and often where and by whom they are treated for their illness. I would consider the chance of someone constructing a false identity as a diabetic, with all the details and inside knowledge about the illness, to be very small.

In the following passage, I will briefly describe some of the most important findings from the study.

Main Results from the Study

By closely following the articulation and stories told and written by youth about diabetes, new perspectives were drawn in relation to experiences of chronically ill youths. By focusing on concepts often overlooked in care and treatment such as gender, body, existential and faith perspectives, a collective story was drawn about what diabetes can also be, a story often marginalized and oppressed.

Richardson (1990, 1997, 2000) promotes the way that we may write to represent the voices of our research participants. Among others, she suggests poetic accounts. By developing condensed poetic accounts (Richardson 1990,1997, 2000) of the empirical material and combining this with the Internet based communication, new ways were developed, both in relation to qualitative methods and presentation, and potential meeting points between the professionals and the youths.

The study showed that by working with theoretically founded research and experimenting at the same time, new and relevant research can be produced, research that is not only related to a narrow group, but to a broad range of clinical and theoretical fields. Hence an outline of a new understanding of diabetes was drawn up and it was (among other things) concluded that:

Diabetes is a Lived Collective Experience

The point with focusing on the collective, rather than the individual problems is basically to stress that, even though diabetes is something the individual must live with in his/her every day life, there are many things that bind them together. Diabetes is not just a problem if the individual makes it one, it is an illness which sometimes takes up much space and sometimes less, but it is never a stable unproblematic condition.

When Diabetes is an Event in Youth

When the health care system mediates the significance of diabetes to youths, this is done on the basis of an understanding of youth as individualized and problematic. In spite of this, young people often regard the information offered as generalized and too optimistic. The consequence can easily be that the individual youth feel marginalized and isolated with his or her diabetes and that he or she also have to control this part of life. If one fails, the fault is their own.

Offers and suggestions of changes in the everyday life of youths must therefore be better suited to the needs and actual economic and social life situations than is the case now. It is also important to recognize the fact that youths today obtain knowledge in different ways than previous generations, for instance via electronic medias, and this must be reflected in the offers given.

Diabetes is an Event that Takes Place Over Time

Even though the significance of diabetes changes over time, this does not mean that it becomes less important. It changes character and has different meanings depending on where in life the individual is. The help, supervision or help-to- self-help needed by the individual can not be given once and for all. Consequently, standardized educational programs seldom serves as more than as a general frame created by professionals where they can deliver the knowledge they have and express their ideas as to what needs people with diabetes have.

Diabetes is a Gendered Event

It is very important that knowledge of gender as more than a biological category is drawn into education and training of health care professionals, as gender has significant importance in relation to how diabetes is understood and lived and for the kind of help one gets and needs.

Diabetes is a Bodily Event

Like gender, the body must be understood as more than the arena for the biological destruction initiated by the diabetes. The body is many young peoples` window to the world and is read by the surroundings as being under control or not. But a well-trimmed body can sometimes cover a vulnerable and confused inner condition not acknowledged or understood by professionals.

Diabetes is an Existential Event

Diabetes is not a choice and irrespective of any positive side effects there might be, it is an intense blow for young people to embody a lifelong illness. For some the diagnosis can cause massive psychological problems; problems sometimes not even observed, let alone resulting in professional support.

Diabetes is Faith

It is important to be aware that many people consider diabetes a matter of faith. Regardless of scientific medical explanations, some of the young people create their own explanations why they have got diabetes, explanations they need to be able to share with others without being ridiculed.

Diabetes is a Part of the Future

The youths take their diabetes seriously, but they also know for a fact that even the most correct lifestyle cannot guarantee that they do not develop serious complications. It is therefore important to create a safe environment where worries about worst case scenarios can be expressed. Several young people in this project have suggested that adults with severe diabetes complications be part of patient education, in order to give the them an opportunity to see what might happen, and also to learn how one can live with such complications.

CONCLUDING WITH SOME ETHICAL IMPLICATIONS OF ONLINE RESEARCHING

Since ethics is a matter of human relations/interactions, it seems to me that the *questions of ethics* in research on the Internet depends on whether interaction via the Internet creates new forms of human relationships that demand new ways of acting ethically. In other words, if research in cyberspace is regarded as something special, new ethical guidelines should be constructed for its use. If cyberspace is regarded as an extension of existing interaction and communication research, it should be possible to extend the current ethical practice to virtual space. For example Gotved (2000: 83) claims that:

> Cyberspace is closely connected to the space of everyday life, and even though the means of expression vary over a broad spectrum, they can at the same time be captured by more or less the same ethical guidelines. Not that we shouldn't relate to the special, but on the contrary, that the nature of the special derives from and is defined in relation to the well known.

In this work, my main ethical considerations had to do with respect for the participants in the study. By using the inspiration from the *free association narrative approach*, the youth primarily formulated questions they answered themselves. I promised them anonymity in the project. I always responded to writings like "This is really hard to tell" with a request not to go on if it became too hard. It never did, because responses always came back explaining to me that even though it was hard, it was also good. I answered the e-mails I received within 24 hours. All the informants declared that I could contact them any time for further questions, and none has contacted me with questions or problems. A few has sent me virtual Christmas cards, and some have my e-mail address on their personal mailing list. This means that I sometimes receive jokes, small comic strips and so on. I could not see what went on in the room where the individual young person sat and wrote to me, or what went on in their minds after they sent me their e-mails, but I do not consider this any different than my lack of knowledge of what happens when I leave the house of one of my other informants.

Many of the early adaptors of the new technologies, whatever they may look like and are capable of, are young people. If we, as youth researchers, wish to understand what goes on in young peoples lives, we need to use and understand the same communication tools, and if we happen to be lucky enough to work with young peoples' health as well, I would say it is a necessity.

REFERENCES

[1] Danish Diabetes Association/Diabetesforeningen, 1998, *Sukkersyge- en sygdom i eksplosiv vækst*, rapport nr. 1.

[2] Charmaz, K., 1991, *Good Days, Bad Days: The Self in Chronic Illness and Time*, Rutgers University Press, New Brunswick.

[3] Giddens, A.,1991, *Modernity and Self-Identity: Self and Society in the Late Modern Age*, Polity, Cambridge

[4] Gotved, S., 2000, *Cybersociology – Same Old Thing in a new Disguise*, Unpublished doctoral thesis, Sociologisk Institut, University of Copenhagen

[5] Holge-Hazelton, B., 2003, *Diabetes- A School for Life*, Unpublished doctoral. thesis, Samfundslitteratur, Copenhagen

[6] Holge-Hazelton, B., 2002, May, 'The Internet: A New Field for Qualitative Inquiry?', *Forum Qualitative Sozialforschung / Forum: Qualitative Social Research* [On-line Journal], vol. *3*, no. 2. <*http://www.qualitative-research.net/fqs/fqs-eng.htm*>

[7] Hollway, W. and Jefferson, T., 2000, *Doing Qualitative Research Differently: Free association, narrative and the interview method*, Sage Publications, London .

[8] Mann, C. and Steward, F., 2000, *Internet Communication and Qualitative Research. A Handbook for Researching Online*, Sage Publications, London

[9] National Board of Health, 1994, *Sundhedsstyrelsen,* Diabetesbehandling i Danmark-fremtidig organisering, Redegørelse.

[10] Richardson, L., 1990, *Writing Strategies: Researching diverse audiences*, Sag Publications, Thousand Oaks, California

[11] Richardson, L.,1997, *Fields of Play. Constructing an Academic Life*, Rutgers University Press. New Brunswick, New Jersey

[12] Richardson, L., 2000, 'Writing: A Method of Inquiry', in N.K. Denzin and Y.S. Lincoln (eds.), *Handbook of Qualitative Research*, pp. 923-948, Sage Publications, London.

[13] Schutz, A., 1973, Collected Papers 1. The Problem of Social Reality,Martinus Nijhoff/, The Hauge.
[14] Van Manen, M., 1997, Researching Lived Experience: Human Science for an Action Sensitive Pedagogy, The Althouse Press, London, Ontario

In: Health Research in Cyberspace
Editor: Pranee Liamputtong, pp. 171-191

ISBN 1-59454-819-6

Chapter 11

ONLINE DATING AND MATING – SOME RESEARCH EXPERIENCES

Danielle Couch and Pranee Liamputtong

LURID WEBSITE LAYS BARE FAMILY SECRETS

Joe and Maria Korp appeared to be a quiet suburban couple to their neighbours.

Joe, an amiable bloke, was polite and always up for a chat. Maria loved pottering around in the garden and feeding the family pets.

But the Korp couple had a secret.

In late January, details of their sex lives appeared on a website for suburban swingers.

The advertisement on the lurid introduction website leaves little to the imagination.

The Herald Sun will not reveal full details because of their explicit nature.

The website describes itself as Australia's largest on-line adult dating site with the motto: "It's the fun, easy and safe way to meet men, women and couples who are looking for love, relationships and casual encounters."

On the Korps' extended posting -- which includes several photos of Maria -- the couple's likes and dislikes are listed.

Under the user-name title "Cple (Couple) for Fun", the posting says the husband and wife are looking for "discreet relationships".

The posting states: "Happily married couple looking to have fun with another lady or couples. We like to meet and get to know each other before taking the next step.

"We are not asking for Beauty Queens but it is always nice to meet, talk things through and see if everyone is comfortable.

"Looking for a woman or couples who would like to relax in a friendly atmosphere and if the chemistry is right, have some real fun."

On their biographies, the couple are listed as Latino non-smokers who enjoy a social drink.

The couple were placed on the introduction website on January 31 as premium members.

Their posting was last viewed on the day Mrs. Korp went missing.

Homicide detectives are investigating any connection between the website and Mrs Korp's disappearance after being alerted by the Herald Sun yesterday. Det-Insp Steve Francis said the sex site link would be treated as an avenue of inquiry…

(Anderson and Hodgson, 2005: 1)

A Personal Introduction to Online Dating and Mating – Danielle Couch's Reflections

Eighteen months prior to the above excerpt running in a Melbourne newspaper, Danielle had joined the website the above article refers to. One evening, whilst driving, she heard an advertisement for an adult online dating website. Faced with the prospect of heading home to continue work or checking out the website, she quickly opted to investigate the site. Pitching itself as a site for matchmaking adults, it was possible to register for free and set up a profile.

Having a profile involved registering with an online name (handle), providing an email address (for the website's administration purposes) and password and then providing an array of details about herself. These details included basic demographics such as: her state of residence, suburb, postcode, age, ethnic background; physical descriptors, including her height, weight, hair colour, body hair and body type; behaviour descriptors, including smoking and drinking habits; and sexual descriptors. The sexual descriptors included: nominating her sexuality, relationship status, sexual interests, such as spanking (light or hard), oral sex (giving or receiving), anal sex (giving or receiving), one on one sex, group sex, erotic picture swapping, erotic email and numerous other options; whether she was registering as a single person, couple or group; and whether her interests were in male, female, transgender, single people, couples and/or groups. Danielle could also nominate her safe sex preferences as always, sometimes or never practise safe sex. She had the option to post pictures of herself in her public gallery (viewable by all of the website users) or in her private gallery (where she could control who had viewing access to her photos).

Danielle decided to set herself up, and she was soon receiving winks (a simple gesture indicating interest from another user) and emails. The ratio of men to women on the website was about 7:1. She was receiving plenty of attention and began exchanging emails, chatting and contemplating arranging her first dates. Her first foray into the online dating and the response she was receiving created a desire to know more about this phenomenon, so she joined another site, but one that was more focused on romance and relationships (be they friendships short term or long term). Danielle found the amount of attention she was receiving was very flattering - she had certainly never been in this demand before!

The excerpt from a newspaper article below suggests the experience of being overwhelmed by the degree of contact is not uncommon when one starts online dating (Jackman, 2004: 1) :

Suddenly, what was meant to be a whimsical romantic foray had become an administrative and logistical nightmare. "I feel like an air traffic controller," Holmes emails, late one night. "It's like I am trying to keep dozens of planes aloft, trying to keep them happy with little titbits of fuelled reassurance, juggling their interests and positions, nudging some closer to the landing approach … and occasionally plucking one out of the sky to land on my dating runway".

> "But … many have crashed. I've long forgotten some of them and they've left my radar screen for ever. Some have gotten the shits with their place in the 'holding pattern' and zoomed off to another controller…"

After using the adult online dating website for a while and perusing other users' profiles, Danielle became aware that some people specifically noted that they were "clean and healthy" and looking for the same in their prospective sexual partners. Or, they would note they were DandD (drug and disease) free and seeking same. Working in public health, these descriptions caught her attention.

RATIONALE AND GETTING STARTED

The internet has been referred to as an "erotic oasis for obtaining sex online or in person" (Ross et al., 2000). It allows people to find and screen large numbers of potential partners in a short amount of time (Weinreich, 1997). It has been found that the use of the internet to seek sexual partners is a risk environment for sexually transmitted diseases (STDs), as it can act as a rapid, efficient medium for arranging sexual contact, which in turn may result in more efficient STD transmission (Bull and McFarlane, 2000). In a study conducted to compare the risk of STD transmission for persons who seek sex partners through the internet in comparison with the risk for persons not seeking sex partners online, it was found that the online persons had a greater number of partners than the offline persons, were more likely to have had an STD previously, were more likely to have used a condom during their last sex encounter and were more likely to have participated in oral and anal sex, rather than vaginal sex, more likely to be men, and more likely to be men who have sex with men (McFarlane et al., 2000).

In relation to women specifically, North American research highlighted that women also use the internet as a method of seeking sexual partners, and that those who did use the internet to find sexual partners were more experienced with testing for STDs and were more likely to be white and older than those who have never met a sexual partner online. Additionally, these women had larger totals of lifetime partners, they more frequently used condoms but they did not regularly use condoms, they engaged in vaginal, oral and anal sex with internet partners and had reported high rates of STDs (McFarlane et al., 2004).

Discussing her thoughts with Pranee (as a supervisor), we decided to undertake a qualitative research project which involved analysis of a selection of personal profiles on the adult online dating website, with a particular focus on the health related content within individuals' profiles, or lack thereof. Unfortunately, after scoping this idea, developing the research proposal and submitting the ethics application, the website we were interested in using changed its terms and conditions to explicitly prohibit the use of its content for study and research purposes.

Around this time, we also noticed that individuals had started posting warnings on their profiles targeted at researchers from a particular university stating they would take legal action if any details from their profiles were used for research purposes. We were not able to determine what the research was that was so offending and affronting to many of the website's members, but it made clear the need to investigate online dating and sexual behaviours using a different method and one that gave those being studied the opportunity to be involved in a far more participatory manner.

Through Danielle's personal use of online dating websites, we came to realise that it was common practice amongst website users to move away from the website to freely available chat programs such as MSN Messenger or Yahoo! Messenger, which allow users to chat in real-time (synchronously) online via text (and increasingly via voice and video). Moving communications away from the website did not necessarily mean that a date would eventuate between a contact and Danielle or even that there would be extensive chat between them, but what it did allow was a way to circumvent the fees related to communicating through fee-based online dating websites and to avoid the clunky private chat options offered by the site.[1] Using online chat can feel just like having a conversation with someone, although it involves a lot of keystrokes rather than talking. Danielle was already a regular user of chat programs, and as, like many people, she had found them a useful method for keeping in contact with family and friends and also liaising with work colleagues when working offsite.

Discussion between Pranee and Danielle about emerging methods of online research led to the discussion of using chat as a method to explore how people were using online dating, their engagement with those they met online and offline, particularly in a sexual context, and how they thought about online dating in relation to risk and safety. It seemed very appropriate as it was a method of communication that many online daters were already comfortable with and using regularly for dating purposes; and the internet is becoming recognised as a useful tool for exploring HIV risk behaviours, with particular relevance to isolated and hard to reach groups (Davis et al., 2004). Therefore, the second rendition of the research proposal and ethics submission was based on undertaking online in-depth interviews, conducted via chat, to explore peoples' experiences of online dating.

When working through the practicalities of how we would conduct the study, it occurred to us that getting the signed consent forms from each participant would be difficult. Sending someone an electronic consent form and then expecting them to post back a signed copy was not going to be suitable for a study conducted online, nor would it fit with how people use chat technology. To manage this, we planned to use the file transfer capability available in the chat programs to send the information and consent form (and if this could not be achieved we could email the form). When the potential participant had reviewed the form we asked he or she to advise their consent in the chat window or via email (see also Chapter 2 in this volume).

Once the study had commenced we found some people to whom we emailed the consent form to would consent via return email and others would open a chat when we were next online concurrently and advise via chat that they consented to participate. Being concurrently online with the potential participants when the consent form was sent allowed potential participants to ask any questions they might have and clarify issues of confidentiality and how long the interview might take. In the instance below, we were also able to answer questions and concerns of the partner of the potential participant.

> Asked BeachBelle to participate. I have emailed her the consent form. She will check it out and let me know. Might have some other contacts too. Have spent quite a bit of time

[1] Private chat is online chat between two people, or perhaps a small group, as opposed to the chat rooms that are hosted by various websites where many people can enter the room the room at random and chat with many others all at the same time.

explaining the process to her as I am very keen to have her support and participation, as I think she is very well networked in the 'scene'. Her husband also had a question re why there were no set questions. I endeavoured to explain and have also sent a website link that is quite theoretical, but should hopefully demonstrate that we are not making up this research style!!! (Memo, 06/03/2004)

Recruiting Participants

To be included in the study, a potential participant needed to have used online dating as a method for seeking partners and/or sexual interaction. Snowball sampling was used, recruiting participants through contacts previously made through Danielle's personal use of online dating websites, and through her contacts' contacts.[2] For a project such as this, snowball sampling was reasonable as it is a useful sampling strategy for participants who may be hard to reach directly, but may be well networked (Liamputtong and Ezzy, 2005).

Danielle's current contact list has 170 people on it, some of which she has exchanged only a few words with and some with whom she has developed an ongoing, but sporadic purely chat relationships with, along with some family members and friends. Some of these contacts are online seven days a week and some are rarely online at the same time as her. Danielle has no idea who some of them are – they may have only exchanged a few brief words in the past – but some she knows very well, both online and offline.

Additionally, because her chat email address closely matches the name she uses on her profiles on two online dating sites she has experienced people guessing her chat address and adding her to their contact list. When the option to accept these new contacts is presented she has accepted, assuming they might have been someone she had corresponded with previously only to find in an initial chat that she had never had any contact with this person before. To be added to someone's contact list, you have to accept their invitation; declining their invitation means you will not be added to their contact list and they will not be able to chat with you. This provides each chat user to control who they make themselves available to via chat. Furthermore, each chat user has the option of blocking contacts if they no longer wish to be contactable by that contact. This can prove very useful for protecting oneself from abusive or threatening or inane chatters.

Danielle's list of contacts provided a starting point for recruiting participants. She asked people she had met through her own use of online dating to introduce us to some of their contacts who could perhaps be interviewed. Having the credibility of being a fellow online dater added legitimacy to the recruiting, so that potential participants did not feel they were being studied, but rather one of their own was investigating this area. This was particularly important after the media blitz that surrounded the Korp case – the case which introduces this chapter.

On other occasions, Danielle changed her online handle to reflect the desire to interview people. For example, she changed her handle to:

- Let's talk about sex and online dating

---

[2] Contact is the term used in most chat programs to refer to people that have been added to an individual's contact list or address book – that is people accessible through use of the chat software.

- Anyone want to talk about online dating and sex???
- I'm looking for people to interview
- Introduce me to your friends

Over time some of the people in her contact list became obvious candidates for possible participation in the research. For example, with three of the participants a sporadic friendly online chat relationship had developed – say hi when both online, how's your week going? How's work? How are you children? What did you get up to on the weekend? Questions and conversation typical of many social relationships. The contacts would provide updates on how their dating was going - this kind of information would come up when chatting about weekend plans or what happened on a previous weekend. Chatting about current dating experiences in chat amongst other online daters and contacts is common. People are aware that if someone still has their profile up on a dating website they are still in the dating marketplace, so it perhaps allows for greater dialogue and transparency in that dialogue about how people's dating experiences are progressing. When using chat for personal reasons Danielle is frequently asked "how is the website going". It seems many seek to discuss their dating experiences with others as a way of validating their own experiences or to measure if their experiences are comparable to others' experiences. Some contacts volunteered to participate, wanting to share their experiences of online dating.

To broaden opportunities for participation, we had also hoped to place details of the research and how to participate on the community notice boards of the adult online dating website.

USING THE INTERNET TO MEET PEOPLE? WE WOULD LIKE TO HEAR FROM YOU

Hello,

As a fellow online dater, I am interested in exploring sexual behaviour and online dating as part of my thesis.

The research project will aim to examine the use of the internet and online adult dating to meet sexual partners, and to gain insights into the sexual interests and behaviours of people using the internet to meet sexual partners.

I am very keen to hear the thoughts of other people who are online dating users, and I would like to undertake *confidential* online interviews with anyone interested in being involved. The interview would take place via chat software (e.g. MSN Messenger)

I will provide an information sheet on the project and a consent form. You will be able to opt out of the interview at any point.

I hope that the interview process will be insightful for all parties involved, so that we all get something out of the experience.

If you would like to be involved or would like further information please contact me at: [email address].

Thanks,

Danielle Couch

The advertisement was submitted to the website, but it was unfortunately rejected with no explanation provided. The advertisement was submitted after the media frenzy which accompanied the disappearance of Maria Korp and the subsequent case. Much of the media attention on the Korp case focussed on the sex or swingers website that Maria Korp was allegedly involved with, which was the site we wanted to recruit our potential participants from - the same site that had explicitly prohibited use of its content for research purposes, and the same site where a number of users had already been upset by other researchers. Thus, although disappointing, it was not too surprising that the website managers were not amenable to us using their site to recruit participants.

The participants in the project have been all Australian and predominantly Victorian. This is not surprising given how participants were found - we commenced sampling through contacting people Danielle had met through her own use of online dating. As she lives in Melbourne, Australia, she has only sought out potential partners that also reside in Melbourne, Australia, and these people have also sought other in close geographical proximity. This is not surprising as the purpose of online dating is, of course, to potentially meet the person you commence communication with, and the likelihood of meeting is substantially improved by residing in the same city!

FEELING EXPOSED

Sending through the information and consent form to potential participants made us feel exposed at times, as it made us into a real people who could not hide behind their chat program email addresses and handles. As is normal practice our full names and university details were provided on the consent form. This is much more information than Danielle would normally comfortably provide to a new online chatting contact, although she hoped that by 'exposing' herself in this way in the research she would gain the confidence and trust of those being asked for interviews (Liamputtong and Ezzy, 2005; Liamputtong, in press). One of the research participants shared this feeling of risk of exposure: he noted "that's why we have hotmail accounts, I guess," when referring to receiving unwanted information from people related the adult online dating website. When Danielle admits that she feels exposed when sending out the consent form, Elipse advises "Yes...I wouldn't share that email with people you haven't met."

8:07:43 PM	Miss Spectra	*I sent you the info and consent form from my real email addy, so have a look and if you change your mind re being interviewed online let me know. :)*
8:11:56 PM	Elipse	I'll ask others first. You know, there are some things happening on [adult online dating site] which are annoying me
8:12:41 PM	Elipse	First, there are Prostitutes, then there are people who have set up theri own Net Sites in opposition to [the romantic online dating site] and on [the adult online dating site], and are poaching innocent people
8:12:54 PM	Elipse	you receive/send a message, then never hear
8:13:31 PM	Elipse	then the next thing you know - Bingo...in comes an Invitation from the on [adult online dating site] email address
8:13:48 PM	Elipse	Thats how I know and thats why we have hotmail accounts accounts, I guess

8:13:54 PM	Miss Spectra	*i track receive emails re online dating from some news services. in the states a lot are moving to criminal checks of memebrs.*
8:13:56 PM	Elipse	It pisses me opff
8:14:00 PM	Miss Spectra	*a whole new business!*
8:14:09 PM	Elipse	Yes
8:14:13 PM	Miss Spectra	*ah, okay.*
8:14:35 PM	Elipse	Enough of my whinging
8:14:44 PM	Miss Spectra	*yes, it's funny. i was just writing in my study notes how i feel exposed when i send info from my "real" email ady like i just did to you*
8:14:53 PM	Miss Spectra	*so i know how you feel!*
8:15:14 PM	Miss Spectra	*hotmail anonyminity gives a certain comfort leve;*
8:15:17 PM	Elipse	I might go and watch the Idiot Box in front of the fire for a while
8:15:20 PM	Miss Spectra	*level and exposire level*
8:15:26 PM	Miss Spectra	*oaky, enjoy*
8:15:35 PM	Elipse	Yes...I wouldn't share that email with people you haven't met

USING CHAT

One of benefits of interviewing via chat and being regularly online is the ability to follow up on issues, thoughts and questions that you may have during the research process. Whilst writing this paragraph about the geography of the sample, we were able to test our assumption by asking two of the participants, Anton and Elipse who were signed into the chat program while we were writing.

Both Anton and Elipse had their statuses set to away on the chat program (chat programs generally allow users to set their status to online, away, out to lunch, busy, be right back or on the phone). Seeing this, we thought they might not be there or they might have just set it to that to give them the freedom to respond to chat requests at their leisure (or not at all), rather than feeling obliged to respond.

Anton responded promptly to our question about geography, as indicated by the lapse in time between Danielle's (Miss Spectra's) request and his response:

29/05/2005	1:17:10 PM	Miss Spectra	*hey Anton, quick research question for you.... as i'm writing something about research online at the moment and the online dating/sex research...*
29/05/2005	1:17:17 PM	anton...	**hit me**
29/05/2005	1:17:19 PM	Miss Spectra	*How does geography impact on people you contact through online dating?*

29/05/2005	1:17:35 PM	anton...	**if its going 2 be 2 far,then she wanna be hot**
29/05/2005	1:17:44 PM	anton...	**other wise 4get it**
29/05/2005	1:17:56 PM	anton...	**half hour in any direction**
29/05/2005	1:18:00 PM	Miss Spectra	*ok...*
29/05/2005	1:18:10 PM	anton...	**maybe hour**
29/05/2005	1:18:13 PM	Miss Spectra	*so how about interstate or regional?*
29/05/2005	1:19:12 PM	anton...	**nope**
29/05/2005	1:19:12 PM	anton...	**no way**
29/05/2005	1:19:12 PM	anton...	**only if i was going there in the first place**
29/05/2005	1:19:12 PM	anton...	**stop by 4 a shag**
29/05/2005	1:19:13 PM	anton...	**then on my way**
29/05/2005	1:19:13 PM	anton...	**:D**
29/05/2005	1:19:22 PM	Miss Spectra	*:)*
29/05/2005	1:19:25 PM	Miss Spectra	*cool.*
29/05/2005	1:20:27 PM	Miss Spectra	*i had another thought the other day too, I know you have told me you have been to parties/events organised thru [adult online dating website] before. has this extended your network of sexual partners further than just those you had alrady contacted thru the site?*
29/05/2005	1:20:50 PM	anton...	**no,they were all pigs**
29/05/2005	1:21:19 PM	anton...	**didnt want any of them'**
29/05/2005	1:21:19 PM	anton...	**quite disgusting really**
29/05/2005	1:22:01 PM	Miss Spectra	*okay, thanks for clarifying, i appreciate it. :)*
29/05/2005	1:22:10 PM	anton...	**anytime danielle**

The conversation with Anton lasted five minutes, but while we were waiting for responses from Anton we was editing and discussing other parts of the research. Multi-tasking is the norm for most people using chat. Anton would have been doing other things - in fact to establish whether or not this assumption was again true, Danielle asked him:

29/05/2005	1:32:37 PM	Miss Spectra	*another quesiton for you... what are you doing at the moment? on your PC or generally? and what else were you doing when i asked you those couple of questions re the research?*
29/05/2005	1:33:30 PM	anton...	**i play puter games if i'm not hunting chicks danielle**

29/05/2005	1:33:51 PM	Miss Spectra	*:) thanks Anton*
29/05/2005	1:34:01 PM	anton...	**no stress kid**

Elipse took time to respond, and as the transcript below reveals, this was because he was away from his computer (again, note the lapse in time from when we posed the question to when Elipse responded). We also checked with him what else he might be doing whilst logged into chat – his transcript reveals initially he was fixing his pergola, that's why his response was tardy, but he also informs Miss Spectra that he usually checks emails when logged into "msn" – the chat program he uses.[3]

29/05/2005	1:09:00 PM	Miss Spectra	*:)*
29/05/2005	1:09:48 PM	Miss Spectra	*Hello, just in the middle of writing some stuff re research and have a quick question for you if you're around.... How does geography impact on ppl you contact thru online dating?*
29/05/2005	1:35:24 PM	Elipse	Hello
29/05/2005	1:35:37 PM	Elipse	I'm just out still working on my Pegola
29/05/2005	1:35:55 PM	Miss Spectra	*okay. keeping busy. :)*
29/05/2005	1:36:01 PM	Elipse	Geography is important
29/05/2005	1:36:11 PM	Elipse	I'll answer whatever questions you have
29/05/2005	1:36:46 PM	Elipse	I don't travel fruther past Shore St, Milford Grove, Shannon St or St Villar St
29/05/2005	1:36:47 PM	Elipse	lol
29/05/2005	1:36:49 PM	Miss Spectra	*thanks. I am just testing an assumption re my sample.*
29/05/2005	1:36:54 PM	Elipse	only joking
29/05/2005	1:37:10 PM	Elipse	30 minute drive is enough for me
29/05/2005	1:37:11 PM	Miss Spectra	*so hpow is geography important?*
29/05/2005	1:37:26 PM	Elipse	21 sets of traffic lights max.
29/05/2005	1:37:26 PM	Miss Spectra	*okay. so what about interstate or regional?*
29/05/2005	1:37:32 PM	Elipse	WHAT ?
29/05/2005	1:37:39 PM	Elipse	Forget it
29/05/2005	1:37:46 PM	Elipse	I used to see someone who lived in Clyde
29/05/2005	1:37:53 PM	Elipse	35 - 40 minute drive
29/05/2005	1:37:55 PM	Elipse	too far
29/05/2005	1:38:16 PM	Elipse	If its interstate, then all you have is a fun-time buddy
29/05/2005	1:38:24 PM	Elipse	thats no relationship
29/05/2005	1:38:39 PM	Miss Spectra	*okay. thanks for clarifying. :)*
29/05/2005	1:38:56 PM	Elipse	Hey...have you cleared the outstanding 2.5 remaining interviews ?
29/05/2005	1:39:14 PM	Elipse	That lady Jane wants to come and see me
29/05/2005	1:39:14 PM	Miss Spectra	*no, not yet, busy writing chapter for book about process of online dating...*
29/05/2005	1:39:28 PM	Elipse	I think she lives in Kilmore or somewhere
29/05/2005	1:39:37 PM	Elipse	Oh
29/05/2005	1:39:51 PM	Miss	*tell me, when you are chatting online to a person, are you generally*

[3] The typographical errors in these transcripts have been left in to demonstrate what real chat is like.

		Spectra	*chatting soley to them or doing other things?*
29/05/2005	1:39:59 PM	Elipse	Yes, i do like the within 5km of [my home] which I can flag on [romantic website]
29/05/2005	1:40:09 PM	Miss Spectra	*oops, no writing chapter about process of doing research online!!!!*
29/05/2005	1:40:32 PM	Elipse	make up your m ind please
29/05/2005	1:40:53 PM	Miss Spectra	*okay, thanks. I wanted to check out these things, so i can put your thoughts in chapter i am writing. clarifying one of my assumptions*
29/05/2005	1:40:56 PM	Elipse	I log onto my Email and msn at the same time
29/05/2005	1:41:06 PM	Miss Spectra	*ok*
29/05/2005	1:41:11 PM	Elipse	What was your assumption ?
29/05/2005	1:42:32 PM	Miss Spectra	*that my sample of interviewees are all Victorian and mainly Melbourne based. I was thinking htis is because i have interviewed my contacts and thru them and that ppl are more likely to make contact with ppl wihin a certain geographic proximity as it faciltiate meeting.*
29/05/2005	1:42:55 PM	Elipse	Yes
29/05/2005	1:43:14 PM	Elipse	There is another lady who I'd been in contact with who seems to work all over Victoria
29/05/2005	1:43:26 PM	Elipse	and she seems to have Bonk Buddies scattered around
29/05/2005	1:43:43 PM	Elipse	or she just treats every one of them as if it were her last
29/05/2005	1:44:08 PM	Elipse	So, geography is noit an issue for her

The transcripts also demonstrate the close rapport that we have established with these participants, and their level of participation in the research. The immediacy of feedback for researchers, when such a rapport is established, can be incredibly beneficial for theory development and for inductively working through any issues raised in the research (see also Chapter 1 in this volume).

Chat programs offer a range of functionality, some of which include the ability to store a conversation history of previous chats. Any chat user can enable this on the chat program. Conducting the interviews with chat history enabled ensured that when consent was provided in the chat dialogue there is a written record of this consent in the conversation history. If working in a Windows environment, these conversation histories are generally stored on a user's hard drive in the Received Files folder. These conversation histories can act as the interview transcripts, which can printed for analysis or copied into other programs if the transcript is to be analysed with software.

NON-LINEAR CHAT

With the speed of chat and because you are not seeing the other person whilst chatting, it is common to have two threads of conversation going with one person at one time. Chat does not always follow the conventional norms of turn-taking, nor is it always linear (Daviset al., 2004). This can be confusing when first encountered but quickly becomes a normal way of communicating – perhaps because people are often chatting to several people at one time, hence, jumping from one topic to another becomes comfortable, even in a conversation with only one person.

During the research, when interviewing, this happened. We would think an interviewee had finished answering a question and so we would move onto the next area of the interview only to find that they were still answering the previous question. They might then answer the next question asked while we went back to probing them on their previous response. As generally you cannot see your participant, it is difficult to determine what they are up to.

The lack of visual contact and non-verbal reinforcement has been noted as compounding the noticeable slowness of interviewing online (Mann and Stewart, 2002). As Markham (1998: 70) points out, "because writing takes much longer than talking, being a good interviewer means being patient"(Markham, 1998). Typing takes longer than speaking, and so responses take longer to iterate. Additionally, the interviewer must account for the fact they cannot see the participant's face, so need to be aware that they may be missing the visual cues of reflection and contemplation (see Chapter 1 in this volume). Although as an online interviewer, you need to be aware that your participants may be very busy "multi-tasking" during the interview.

When someone you are chatting with has a webcam and they are using it, you can see them in much the same way you would in a regular conversation, hence, you can see when they sit back and pause to think or have a sip of their drink or turn around to talk to someone else who may have entered the room they are in before returning to type their message to you. Watching people using chat via web cam using chat is a good way to become familiar with the various manners in which people use chat. You realise that the person you are chatting to is in another environment, with potentially numerous other things going on around them – they are not necessarily dedicated solely to their keyboard patiently awaiting the next chat comment or question to pop up on their screen. They might be playing computer games, talking on their phone, wandering off to the fridge to get a drink or turning around to talk to someone that is physically in the room with them, or they might be busy in other chats....

> I have asked BeachBelle again if she would like to participate and she is keen, so I have commenced the interview. She has told me she is in four chats and has a guy masturbating on webcam for her at the moment, so she might be a little slow in responding. I was originally introduced to BeachBelle via one of my online dating contacts. Ii have been keen to interview her for a while as I would like more female participants. just not certain how well the interview will go if she is really distracted... A pro or a con - she can multitask while being interviewed and so can I, but if she is doing something more interesting in another window, the responses to me might suffer... (Memo, 25/04/2005).

Online interviewing is different and as such the interview methods and techniques need to be adapted to the situation. It has been noted that researchers need to adopt some of the conventions of chat when conducting online interviews (Davis et al., 2004). To us, this is given, for example when you conduct telephone interviews you use the telephone in a manner similar to how you would when making a telephone call and when you conduct face-to-face interviews you follow the social norms appropriate to the environment. The same is, of course, relevant for online interviews. As such interviewers need to be comfortable with being online and using chat as a normal communication method before assuming they can start effectively interviewing online. The ability to interpret what is being communicated online will also be affected by the interviewers familiarity with the space and context. The interview notes, given below, relating to one of the first interviews we conducted online show some of the early learning experiences in terms of adapting to the interview environment.

> 10:24pm
> Really hard to provide feedback or just encourage continuation of the interview without entering the conversation. If I just stick with "Yes" "A-ha" ""I see" as responses it makes the interview seem stilted as the medium is all about chat!!! and conversation = interaction 2-ways. Yet I am conscious of trying not to lead the interview or to put to much of "me" into it. (Memo, 17/02/2005)

Concurrent Interviews

There is the potential as a researcher to be talking with more than one research participant at once, although we would not recommend it. It occurred once during this research project. Danielle was faced with the dilemma of being in the midst of one interview when another contact introduced one of their contacts as a potential participant, and this potential participant was ready and keen to be interviewed right then and there. Danielle was torn between whether she should tell this potential participant we could do the interview another time and risk losing her interest and availability or endeavouring to undertake two interviews simultaneously. She opted to do the two interviews at once, as previously other potential interview opportunities had been missed when an opportunity had not been taken when it presented itself.

Fortunately, the person Danielle was in the midst of interviewing was busy at work, so he was also multi-tasking throughout the interview, and as a result of this, his responses were slow. This gave Danielle a little more time to respond to him with follow up questions. At the same time she started interviewing the woman who was responding very rapidly to all of the interview questions. While both interviews were taking place, Danielle also had open her interview log document, to which she added relevant thoughts, ruminations and details as the interviews were progressing.

> 8:56pm
> Fairly succinct answers. Working at same time as responding to me. Good he was slow as I was interviewing Bally hoo at same time and she was very fast. Felt like he didn't feel comfortable exposing himself through answering qus. So probably not the most in depth answers… (Memo, 21/02/2005)

Emoticons and Acronyms

Most of the interview transcripts are littered with emoticons, which are symbols that can be typed using characters to create more expressive and efficient communication. For example, :-) and :) are used to represent a grin or smile, ;-) a winking smile and :-(a sad face. :D is a big grin and :p is sticking one's tongue out.

With advances in chat software, emoticons are becoming increasingly graphic. What started out as a combination of characters and punctuations marks attempting to represent emotions, feelings and expressions are quickly being replaced by cartoon like faces and various animations. The chat user has the option to select from a menu of emoticons and insert these into chat conversations at will.

Acronyms are also very common in chat as they speed communication – they are much quicker than typing whole phrases, and again, can be used to quickly inject emotion into chat, such as:

- brb = be right back (this one gives the participant (or researcher) an opportunity to make a cup of tea, use the bathroom or answer a telephone call).
- lol = laughing out loud
- lmao = laughing my arse off
- btw = by the way

A quick web search can provide any user with a glossary of emoticons and acronyms commonly used online.

Interviewees might use emoticons acronyms to demonstrate humour, feelings such as happiness and sadness, curiosity or ire. When conducting interviews, we have found emoticons useful for providing encouragement and visual recognition that we had 'heard' what the interviewee was telling us and so emoticons could act as a prompt for the interviewee to continue with their stream of thought or chat without being interrupted by words. Emoticons can be used to replace the nods on encouragement that one might use in a face-to-face interview. See also Chapter 13 in this volume.

PERSONALISATION OF THE CHAT ENVIRONMENT

Some chat programs allow users to post a picture that will appear when they are in a chat window. People can choose to display whatever picture they like. There are pictures included as part of the chat program, but users also have the option of selecting from pictures they might have available on their personal computer, such as their own digital photos. When Danielle chats, she has a picture of herself visible as part of the chat window, so people can see a visual representation of her. Other examples of pictures people use are digital photos of their pets, their genitalia, cartoons, or photos of themselves with their face hidden, cropped off or blocked out if they are concerned about revealing their identity.

Additionally, most chat programs also allow users to change the colour and font of their text, which can allow users another avenue for expression of personality and mood. In one interview Danielle was using the same font type and colour as the interviewee, Bally Hoo, which was causing some confusion:

Bally Hoo	hey we have to change colors im getting confused
Bally Hoo	lol
Bally Hoo	hang on
Bally Hoo	thats better [when her text changed from pink to blue]
Danielle	ok!!

When using chat it is also possible to change your handle - a handle is a nickname that an individual chooses to use when appearing online in chat. A handle may be similar to a user's email address or it may be completely different. Some people choose never to use handle and appear in chat solely by their chat email address or by their first name.

Changing one's handle allows people to reflect their mood, what is going on in their life or a message they are trying to convey. Some examples of handles are:

- Mondayitis ☹
- Bombing For Peace is Like Fucking for Virginity
- Girls drive me nuts
- In Sydney on February 1
- So snowed under with paper work
- coolangatta kid

It is common for people to regularly change their handle depending on how they feel and what they might be trying to express at a particular time). For example, one of Danielle's chat email addresses starts with spectraelectra@.... Danielle changes her handle regularly and some of the names she had used include:

- Miss Spectra
- Studious Spectra
- Spectra from Planet Electra
- Spectra is sleeping
- miss spectra reading transcripts
- poor dog next door is howling

And as previously mentioned, changing one's handle can be a useful method for attracting potential participants. Using the handle *Introduce me to your friends* created some interest in Danielle's contact list and facilitated the introduction to some contact's contacts which resulted in interviews.

Introductions

As noted earlier, the sampling strategy involved having already known contacts introduce us to their own other contacts. Anton proved a great recruiter. In the chat excerpt below, he introduces two potential participants, and for a little while there are four of us in the one private chat.[44]

Time	Speaker	Receiver	Chat
6:40:52 PM	Anton	Miss Spectra Electra	hows your sex survey going?

[4] It is possible to bring numerous people from a contact list into a chat together, by inviting others into a chat that you may already be having.

6:40:57 PM	Miss Spectra Electra	Anton	what did you get up to?
6:41:03 PM	Miss Spectra Electra	Anton	still need to interview ore ppl.
6:41:08 PM	Anton	Miss Spectra Electra	went 2 a party
6:41:13 PM	Miss Spectra Electra	Anton	know anyone who might be interested?
6:41:14 PM	Anton	Miss Spectra Electra	o.k
6:41:16 PM	Miss Spectra Electra	Anton	need some women!!!
6:41:21 PM	Anton	Miss Spectra Electra	just thinking that
6:41:27 PM	Anton	Miss Spectra Electra	1 sec i'll ask
6:43:57 PM			Leah has been added to the conversation.
6:44:06 PM	Anton	Miss Spectra Electra, Leah	say hi 2 danielle Leah
6:44:14 PM	Miss Spectra Electra	Leah, Anton	Hi Leah!
6:44:18 PM	Miss Spectra Electra	Leah, Anton	nice to meet you.
6:44:55 PM	Anton	Miss Spectra Electra, Leah	Leah
6:44:58 PM	Anton	Miss Spectra Electra, Leah	where are u
6:45:40 PM	Miss Spectra Electra	Leah, Anton	probably busy with something else for the moment
6:45:48 PM	Anton	Miss Spectra Electra, Leah	god knows
6:46:07 PM			Bally Hoo has been added to the conversation.
6:46:13 PM	Leah	Miss Spectra Electra, Bally Hoo, Anton	hiyaaaaaa
6:46:23 PM	Bally Hoo	Miss Spectra Electra, Leah, Anton	hiyaaaaaaaa
6:46:26 PM	Miss Spectra Electra	Bally Hoo, Leah, Anton	hi
6:46:28 PM	Leah	Miss Spectra Electra, Bally Hoo, Anton	hi bally
6:46:29 PM	Bally Hoo	Miss Spectra Electra, Leah, Anton	roped 2 of us in ants ?? lol
6:46:35 PM	Miss Spectra Electra	Bally Hoo, Leah, Anton	lol
6:46:36 PM	Anton	Miss Spectra Electra, Bally Hoo, Leah	and this is bally hoo danielle
6:46:37 PM	Bally Hoo	Miss Spectra Electra, Leah, Anton	hey swoooooffffffffffffffffffffffffssss
6:46:40 PM	Miss Spectra Electra	Bally Hoo, Leah, Anton	hi bally hoo
6:46:40 PM	Bally Hoo	Miss Spectra Electra, Leah, Anton	hey danielle
6:46:43 PM	Anton	Miss Spectra Electra, Bally Hoo, Leah	there both demons
6:46:49 PM	Miss Spectra Electra	Bally Hoo, Leah, Anton	Anton is being very helpful
6:46:51 PM	Bally Hoo	Miss Spectra Electra,	im an (A)

		Leah, Anton	
6:46:53 PM	Miss Spectra Electra	Bally Hoo, Leah, Anton	well demons are good!!!
6:46:54 PM	Anton	Miss Spectra Electra, Bally Hoo, Leah	:D
6:47:11 PM	Miss Spectra Electra	Bally Hoo, Leah, Anton	did Anton give you the speil about what i'm doing?
6:47:40 PM	Bally Hoo	Miss Spectra Electra, Leah, Anton	kinda
6:47:43 PM	Leah	Miss Spectra Electra, Bally Hoo, Anton	yeah brifly
6:48:03 PM	Bally Hoo	Miss Spectra Electra, Leah, Anton	is this going to take long ???
6:48:04 PM	Anton	Miss Spectra Electra, Bally Hoo, Leah	she is a good girl u 2 guys :D
6:48:18 PM	Miss Spectra Electra	Bally Hoo, Leah, Anton	i'm doing some interviews re peoples experiences of online dating and sex, basicaly it's an interview via chat I ask some quesitons, you tell me as much or as little as you like
6:48:24 PM	Miss Spectra Electra	Bally Hoo, Leah, Anton	lol. what an intro
6:48:35 PM	Anton	Miss Spectra Electra, Bally Hoo, Leah	always 4 u kiddo
6:48:48 PM	Anton	Miss Spectra Electra, Bally Hoo, Leah	i held back with what i really wanted 2 say
6:48:50 PM	Anton	Miss Spectra Electra, Bally Hoo, Leah	lol
6:48:57 PM	Bally Hoo	Miss Spectra Electra, Leah, Anton	fire away !!
6:49:00 PM	Miss Spectra Electra	Bally Hoo, Leah, Anton	if you are interested I can email thru the official form which explains it all, tells you about how it will be confidential etc
6:49:12 PM	Miss Spectra Electra	Bally Hoo, Leah, Anton	well we might want to do it in a private chat window.
6:49:12 PM	Anton	Miss Spectra Electra, Bally Hoo, Leah	o.k u guys go 4 it, i'm goin 4 a smoke
6:49:13 PM	Bally Hoo	Miss Spectra Electra, Leah, Anton	thats cool, do it now
6:49:15 PM	Leah	Miss Spectra Electra, Bally Hoo, Anton	ok mail me detaols
6:49:19 PM	Leah	Miss Spectra Electra, Bally Hoo, Anton	details
6:49:25 PM	Leah	Miss Spectra Electra, Bally Hoo, Anton	ok
6:49:32 PM	Leah	Miss Spectra Electra, Bally Hoo, Anton	Anton give her my e.mail
6:49:33 PM	Leah	Miss Spectra Electra, Bally Hoo, Anton	ok
6:49:36 PM	Anton	Miss Spectra Electra, Bally Hoo, Leah	o.k
6:50:05 PM	Anton	Miss Spectra Electra, Bally Hoo, Leah	[Leah's email address]
6:50:09 PM	Miss Spectra	Bally Hoo, Leah, Anton	great, and i'll add you to my messenger, we can go from

	Electra	there
6:50:22 PM		Leah has left the conversation.

Reflexivity in the Research

For Danielle, there has been a large degree of reflexivity in the research. Her ongoing use of online dating for personal reasons, in addition to interviewing people who are also online dating has meant that she has been immersed in the field, with her own changing experiences influencing how she thinks about the whole process of online dating, her needs, wants, and expectations and others' needs, wants and expectations.

She is constantly chatting with her other online contacts that she has met through dating, and although she cannot use the chats that are not part of the project, these chats are fundamental to her personal experience and interpretation of online dating. Discussions in personal chats can inspire new directions for questioning in future interviews or prompt different ways to look at the data collected to date.

Danielle has been frequently asked: "What are you looking for from the website?" as a part of the early dialogue with new contacts. Knowing that her own responses to this question vary depending on what else is going on her life provides some perspective in understanding the diversity of responses received when people describe their own online dating experiences during interviews. From her personal experiences of online dating chat Danielle also knows that frank and explicit discussions are often common, and not necessarily unexpected in chat, so it is reasonable to consider that many people using chat for online dating are familiar and comfortable with discussing sex and sexual practices in a chat context, which has meant that most of the interviews have been fairly open and explicit.

Chat Interviewing Practicalities – Our Conclusion

When interviewing via chat there are some benefits for the researcher. As soon as the interview is finished the transcript is immediately available for analysis. All the researcher needs to do is locate the conversation history in their received files and print this or begin working with it using analysis software (see also Chapter 1 in this volume).

Interviews can be conducted at any time; all that is needed is for the participant and researcher to be online at the same time. Many of the interviews in our online dating research were conducted late at night on week nights. When potential participants indicated their interest in being involved, we would either commence interviewing immediately if it suited them, or we would just suggest that we would do the interview sometime soon when we were online concurrently.

Only one interview was scheduled for a particular day/time as going online for many people may be a regular occurrence but it is not always planned; many people log in when they have some spare time rather than at pre-determined scheduled intervals. We made several attempts to line up interviews via email with contacts of contacts. Initial contact would seem positive, but the interviews never eventuated. Although it is not possible to determine why, it may be because an email is easier to disregard or put off, whereas when one starts a chat dialogue it is immediate and more likely to engage the person, as any questions or concerns about the process or research can be answered immediately, and the person is already online chatting, so you are not inconveniencing them by asking them to be available at a pre-arranged time.

Online interviewing can offer safety and convenience for researchers and the participants. Involvement does not require anyone to leave the comfort or familiarity of their own home or office, or wherever they may use the internet. The researcher can conduct the interviews from anywhere, provided a computer is available with the chat program loaded on and an internet connection. It can also offer a greater degree of comfort for the participants, as it can alleviate concerns about disclosure and anonymity (Davis et al., 2004) which is beneficial when conducting sex research (see also Chapters 1 and 7 in this volume). It's easy to continue interviews if they need to be cut short for any reason. This has happened on a couple of occasions, and it has been possible to pick up the interview where they left off a couple of days or weeks later.

Overall, interviewing by chat can be very convenient for the researcher and the participants. A number of the research participants noted that is was also convenience that appealed to them about online dating. Anton noted "its quick and straight 2 the point… 2 me its a bit like shopping at coles [supermarket] or something like that …. u just look whats on offer and go 4 it!" For the researcher too, if you can find a contact online at the right time who is interested in participating, then you can just go for it. It also allows for an equalising of power - if the participant wants to finish the interview or have a break, it is very easy for them to do so.

The potential convenience offered by online interviewing is not a panacea for the resource poor researcher. Like any form of interviewing, the interview will be very much dependent on the interviewer's ability which includes their familiarity with the interview context. It would be unlikely that someone who had never used chat before would be as an adept an interviewer in a chat space as a skilled interviewer that was also a regular user of chat. Familiarity with online social customs, mores and expectations that one develops through regular use of chatting will enhance relationships between the interviewer and participants and the interviewer's ability to interpret what is occurring in an interview. Similar to how one might ease into a face-to-face interview by "settling" into an interview (Liamputtong and Ezz, 2005), an online interview should start with pleasantries that might be unrelated to the interview topic and needs to finish with the common courtesies of thanking the participant for their time and responses and also being available to respond to any thoughts or questions they might have regarding the research process.

Having people added to one's contact list also raised the question of what to do after the interview was done. To remove someone from a contact list, you need to block them (which means they can no longer see you when you are online). For this project, we left that option with the participants. Blocking tends to be only done to one's online contacts when there has been rudeness or offence, thus, blocking participants after their interview was completed felt like the height of online rudeness. They could block us, but we were not going to block them – we left this in their control. This has resulted in some people proactively following up on the state of the research and offering to introduce contacts. Others have continued to be visible when online, but have not initiated any further dialogue. Remaining available also allowed participants to follow up any concerns they might have. For example, some time after an interview, one participant was concerned about his gender, age and location being revealed in the research, as he believed it would make him identifiable, even though this confidentiality had been ensured prior to consenting to participate in this study. We were able to talk through this issue in this post interview chat so that he felt comfortable with the process and his anonymity.

Throughout the research all participants continued to appear sporadically online in the chat contact list, so we felt reassured that they were comfortable with our presence, the research and their role in it. Although if someone stopped appearing online in the chat list, we would have no way of knowing if they have blocked us or if they simply spending less time or no time using the chat program.

In sum, chat interviews provide data that is very different to what an interviewer might gather in a face-to-face interviews, but if chat is a common method of communication to the context being researched then it can offer a useful method for exploring how people participate in that context.

REFERENCES

[1] Anderson, P. and Hodgson, S., 2005, 'Lurid Website Lays Bare Family Secrets', *Herald-Sun*, 15 February. <HERSUN0020050214e12f0005u>

[2] Bull, S. and McFarlane, M., 2000, 'Soliciting Sex on The Internet: What are The Risks for Sexually Transmitted Diseases and HIV?' *Sexually Transmitted Diseases*, vol. 27, no. 9, pp. 545-50.

[3] Davis, M., G. Bolding, Hart, G., Sherr, L and Elford, J, 2004, 'Reflecting on The Experience of Interviewing Online: Perspectives From the Internet and HIV Study in London', *AIDS Care*, vol. 16, no. 8, pp. 944-52.

[4] Jackman, C., 2004, 'One Man's Online Love Story', *The Australian,* 16 February. *<http://australianit.news.com.au/articles/0,7204,8696704%5e15397%5e%5enbv%5e,00 .html>*

[5] Liamputtong, P., in press, *The Sensitive Researcher: Researching Vulnerable People*, Sage Publications, London.

[6] Liamputtong, P. and Ezzy, D., 2005, *Qualitative Research Methods*, 2nd edition, Oxford University Press, Melbourne.

[7] Mann, C. and Stewart, F., 2002, 'Internet Interviewing', in J. Gubrium and J. Holstein (eds.), *Handbook of Interview Research: Context and Method*, pp. 603-627, Sage Publications, Thousand Oaks, CA.

[8] Markham, A., 1998, *Life Online: Researching Real Experience in Virtual Space*, Altamira Press, Walnut Creek.

[9] McFarlane, M., Bull, S.S. and Rietmeijer, C.A., 2000, 'The Internet as a Newly Emerging Risk Environment for Sexually Transmitted Disease', *JAMA*, vol. 284, no. 4, PP. 443-6.

[10] McFarlane, M., Kachur, R., Bull, S.S. and Rietmeijer, C.A., 2004, 'Women, the Internet, and Sexually Transmitted Infection', *Journal of Women's Health*, vol. 13, no. 6, pp. 689-694.

[11] Ross, M. W., Tikkanen, R. and Mansson, S.A., 2000, 'Differences between Internet samples and conventional samples of men who have sex with men: implications for

research and HIV interventions', *Social Science and Medicine*, vol. 51, no. 5, pp. 749-58.

[12] Weinreich, J. D., 1997, 'Strange Bedfellows: Homosexuality, Gay Liberation and The Internet', *Journal of Sex Education and Therapy*, vol. 22, pp. 58-66.

In: Health Research in Cyberspace
Editor: Pranee Liamputtong, pp. 193-207
ISBN 1-59454-819-6

Chapter 12

A LONGER WORKING LIFE FOR AUSTRALIAN WOMEN? – THE BABYBOOMWOMEN@WORK2020 WEBSITE

Monika Merkes

INTRODUCTION

The world around us is changing rapidly and is shaping our aspirations, hopes and fears for the future. Exposure to global markets and changes in the economy, workforce, technology, population and family structures have implications for individuals and communities, for example, in regard to living arrangements, public expenditure and revenue, labour force participation rates, retirement decisions, and consumption patterns.

Longer life expectancy and an increasing proportion of older people in the community are expected to influence fiscal, economic, and social policy and put pressure on government income support systems. These pressures will be exacerbated by older workers leaving the workforce. With an increasing proportion of older people in the population and increasing health and longevity, paid work after the age of 65 years may become an option or a necessity in the future.

An increase in female participation in paid work – though often part-time or casual and without job security – has been noted (Jones, 1998; Hancock et al., 2000; Ginn, 2001). The increased labour force participation of women and a declining male labour force participation might suggest that women's increased access to paid work is balanced by men's increasing responsibility for unpaid work. However, this is not so. Hancock and colleagues (2000: 11) note that the male participation rate has been centred on the loss of full-time jobs, while the increase in female participation has largely been in part-time work. Further, they argue that a growth in two-earner households and no-earner households confirms that the growth in women's labour force participation is not a general trend but hides an increasing polarisation of women's experience along lines of class, education, geography, and ethnicity.

Paid employment has come to be regarded as synonymous with work (Biesecker and von Winterfeld, 2000; Probert, 1998; Williams and Thorpe, 1992). Ginn et al. (2001) present time budget data from Britain indicating that unpaid household work exceeds paid work and would cost up to 120% of GDP if paid at average wages. Mitchell and Thompson (2001) suggest that the costs of caring serve to penalise many women: health costs, relationship costs, career costs and financial costs, both in the short and longer term. Further, as a result of women's greater life expectancy and the age differential in marriages, most men can expect to be supported by wives in old age while most women rely on help from other sources (Scott and Wenger, 1995).

What do these changes mean for the women that are approaching retirement? What are the views of women of the baby boom generation (that is, those born between1946-1964)? What are their hopes and plans for the future? What policies should be developed and implemented to address population ageing?

When this research project started, there was scant research on issues of future generations' work-retirement decision and its policy implications, including implications for unpaid work such as volunteering and caring. Further, existing studies of the retirement experience had largely been based on men's experience of retirement rather than women's.

This chapter draws on a research project that was undertaken for my PhD thesis at La Trobe University, Melbourne. The focus was on Australian women of the baby boom generation, their working futures and the work-retirement decision. This was explored both from the viewpoint of women and from a social policy perspective. The research included focus group discussions, computer mediated communication (CMC) involving a website with four future scenarios for the year 2020, and the analysis of data from a large survey. This chapter concerns itself with the CMC component of this research project. In the following, I outline the methods that I used in undertaking this CMC research and present some of the results.

METHODOLOGY

This section presents the research framework for this project and briefly reviews the literature on the Internet and CMC, ethical considerations, and future scenarios. This is followed by a description of the website.

Research Framework

The way we design research, collect, analyse, and interpret data is conditioned by the way it is theoretically framed and by the researcher's own ideological assumptions and values (Kincheloe and McLaren, 1994). Researchers in the tradition of critical theory «enter into an investigation with their assumptions on the table, so no one is confused concerning the epistemological and political baggage they bring with them to the research site» (Kincheloe and McLaren, 1994:140). Research is political (Wilson, 2001), and it is important for the researcher to acknowledge the political epistemology of her or his research – to elucidate the relationship between the inquirer and the known and to have an awareness of the values that the researcher brings to the research process and the data (Guba and Lincoln, 1994).

This research has been undertaken from a feminist perspective and with a concern for social justice. While there are many different versions of feminism, it has been argued that all the variants of feminism seek to explore the nature and origin of women's oppression and to understand the relationships among different forms of inequality (Broom, 1987). As Olesen (1994: 158) contends, it is «important to centre and make problematic women's diverse situations and the institutions and frames that influence those situations ... in the interest of realizing social justice for women».

The principle of empowerment has been central to the aims of this research, which has aimed to ensure that those who are the focus of the research gain from it. Women have been studied as active subjects and given a voice (Ginn and Arber, 1995; Riley et al., 2003). Further, the policy initiatives that were identified by this research aim at achieving better working futures for women.

Feminist research often starts with one's own experience. It has been argued that starting from one's own experience «is a way the researcher assures herself that she is 'starting from the standpoint of women' » (Reinharz 1992: 259). As a female baby boomer, I was curious and concerned about the future of work, in particular how my generation will deal with decisions regarding work and retirement and how we will financially support ourselves through the later years of life. The CMC component of this study was also motivated by my interest in information technology and curiosity about how CMC could be used in new ways to undertake qualitative research.

The research undertaken for this project addressed two questions and consisted of three studies. The research questions comprised the following: «How do women of the baby boom generation envisage paid work after the age of 65?» and «What are the policy implications of an ageing female workforce?».

Study 1 was concerned with women's views, beliefs, attitudes, and opinions relevant to the research topic. Focus group research was chosen for this part of the research.

Study 2 – dubbed «BabyBoomWomen@Work2020» – aimed to explore current thinking on the research topic in Australia and overseas. Computer-mediated communication was used for this study, and research participants were individuals with a personal or research interest in the topic. They included women and men from Australia and other countries. There was no requirement for the participants of Study 2 to be of any particular age. In addition to the website, Study 2 also included a policy discussion group with female academics and senior administrators, who were members of a women's network. The findings of the focus group discussions and the data from Study 2 were analysed using thematic analysis.

In Study 3, this qualitative component was complemented by an analysis of quantitative data from the Healthy Retirement Project (HRP), a longitudinal study of mature-age workers' expectations as they approach retirement and their adjustment as they retire. The HRP was undertaken by the Lincoln Gerontology Centre for Education and Research, Faculty of Health Sciences, La Trobe University. Analyses focused on women born between 1946 and 1964, contrasting their views with those of older women in the HRP. The focus of Study 3 was on attitudes towards retirement, retirement plans, and the preferred and expected age of retirement.

As noted above, this chapter concerns itself with the CMC component of this research.

The Internet and CMC

This study used the Internet as a tool for data collection. The literature on future scenarios and the Internet as a research tool was taken into account when the *BabyBoomWomen@ Work2020* website was developed. At the inception of this study in 2001, the literature on the Internet as a data gathering tool was scant, in particular regarding qualitative research. As Mann and Stewart (2000: 4) note, «there has been little systematic analysis of how the Internet might be incorporated into qualitative research practices». While there had been little published research on CMC, research methodologies that combine face-to-face and CMC research were even less common. Published accounts of a methodology identical to that used in this study could not be located.

The Internet is a medium that can be experienced in different ways. A computer and keyboard are usually the mediator of people's Internet experience, and there are different ways in which users can explore the Internet, present themselves, and communicate. CMC has been described as «the process of sending messages – primarily, but not limited to text messages – through the direct use by participants of computers and communication networks ... [where] the communication must be done by participants fully aware of their interaction with the computer technology in the process of creating and delivering messages» (Lawley, 1994: para. 5). Two distinct types of computer mediated communication can be identified: synchronous and asynchronous CMC (Riva, 2001). A range of different Internet environments have been noted, such as the World Wide Web (www), electronic mail (e-mail), asynchronous discussion fora (newsgroups), synchronous chats (Internet Relay Chat, or IRC), multi-user dungeons (MUD; i.e., text based virtual environments), metaworlds (3D MUDs; that is, 3 dimensional virtual environments), and interactive video (Riva and Galimberti, 2001; see also Chapter 1 in this volume).

The environment created by the Internet is often referred to as cyberspace:

> A universe made up of things that can be seen and heard, but they are neither physical objects nor necessarily a representation of physical objects. They are built of information coming partly from operations of the physical world, but largely from the accumulation and exchange of knowledge arising from human initiatives in the fields of culture, science, and art (Riva and Galimberti, 2001: 1).

The Internet is an excellent medium for quick and inexpensive communication with individuals who are geographically distant. It offers opportunities to reach informants that may otherwise be more difficult and costly to locate. CMC crosses time and space barriers, and in its asynchronous forms people can choose their own time and place to respond to a research request. It provides a safe environment, in particular for women, older people, and people with disabilities who may otherwise have to travel to participate in a research project. CMC allows easy handling of data and does not require transcription as the text is already provided.

There are a range of challenges for researchers who use CMC. These include computer literacy, recruitment of research participants, and finding e-mail addresses, as directories are incomplete. Not everybody feels comfortable with this type of communication and therefore the sample may be unrepresentative. Access and gender as well as access and age are issues, as to date more men than women and more young people than older people use the Internet (Kennedy et al., 2003; see also Chapter 2 in this volume).

The methodologies of studies using the Internet as a research tool that are discussed in published articles include e-mail surveys, web-based surveys, and online focus groups. Compared to paper-based surveys, there are advantages and disadvantages in using CMC. For example, the cost of an e-mail survey is estimated to be between 5% and 20% of a paper survey (Sheehan, 2001; see also Chapters 6 and 7 in this volume). The costs of e-mail and web-based surveys decrease significantly as the sample size increases. In addition, «people tend to provide longer open-ended responses to e-mail than to other types of surveys, and responses to e-mail surveys tend to be more candid than responses to mail or phone surveys» (Sheehan, 2001).

Using the Internet as a tool for survey research offers exciting new possibilities to the researcher (Sade-Beck, 2004; see also Chapter 7 in this volume). However, the limitations of this methodology need to be understood. For example, it is not possible to access samples representative of the general population because Internet access and use vary for different populations. Riva (2001) argues that people who participate in online research are self-selected and by no means randomly representative of the general population. In particular, they are usually skewed toward the high end of the socioeconomic and educational spectrum.

Both researcher and respondents must have a certain degree of computer literacy to implement a web-based survey. Technical knowledge such as expertise in Hypertext Markup Language (HTML) or web development software is required to set up a web-based survey. In addition, the survey has to be promoted and the website registered with search engines. The target population must be technologically competent enough to use the Internet and be able to have access to computers and the Internet. The difficulty to determine the authenticity of respondents to web-based surveys presents another issue as Internet users can participate in a survey anonymously. However, the same is true for paper-based surveys unless the researcher can observe their completion.

Determining the response rate of online surveys can be difficult (see Chapter 7 in this volume). Smith (1997: Discussion section, para 2) argues that

> The primary problem with web-administered surveys is there is no precise and reliable means of determining response rate. One could install a 'hit' counter which tracks the number of times a page is called from the server, but these counters do not distinguish repeat from unique visitors, nor do they reflect whether a page is allowed to fully load in the browser.

Declining response rates for all types of surveys have been reported. This is due to growth in the amount of survey research being undertaken and an increase in the number of requests to individuals to complete surveys (Cook et al., 2000; Sheehan, 2001). Response rates to online surveys have been found to be relatively low, for example: 10% or lower (Witmer et al., 1999), 2.3% (Smith, 1997), and 5% (Nicholas et al., 2001). When comparing different online surveys, factors associated with higher response rates included the number of contacts, personalised contacts, and pre-contacts (Cook et al., 2000). While it has been argued that it is unacceptable to send unsolicited e-mail surveys as they may be regarded as spam, post-notification, or follow-up contact, has been found to have positive effects on response rates to both postal mail and e-mail (Sheehan, 2001).

Sheehan (2001) points out that the longer the survey, the more likely it is that the response rate will be low. Smith (1997) also notes that length is an issue for e-mail questionnaires. Conversely, a meta-analysis of response rates in web-based surveys found that survey length is not associated with response rates (Cook et al., 2000). Similarly, Witmer and others (1999) suggest that response rates for online surveys may not be particularly sensitive to questionnaire length.

Sheehan (2001) notes that other elements like respondent contacts and topic salience may also have an influence on response rates, while Cook and colleagues (2000) find that when the topic of web-based surveys is less salient, response rates tend to be both slightly lower and also more highly variable. «Salience of an issue to the sampled population has been found to have a strong positive correlation with response rate for postal, e-mail and WWW-based surveys» (Sheehan 2001, Issue salience section, para. 1).

Ethical Considerations

The World Wide Web provides a rich source of easily accessible data for social researchers. However, there are ethical considerations, for example how researchers collect data, treat their informants, and publish their findings. Online research takes place in an environment with largely customary, as opposed to legally enshrined, laws. Consequently, self-regulation and responsibility become issues of concern for the online researcher (Mann and Stewart, 2000).

Internet researchers come from different backgrounds and disciplines and bring with them a range of different codes of ethics which do not necessarily adapt well to this medium. Some of the questions raised by Internet researchers (Frankel and Siang, 1999; Jones, 1994; Kraut et al., 2003) include the following:

- Are issues of privacy and dignity in virtual communities significantly different from those in non-virtual communities?
- Under what circumstances can one ethically analyse postings to a mailing list or newsgroup?
- Is it necessary to ask permission of list members first, or of those that the researcher would like to quote?
- Is it necessary to ask permission of the list administrator or moderator?
- Does it matter whether the list or newsgroup is publicly archived? Is «private» information private if it is freely available online?
- Does it matter whether the subject matter of the list is sensitive, or whether its members can be considered vulnerable?
- Does purely statistical analysis have to meet different ethical standards than content-based analysis?
- What constitutes informed consent?
- Should people have access to the data collected about themselves?
- Who owns messages posted to newsgroups or e-mail lists? Are there copyright issues?

- Should ethical standards be universally applicable - irrespective of culture, nation, and race?

To date, there is no universal agreement on the ethics of research that involves CMC. Online research is further complicated by issues of anonymity and pseudonymity (Jacobson, 1999; Ess and AoIR ethics working committee, 2002; see also Chapter 1 in this volume). However, the Association of Internet Researchers provides guidelines «on what may – and what may not – be defended as ethical behaviour» (Ess and AoIR ethics working committee, 2002: 3). Further, the American Psychological Association has identified ethical principles including competence, integrity, professional and scientific responsibility, respect for people's rights and dignity, concern for others' welfare, and social responsibility (Kuntze et al., 2002).

The BabyBoomWomen@Work2020 website included a consent form which provided details about the research project and the researcher. The research respondents were advised that their comments and name – if provided – might be publicly displayed unless they indicated to the researcher that they did not wish this to occur. The website was set up in such a way that potential research participants were directed to the consent form before participating in the research.

FUTURE SCENARIOS

Scenarios are a tool of futures research and apart from research have been utilised in a range of ways for the purposes of planning, change management, and policy development. Other futures methods include forecasting, modelling, scanning, futures web, imaging (Slaughter, 1995), trend extrapolation, cross-impact analysis, and the delphi method (Weingand, 1995).

Inayatullah (2002) notes that the foundational method in futures studies is the use of scenarios. Bloom and Menefee (1994: 224) describe a scenario as «a description of a possible or probable future. Scenarios have also been described as «contrasting pictures that provide a framework for considering a range of alternative futures» (Slaughter 1996:101) and «stories of credible, alternative futures» (Ramsey, 2000: 55).

Four scenarios for the year 2020 were developed for this study. The year 2020 was chosen because those born in 1955, the mid-baby boomers, will reach the age of 65 years in 2020. At that age, Australians become eligible for the government age pension – however, this may change in the future. The scenarios describe possible future policy environments in which baby boom women engage, or do not engage, in paid and unpaid work.

Scenarios are usually a team effort and are rarely developed by a single individual. For this reason, I chose an existing set of four scenarios and developed it further, focusing on women of the baby boom generation. A set of scenarios developed in 1995 by a group of 400 Australians as part of the Global Scenarios Project (Economic Planning Advisory Commission, 1996) was considered to be well-suited for this purpose.

The four scenarios – *Oztopia*, *Bladerunner*, *Australia on a bad day*, and *The island nation* – were developed by this group of Australians after they identified the two most critical and uncertain dilemmas for the future of Australia. These were the issues of:

- Australia's successful participation in the global economy, global politics, and social responsibilities, or failure to be a global participant and the insularity as a result of this; and
- the development and growth of community and spirituality, or a society which celebrates and rewards individualism and materialism only.

This type of scenarios has been described as driving-force scenarios (Morrison and Mecca, 1989).

The above four scenarios provided the starting point for the scenarios which I developed and created for the BabyBoomWomen@Work2020 website. At the time of writing the scenarios, the first three face-to-face focus group discussions with women who were born between 1946 and 1964 had been completed. In developing the scenarios, I considered the issues raised in these focus groups and in relevant literature. Further, I intended to ensure that Australia's diverse community was represented in the scenarios and chose protagonists from different cultural and linguistic backgrounds as well as a woman with a disability. Apart from these considerations, the stories emerged from my imagination.

The scenarios describe four future environments in which women of the baby boom generation have – or lack – the opportunities and choices to engage in paid and unpaid work. Each scenario starts with a description of the general political and social environment, followed by a description of the living and working circumstances of four baby boom women.

Oztopia describes an Australia that is actively participating in a globalising world, and has developed its spirituality and sense of community. *Bladerunner* is also an active participant in a global world, but its predominant values are individualism and materialism. *Australia on a bad day* describes a country that has failed to compete and participate in the global communities, a free market economy that has brought uncertainty and insecurity for most of its citizens. *The island nation* depicts an Australia with strong shared community values, a weak economy, poor participation globally, and a return to nationalism.

THE BABYBOOMWOMEN@WORK2020 WEBSITE

The website developed for this study included:

- four scenarios for the year 2020;
- a list of questions and an invitation for readers to respond directly via e-mail to the researcher, participate in a discussion board on the website, or respond to the questions online (this option was added in June 2001);
- a consent form;
- a «What's New» page;
- references and hyperlinks to relevant organisations and publications;
- information about the non-CMC components of the research;
- information about myself; and
- a response rate survey, which sought feedback from those readers who had visited the website but did not participate in the research.

Since completion of the study, the four scenarios and other information about the research have been displayed on my personal website at *http://member.melbpc.org.au/~monika*.

The questions displayed on the website about the four scenarios included the following:

- How likely are the scenarios?
- What aspects are likely?
- What aspects are less likely?
- What are the factors that make them more or less likely?
- Which scenario(s) do you prefer?
- What (if any) other elements would you include in your preferred scenario(s)?
- What factors will contribute to achieving your preferred scenario(s)?
- What will be the major challenges to achieving your preferred scenario(s)?
- What factors could prevent your preferred scenario(s) from becoming a reality?
- What overall strategies should be adopted to achieve your preferred scenario(s)?
- What action has to be taken now or in the near future to achieve your preferred scenario(s) or elements of your preferred scenario(s)? (for example, in the areas of taxation, finance/savings, health, support services, education, training, housing, transport, retirement policy, and pension policy).

Readers were asked to read the consent form including a statement that participation in the research implies consent. Next, they were encouraged to read the four scenarios and the questions listed above. The list of questions was headed by the following text: «Please comment on any of the questions. You are not expected to comment on all questions. Any comment is welcome. Alternatively, feel free to comment on other aspects of the scenarios, the research, or this website». Three alternative ways of responding were offered: e-mail, an online discussion board, and an option to respond to the questions online, which involved the use of text boxes and a «Submit Form» button.

The postings to the website and e-mails in response to the website comprised the data for this study. The website was available at http://www-sph.health.latrobe.edu.au/bbww from 8 March to 8 July 2001, and at http://HS053287.health.latrobe.edu.au/bbww/ from 16 July 2001 to March 2002. The change in URL resulted from a decision by the Faculty to change servers and was out of my control.

The website was promoted through registration with search engines; postings to email lists with a focus on policy, research, women, health, media studies, Internet research, and futures studies; emails to individuals and newsgroups; and registration with other websites for the purpose of providing a hyperlink to the study's website.

RESULTS

This section describes the data received in response to the *BabyBoomWomen@Work2020* website, summarises the content of the research participants' contributions, and presents some of the difficulties encountered while conducting the research.

Description of the Data

The data included postings to the website's discussion board, e-mails, e-mail attachments, and postings in response to the online survey and the response rate survey. As several research participants were friends, acquaintances, or work colleagues, some e-mails in response to the website also included information that was not related to the study's objectives.

Further, I entered into an exchange of e-mails with several research participants. Not every single e-mail in such an exchange included a new comment or thought. For example, some people asked questions about the research without commenting on it. To make a clear distinction between contributions that were considered as data for the purposes of the study and communications with research participants that were unrelated to the study or did not provide relevant data, I developed criteria for the inclusion of data relevant to the research.

All contributions in response to the website were «appropriate» comments, that is, they commented on the topic of the study and/or the methodology and were friendly in tone. There was a total of 67 responses to the website and the total number of participants was 50. Twelve individuals sent more than one response. Thirty-three respondents were women, 11 were men, and for 6 individuals this could not be identified as they did not provide details such as their first name.

Of the 50 research participants, 11 were known to me in person prior to the research. These were friends, acquaintances, work colleagues, or fellow students. During the data collection period, I met four research participants previously unknown to me. Thirty-five contributors to the research were not personally known to me. As far as the country of origin could be identified, the research participants were from Australia, Canada, Sweden, Switzerland, the UK, and the US. The country of origin was identified through the participants' e-mail address, or by information provided in the text of the message (such as «here in Canada»), or the e-mail signature. The research participants known to me were of different cultural and linguistic backgrounds, including French, German, Italian, Chinese, Irish, and British.

What the Research Participants Wrote

The research participants did not believe that the scenario features they liked would become a reality in the future. The preferred future was not considered probable. Oztopia with its inclusive, spiritual, and community-minded society was the preferred scenario. However, one person wrote that the highly developed application of technology also would make it a «slightly creepy place». In contrast, some features of Australia on a bad day and Bladerunner were considered to be already in existence and would continue and become worse. These included increasing inequality, a lack of vision and leadership, fear, and decreasing government support for education and research.

The research participants provided a wide range of suggestions for policy change. Many of these were identical to those made in the focus groups and touched on the areas of work, education, health, incomes, housing, and community values. A work-life balance, flexible work practices, and a reflection of Australia's growing cultural diversity in the work place were considered as essential. The following suggestions for policy change were offered:

- more flexible workplaces, such as flexi-time, purchased leave, compressed weeks, and working from home;
- attraction, retention, and appreciation of older workers;
- affordable or free education and training for people of all ages;
- promotion of holistic health, exercise, and healthy food;
- environmentally sustainable agriculture and development;
- increased assistance with saving for retirement for women;
- broadening of the debate on retirement incomes;
- introduction of a minimum and maximum income;
- changes to the superannuation system, such as increased compulsory contribution, decrease of taxes on superannuation savings, and a government guarantee for superannuation savings;
- introduction of an insurance based retirement savings system;
- broadening of community living options;
- a value shift towards a more inclusive community; and
- more compassion for asylum seekers.

EMERGING ISSUES

This CMC study achieved only a small number of respondents (n=50) and responses (n=67) despite a hit rate of over 3,000. However, it yielded a large quantity of data as some participants sent me lengthy e-mails and attached articles and papers that they had written on the topic. While the small number of research respondents was disappointing, similarly low response rates have been reported in the literature (see above). Further, the discussion board on the website did not generate a discussion. Instead, participants posted messages that did not refer to the postings of other participants. This might have been due to my lack of skills in online moderation or to the participants' potential lack of familiarity with online discussions.

There are several possible reasons for the low response rate to this CMC study. Smith (1997) notes a degree of suspicion in stranger-to-stranger communication in cyberspace, even when the topic is of mutual interest. Further, the material on the website was lengthy and complex, and may have required more time and focus on the topic than the participants were prepared to offer. A response rate survey on the website aimed to find out why people who visited the website did not participate in the research. Too much to read, not enough time, a preference for face-to-face discussion, and no incentive to participate were provided as reasons for non-participation.

The respondents to the study were by no means representative of the general population. The nature of the research tool – the Internet – does not allow for verification of sex, age, or any other attributes of research participants, and the use of the Internet is not common in all populations groups. Although all responses were relevant to the topic, some were not useful as data. For example, some respondents asked questions but did not comment.

While the use of the Internet is increasing, not all people have equal access to this technology. In Australia, people on lower incomes, those who live in regional or rural areas, women and older people are less likely to use the Internet (Australian Bureau of Statistics, 2000). Therefore, those who participate in online research do not represent the voices of the general population. I anticipated that the individuals who participated in this online research study would be likely to have tertiary education and a personal or professional interest in the topic. This was considered as acceptable, as this was one of three studies. The other two studies attempted to reach research participants from a broad range of different socioeconomic and cultural backgrounds.

Through the website, this research project became known to people in Australia and other countries who were interested in the topic or were undertaking research in related areas. This would not have been possible without the website, and the resulting international networking was an unexpected benefit of the research.

When I started this project, there was little IT support provided by the university for student projects. However, I had been a member of the Melbourne PC User Group – a group of more than 11,000 people with an interest in personal computers – for several years and participated in its newsgroups. With online tutorials on web development and the help of fellow User Group members I taught myself HTML and subsequently developed and maintained the *BabyBoomWomen@Work2020* website. In the process, I learned much about web development and I still keep learning.

CONCLUSION

This chapter reports on the CMC component of a research project that used qualitative and quantitative, online and face-to-face methods to explore the views of Australian women of the baby boom generation, their working futures, and the work-retirement decision as well as the social policy implications of an ageing female workforce. The research included focus group discussions, CMC involving a website with four future scenarios for the year 2020, and the analysis of data from a large survey.

This research project crossed research fields and used an eclectic mix of methodologies to examine the research questions from different angles and in different ways. The methodology comprised common data collection tools – focus group discussions and a survey – with more innovative and less well documented ways of collecting research data (i.e., an Internet website and future scenarios).

The BabyBoomWomen@Work2020 website was available online between March 2001 and March 2002. The website's main features were four future scenarios for the year 2020 and a set of questions relating to the scenarios. Visitors to the website were invited to identify probable and preferable elements of the scenarios, policy issues, and possible solutions. Postings to the website's discussion board, e-mails, e-mail attachments, and postings in response to an online survey and a response rate survey comprised the data for this study.

The website generated rich data, in particular some respondents sent lengthy emails, articles and papers that they had written on the topic. However, the overall number of respondents (n=50) and responses (n=67) was relatively low. The text on the website that participants were expected to read was lengthy and complex, and may have required more time than most visitors to the website were prepared to offer. Thus, the people who contributed their views were likely to be those with a particular personal or research interest in the topic.

The participants in this research offered a wide range of ideas, suggestions for change, and strategies for achieving equality and equity for women. In regard to social policy changes, three areas were considered of particular relevance: prolonging working lives, improving income systems, and achieving a balanced life.

The Internet is increasingly used as a tool for gathering research data. However, the literature on CMC research is scant, in particular regarding qualitative research. Research methodologies that combine face-to-face and CMC research are even less common and less well documented. More research with a mix of methods is required to determine the characteristics of qualitative research that are well suited to the Internet environment. Further, research projects that do not use the Internet as a research tool may also benefit from a website that promotes the research and raises awareness about the research topic as was the experience with this study.

REFERENCES

[1] Australian Bureau of Statistics, 2000, *Increasing Use of the Internet and Home Computers*, Commonwealth of Australia. *<http://www.abs.gov.au>*

[2] Biesecker, A. and von Winterfeld, U., 2000, 'Vergessene Arbeitswirklichkeiten', in U. Beck (ed.), *Die Zukunft von Arbeit und Demokratie*, pp. 269-86, Suhrkamp, Frankfurt am Main, Germany.

[3] Bloom, M. J. and Menefee, M. K., 1994, 'Scenario Planning and Contingency Planning', *Public Productivity andandandandand Management Review*, vol. 17, no. 3, pp. 223-30.

[4] Broom, D. H., 1987, 'Another Tribe: Gender and Inequality', in C. Jennett and R.G. Stewart. (eds.), *Three Worlds of Inequality*, pp. 264-81, MacMillan, Melbourne.

[5] Cook, C., Heath, F. and Thompson, R. L., 2000, 'A Meta-Analysis of Response Rates in Web- or Internet-Based Surveys', *Educational andandandandand Psychological Measurement*, vol. 60, no. 6, pp. 821-36.

[6] Economic Planning Advisory Commission, 1996, *The Global Scenarios. Developing a Scenario for Australia in an Emerging World*, Parkes, ACT.

[7] Ess, C. and AoIR ethics working committee, 2002, 'Ethical Decision Making and Internet Research', *Association of Internet Researchers. <http://www.aoir.org/reports/ethics.pdf>*

[8] Frankel, M. and Siang, S., 1999, *Ethical and Legal Aspects of Human Subjects Research in Cyberspace*, Scientific Freedom, Responsibility and Law Program, Directorate of Science and Policy Programs, American Association for the Advancement of Science, Washington, DC 20005. *<http://www.aaas.org/spp/dspp/sfrl/projects/intres/main.htm>*

[9] Ginn, J., 2001, 'Risk of Social Exclusion in Later Life: How Well do the Pension Systems of Britain and the US Accommodate Women's Paid and Unpaid Work?' *International Journal of Sociology andandandandand Social Policy*, vol. 21, no. 4-6, pp. 212-44.

[10] Ginn, J. and Arber, S., 1995, "Only Connect': Gender Relations and Ageing', in S. Arber and J. Ginn (eds.), *Connecting Gender and Ageing. A Sciological Approach*, pp. 1-14, Open University Press, Buckingham.

[11] Ginn, J., Street, D. and Arber, S., 2001, 'Cross-National Trends in Women's Work', in J. Ginn, D. Street and S. Arber (eds.), *Women, Work and Pensions. International Issues and Prospects*, pp. 11-30, Open University Press, Buckingham, Philadelphia.

[12] Guba, E. G. and Lincoln, Y. S., 1994, 'Competing Paradigms in Qualitative Research', in N.K. Denzin and Y.S. Lincoln (eds.), *Handbook of qualitative research*, , pp. 105-17, Sage Publications, Thousand Oaks.

[13] Hancock, L., Howe, B. and O'Donnell, A., 2000, *Reshaping Australian Social Policy: Changes in Work, Welfare and Families*, Growth 48, Committee for Economic Development of Australia.*<http://www.ceda.com.au/New/Flash/html/publications.html>*

[14] Inayatullah, S., 2002, *Questioning the Future. Futures Studies, Action Learning and Organizational Transformation*, Center for Futures Studies, Tamkang University, Tamsui, Taipei, Taiwan.

[15] Jacobson, D., 1999, 'Doing Research in Cyberspace', *Field Methods*, vol. 11, no. 2, pp. 127-45. *<http://people.brandeis.edu/~jacobson/Doing_Research_Cyberspace.pdf>*

[16] Jones, B., 1998, 'Redefining Work: Setting Directions for the Future', *Journal of Occupational Science*, vol. 5, no. 3, pp. 127-32.

[17] Jones, R. A., 1994, 'The Ethics of Research in Cyberspace', *Internet Research*, vol. 4, no. 3, pp. 30-35. *<http://www.mcb.co.uk/services/articles/liblink/intr/ethics.html>*

[18] Kennedy, T., Wellman, B. and Klement, K., 2003, 'Gendering the Digital Divide', *ITandandandandandSociety*, vol. 1, no. 5, pp. 72-96. *<http://www.stanford.edu/group/siqss/itandsociety/v01i05/v01i05a05.pdf>*

[19] Kincheloe, J. L. and McLaren, P. L., 1994, 'Rethinking Critical Theory and Qualitative Research', in N.K. Denzin and Y.S. Lincoln (eds.), *Handbook of Qualitative Research*, pp. 138-57, Sage Publications, Thousand Oaks.

[20] Kraut, R., Olson, J., Banaji, M., Bruckman, A., Cohen, J. and Couper, M., 2003, 'Psychological Research Online: Opportunities and Challenges', *APA-Internet Version* 3.3, no. 9/30/2003. *<http://www.apa.org/science/apainternetresearch.pdf>*

[21] Kuntze, M. F., Stoermer, R., Mueller-Spahn, F. and Bullinger, A. H., 2002, 'Ethical Codes and Values in a Virtual World', *CyberPsychology andandandandand Behavior*, vol. 5, no. 3, pp. 203-06.

[22] Lawley, E. L., 1994, 'The Sociology of Culture in Computer-Mediated-Communication: An Initial Exploration'. *<http://www.itcs.com/elawley/bourdieu.html>*

[23] Mann, C. and Stewart, F., 2000, *Internet Communication and Qualitative research. A Handbook for Researching Online*, Sage Publications, London.

[24] Mitchell, M. and Thompson, M., 2001, 4-6 July 2001, *Changing Conceptions of Informal Care in Australia.* Paper presented at the National Social Policy Conference, Sydney.

[25] Morrison, J. L. and Mecca, T. V. (eds), 1989, *Managing Uncertainty: Environmental Analysis/Forecasting in Academic Planning.* Agathon Press, New York.

[26] Nicholas, D., Huntington, P., Williams, P. and Blackburn, P., 2001, *Digital Health Information Provision and Health Outcomes*, The Internet Studies Research Group, Department of Information Science, City University, London,

[27] Olesen, V., 1994, 'Feminisms and Models of Qualitative Research', in N.K. Denzin and Y.S. Lincoln (eds.), *Handbook of qualitative research*, pp. 158-69, Sage, Thousand Oaks.

[28] Probert, B., 1998, *Working Life. Arguments About Work in Australian Society*, Penguin Books Australia, Ringwood, Victoria.

[29] Ramsey, N., 2000, 'Thinking in the Future Tense', in H. Wilkinson (ed.), *Family Business*, pp. 54-63, Demos, London.

[30] Reinharz, S., 1992, Feminist Methods in Social Research, Oxford University Press, New York.

[31] Riley, S., Schouten, W. and Cahill, S., 2003, 'Exploring the Dynamics of Subjectivity and Power Between Researcher and Researched', *Forum: Qualitative Social Research*, vol. 4, no.2.<*http://www.qualitative-research.net/fqs-texte/2-03/2-03rileyetal-e.htm#g2*>

[32] Riva, G., 2001, 'The Mind Over the Web: The Quest for the Definition of a Method for Internet Research', *CyberPsychology andandandandand Behavior*, vol. 4, no. 1, pp. 7-16.

[33] Riva, G. and Galimberti, C., 2001, 'The Mind in the Web: Psychology in the Internet Age', *CyberPsychology andandandandand Behavior*, vol. 4, no. 1, pp. 7-16.

[34] Sade-Beck, L., 2004, 'Internet Ethnography: Online and Offline', *International Journal of Qualitative Methods*, vol. 3, no. 2. <*http://www.ualberta.ca/~iiqm/backissues/3_2/pdf/sadebeck.pdf*>

[35] Scott, A. and Wenger, G. C., 1995, 'Gender and Social Support Networks in Later Life', in S. Arber and J. Ginn (eds.), *Connecting Gender and Ageing. A sociological approach*, pp. 158-72, Open University Press, Buckingham.

[36] Sheehan, K., 2001, 'E-mail Survey Response Rates: A Review', *Journal of Computer Mediated Communication*, vol. 6, no. 2. <*http://www.ascusc.org/jcmc/vol6/issue2/sheehan.html*>

[37] Slaughter, R., 1995, *Futures. Tools andandandandand Techniques*, Futures Study Centre and DDM Media Group, Melbourne.

[38] Slaughter, R. A., 1996, 'Futures Concepts', in R.A. Slaughter (ed.), *The knowledge base of futures studies*, pp. 87-124, DDM Media Group, Hawthorn, Victoria.

[39] Smith, C. B., 1997, 'Casting the Net: Surveying an Internet Population', *Journal of Computer Mediated Communication*, vol. 3, no. 1. <*http://www.ascusc.org/jcmc/vol3/issue1/smith.html*>

[40] Weingand, D. E., 1995, 20-25 August, *Futures Research Methodologies: Linking Today's Decisions With Tomorrow's Possibilities*. Paper presented at the 61st IFLA General Conference, Istanbul, Turkey. <*http://www.ifla.org/IV/ifla61/61-weid.htm*>

[41] Williams, C. and Thorpe, B., 1992, Beyond Industrial Society, Allen andandandandand Unwin, North Sydney.

[42] Wilson, G., 2001, 'Conceptual Frameworks and Emancipatory Research in Social Gerontology', *Ageing andandandandand Society*, vol. 21, pp. 471-87.

[43] Witmer, D. F., Colman, R. W. and Katzman, S. L., 1999, 'From Paper-and-Pencil to Screen-and-Keyboard. Toward a Methodology for Survey Research on the Internet', in S. Jones (ed.), *Doing Internet research*, pp. 145-61, Sage, Thousand Oaks, California.

In: Health Research in Cyberspace
Editor: Pranee Liamputtong, pp. 209-228
ISBN 1-59454-819-6

Chapter 13

NARRATIVE RESOURCES AND IDENTITY IN AN ONLINE SUPPORT GROUP FOR MULTIPLE SCLEROSIS

Monique Solomon

RESOURCEFULLY RESTORYING THE SELF ONLINE

Participation in an online support group is a social and personal act of resourcefully restorying the self. This chapter looks at how members of an online support group for Multiple Sclerosis (MS) draw upon medically and socially recognised discourses to present themselves as they story their experiences in spontaneous conversations on an online message board. In their posted messages, members invoke larger culturally available narrative resources and learn to engage the locally available narrative resources that emerge and develop from their online participation. Members actively and purposefully construct identity for those who will read their messages, as well as for themselves. Once posted, a message becomes a narrative record of the work of restorying the self. It can be reflected upon, responded to, rejected, challenged or embraced. The textual nature of online messages makes them important examples that reflect how individuals draw on narrative resources to accomplish identity online.

Although people with chronic illness are increasingly turning to the Internet for information and emotional support, "research exploring the development, use, and functions of illness-related groups online…remains limited" (Scheerhorn, 1997: 176). Few studies have addressed the relationship between grand narratives about illness and illness narratives "constructed by the afflicted themselves" (Hyden, 1997: 64). There have also been no comprehensive comparative studies regarding how illness narratives vary depending on the social context (Hyden, 1997). Studying online support groups speaks to the value of these groups as indicators of "how ideologies of health and illness reflect society's conflicting interests concerning disease prevention and the care of the sick" (Radley, 1994: 204). The online context affords a centralised position for observing and uncovering the socially valued narratives for talking about the self and illness. In this study, I address the relationship between social narratives and personal narratives and attend to narratives as they are storied by those who have chronic illness.

Narrative, Identity and Chronic Illness

Experiencing a chronic illness such as MS is a "call to restory the self" and rework identity not only in terms of the physical and embodied changes and challenges that accompany chronic illness but also in terms of social and cultural attitudes, values and beliefs surrounding illness (Frank, 1995). Chronic illness produces a change in social status. As Charmaz (1983: 168) contends, "chronically ill persons frequently experience a crumbling away of their former self-images without simultaneous development of equally valued new ones". Illness narratives hold the potential to rearticulate the illness experience and reconfigure social identity where the major disruptions produced by chronic illness have affected core components of identity, such as social roles and relationships (Hunt, 2000: 89).

In an effort to achieve a better understanding of how the experience of chronic illness is storied into our identity, we are encouraged to look at the whole story, analysing the structure and the content of a story as well as the available narrative resources that are drawn upon to create the story. By examining specific narrative texts online, we can recognise culturally relevant narrative resources drawn upon for accomplishing identity. Narrating experiences in terms of such things as social roles and relationships, and interpreting the "biographical disruption" (Williams, 2000) that results from chronic illness in terms of wider cultural narratives, reconstitutes identity (Riessman, 1990). Personal narratives are, thus, not only representations of experience but also active practices that help to socially construct experience and consequently help to restory the self as it is lived in the wider social and cultural world. In order to explore how identity is restoried in terms of chronic illness, this chapter considers together, the narrative resources available, and the artful activity used to story experience. In this way, we may consider how personal narratives engage with and integrate the contexts of larger discourse to accomplish identity.

Researching Online Support Groups

The application of qualitative methodologies to the study of chronic illness aids in "exploring the subtleties and personal meanings that inhere to living with a chronic illness" (Conrad, 1990: 1257). Studies of online support groups indicate that they have a number of powerful and positive benefits. Online groups have been shown to have supportive benefits that align with "key life functions" of support as identified in face-to-face support groups including self care, mobilisation, communication, socialisation, employment (Braithwaite et al., 1999). Online support improves chances for outreach by addressing the social challenges of illness such as, living a restricted life, existing in social isolation, experiencing discredited definitions of self, and not wanting to become a burden to others (Charmaz, 1983). Further, it helps people with mobility-related challenges, or those who struggle with social and emotional challenges of face-to-face communication, to gain a sense of universality and community support while receiving information and learning from others (Braithwaite et al., 1999). As Conrad (1990: 1260) notes, "we need to study how people manage their illness in their everyday lives (for this) brings greater understanding to the specific illness and contributes to the general understanding of illness experience". By researching the social and personal narratives that members of an online group draw on to accomplish identity, we discover "opportunities for studying ongoing, everyday supportive interaction" (Braithwaite et al., 1999: 124).

Internet chat rooms and message boards provide a valuable site for studying illness narratives. They provide a contained, textual context that is conducive to studying narrative practices and everyday supportive interactions. Unlike traditional research in face-to-face support groups, members of online groups remain relatively anonymous to other members of the group and the researcher (see also Chapter 1 in this volume). The identity of members in the group is thoroughly composed in the choices they make about the content and format of their messages. Messages become mini-autobiographies that implicate a certain identity for the author. Here the self is thoroughly presented in a textual and narrative form that precludes other personal identifiers (that is, appearance, gestures, tone of voice).

By observing online message board postings, this study attends to illness narratives as they are practiced by "the afflicted themselves" (Hyden, 1997: 64). Rather than use an interview method involving formal questions between researcher and subject, this study concentrates on the conversational interactions between group members who share the common experience of having a chronic illness. This was decided based on the supposition that posing interview questions would change or influence the narrative style, and thus the types of narrative resources, that members of the group would drawn upon to talk about their experiences. The messages provided examples of conversational texts happening in real time and highlight the everyday narrative practices that characterise member's experiences of illness and the ways in which members draw on various narrative resources to accomplish identity.

METHOD

The Internet has become a key resource for gaining knowledge and support with regard to health and illness. Statistics Canada (2004) reported that in 2003 almost two-thirds (65%) of Canadian households had at least one member who used the Internet to search for medical or health-related information. Searching for health information on the Internet is now the third most popular use after e-mail and general browsing. For many people with chronic illness, the Internet is likely one of the first places to seek health information following diagnosis or the onset of symptoms. In choosing to explore sites that addressed chronic illness, I began by simply conducting an Internet search using a general search engine (www.google.ca/) just as someone who was newly diagnosed might look for a web site or information. Key words were "googled" to find support groups for chronic illnesses, for example, 'multiple sclerosis support groups'. The search generated thousands of web sites in a matter of seconds. Search parameters identified numerous online health and illness websites for chronic illnesses such as multiple sclerosis, cancer, HIV/AIDS, diabetes. To narrow down the possibilities, only the first few pages of listings were considered.

After a preliminary review of a number of possible sites, it became clear that selecting a site would not be as open as initially thought. According to online site disclaimers, many sites would not allow research or survey activity. Chat rooms and message boards that were sponsored or facilitated by medical organisations or pharmaceutical companies often included many pages of disclaimers. For example, one site listed thirteen message board guidelines including the following regarding online research: "The use of the message boards for gathering information for surveys and research studies is prohibited. You may inform people of a survey and invite them to participate by writing to you personally. Otherwise, these posts will be deleted." Disclaimers and restrictions of this kind speak to a broader discussion about the ethics of online research. According to Bakardjieva and Feenberg (2000: 233) "social life in cyberspace defies the existing procedures for obtaining informed consent from research subjects and groups". As the level and scope of online research continues to develop new ethical bodies are being set up to create guidelines for ethical conduct (Eysenbach, 2001).

While some sites were restrictive, web sites that were created, maintained and facilitated by independent individuals not affiliated with any organisation tended to be more open and welcoming. My personal interest and knowledge of multiple sclerosis led to the decision to focus on a web site for multiple sclerosis (MS). After considering a number of sites, one active online support group for people with MS and their families was selected. The site was founded and facilitated by someone with MS because, as she put it, she had "always worked and needed something to do…" and when asked she expressed surprise at the popularity of the site. At the time of the study the number of registered members in the group had reached 400 (see also Chapter 9 in this volume).

This MS web site offered both a real time chat room for group members and also an open public message board. To post a message on the board, it was necessary to join the group through a major chat room facilitator. However, posted messages could be accessed and read publicly without joining. In this study, care was taken to inform members of the researcher's intentions and the context of the research. With respect for the best interests of group members, full disclosure of the research was provided in an introductory online message posting to the group. The introductory message requested permission from online group members to conduct research regarding the stories and support they shared online. It also indicated that any information taken from the site would be made anonymous and messages that members wished not to be referenced would not be used.

Within twenty minutes of posting the Introductory Message, group members began responding with welcoming permission and encouragement. Once initial contact was made, I remained an observer in the group. I did not pose formal interview questions nor direct the online conversations. The intent of the study was to observe the spontaneous narratives taking place between group members who shared the experience of having MS. It is my supposition that the conversations and subsequent narrative practices shared between group members to story experiences would be influenced or impacted if formal questions were posed to the group.

Online observations took place over the course of two months (eight weeks) between November and January. The site was monitored daily. Posted messages were copied and saved in a word processing document, as they appeared online (i.e., text, grammar, pictures). Over the course of the eight weeks over 150 conversations were collected as posted on the message board. Messages were initially collected and reviewed by the date on which they appeared on the message board. They were sorted and reviewed according to the online titles given by the members (such as "Help with meds", "Newly diagnosed"). Online members who began a new conversational thread gave titles to their message board postings. The titles of the message postings served to inform group members of the topic, indicate the urgency of the message, and pique the interest of readers encouraging them to reply or respond.

Online Group Member's Responses to Introductory Script
Welcome. There are really great people here.
I feel that the more people understand about this disease, the more they can support people touched by MS. Also, the greater the number of people who know about MS, the greater society's push will be for a cure.
MONIQUE, GO FOR IT THE MORE PUBLICITY THE BETTER FOR US. GOOD LUCK
Monique, I think personally what you are doing is wonderful! I'll help anyway I can
Take care and I hope you enjoy the site
I don't know if my experience will help you at all, but if it does, you are more than welcome to use it.
I hope this helps you Monique. I think what you are doing is great.

An initial review of the message postings provided an overall general impression of discursive characterisations and themes. Due to the larger volume of message board postings, a number of message samples were selected that best represented narrative resources that members called upon as they shared stories and support. The message samples in this chapter are presented as they appeared online (such as text, font style and so on) however, they have been edited for brevity, privacy and anonymity. Message samples for the project are discussed as they exemplify the prevalent discursive themes of the messages, the socially meaningful narrative resources used by members, and their implications for accomplishing identity.

RESOURCEFULLY RESTORYING THE SELF: MEDICAL TALK, SOCIAL MEANING, PERSONAL EXPRESSION, AND STORYING THE EXPERIENCE OF MS

Exploring how group members used narrative resources to accomplish their identities prompted consideration of what narrative themes and characterisations people call upon to convey who they are, as well as how narrative resources are practiced in their messages (Holstein and Gubrium, 2000). Holstein and Gubrium's (2000: 94) "analysis of interpretive practice" provided a methodological approach that allowed for flexibility to consider both *how* people tell stories about illness (practices) and *what* is involved in telling the story (narrative resources). The ability to take up the composition of the narrative and the discursive circumstances or contexts from which it is composed provided a unique perspective where we are invited to witness how the self is narratively accomplished. In other words, an analysis of interpretive practice offers a way to integrate how people talk about their experience of chronic illness, what culturally available narrative resources are implicated as they do so, and how these stories work to accomplish identity.

Analytic bracketing does not hold narrative practices or the resources that inform them as a standard discursive reality. Rather, it allows for a deliberation of the active interplay between personal and cultural narratives of illness. It alternately contemplates how people share experiences of illness narratives with what structures and contexts are implicated as they are expressed. Narratives are seen to be experientially real and are taken for what they represent in the moment, for those who are doing the narrating. Employing Holstein and Gubrium's (2000: 95) method of "analytic bracketing" does not aim to limit or define the ways that we talk about illness. It requires us to concentrate on the discursive interplay between resources and construction thus allowing us to glimpse the narrative possibilities for accomplishing identity. In the analysis for this study, online message samples are presented and discussed as they relate to four identifiable thematic narrative resources emerging from the data: medical talk, social meanings, personal expression, and storying the experience of MS.

Medical Talk : Diagnosis, Symptoms, Treatment

The majority of the messages posted by members of the online group exemplified how readily medical discourse has been taken up to accomplish identity. Discussions of diagnosis, symptoms and treatments were the most prevalent narrative resources drawn upon. Members of the online group authenticated membership – and identity – in the group as someone diagnosed, waiting to be diagnosed, or not yet diagnosed. Messages reflected unique experiential understandings of the diagnostic process, the symptoms attributed to MS, and the treatments available. Members sought or offered advice based on narrative resources provided by medical discourse but in doing so transposed the information in a way that made it personal and individual.

About Multiple Sclerosis (MS)

In order to contextualise the narratives presented in this study it is important to provide some background information about the illness that members in the online group are experiencing.

- MS is the most common neurological disease affecting young adults in Canada.
- MS can cause loss of balance, impaired speech, extreme fatigue, double vision and paralysis.
- Canadians have one of the highest rates of multiple sclerosis in the world.
- Every day, three more people in Canada are diagnosed with MS.
- MS was first identified and described by a French neurologist, Dr. Jean-Martin Charcot, in 1868.
- We don't know what causes MS but researchers are closer to finding the answer.

Source: MS Society of Canada *http://www.mssociety.ca/en/information/default.htm*

Diagnosis

Multiple Sclerosis (MS) does not generally come upon people suddenly. Individuals may experience several years of physical discomfort, temporary bouts with disability, or a gradual decline in ability before ever seeking medical advice. The action of seeking medical advice is different for everyone. Generally speaking, it is only when physical discomforts or abilities become severe or do not diminish that a person seeks advice from medical and other health professionals. In some cases, this leads to a quick and clear definition, while in other cases, the 'relief' of having a diagnosis – of giving a name to what ails us – is elusive and frustrating. Faith in the experts to provide an answer often becomes a key focus. Once a diagnosis is made, the reality of this new label prompts a re-evaluation of identity -- a need to restory the self in terms of the medical definition while at the same time retaining a sense of pre-diagnosis identity, integrating new symptomatic descriptions and learning to incorporate new terminology to describe the self.

For members of the online group, diagnosis was a powerful narrative resource for accomplishing identity. Members presented themselves in terms of being diagnosed, not diagnosed, not yet diagnosed, or waiting to be diagnosed. Members most often provided this information in their first time postings (for example, even in my own introductory message posting, I inadvertently identified myself as "not having been diagnosed"). In response to first time postings long-time members responded by providing information about their own diagnosis as a way of welcoming a new member.

Diagnosis

i'm... my nickname is really... i was diagnosed in oct. 2000. i had been having problems for a couple of years before that. i remember thinking i was really out of shape and that if i excercised more my legs would stop feeling so weak. boy was i wrong on that one!! the more i excercised the shakier my legs got. then i decided that i couldn't walk without feeling unbalanced because i was anemic or something. wrong again!! one night while sitting on the couch it felt like one of my kids was dropping cold water on my feet. the kids were no where around. when i told my doctor she decided to do an mri and the rest is history.

Hi... i was dx nov.2000 as of last year... ...like you for years i could not figure out what was wrong with me i never went to see a doctor until my left leg became parylyzed at first i ended up in the emergency room.luckily i was dx right away my neuro said my first outward sign was when i had optic neuritis... ...when i got my dx it sure did answer a lot of questions about how i was feeling for years.i suppose i should have gone to see a doctor sooner but i did not know how to describe what was going on with my body i figured they would think i was nuts !! 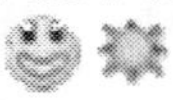

I still haven't received a diagnosis **yet**! ...My two Neurologists (Tweedle Dumb and Tweedle Dumber) still don't know what is wrong. ...(test) showed clear so Dumb said no MS even though I have sevaral lesions..., he said symptoms mean nothing; alot of people have symptoms.

That is good news you can all stop your meds!! You just have symptoms and not MS!!

...All I want is a diagnosis and I can't get one because nothing is wrong. I guess; that's what I'll have on my tombstone - "there was something wrong but we don't know what." I lost my mind but not my humor. When I lose that you'll know it's really bad. ...my friend called yesterday and his brother has Parkinsons and it took 18 years to diagnose; maybe there **is** hope for me! I only have to wait 17 more years; I am sure it will fly by.

In the first message, sample group members introduce themselves using narrative resources referring to family roles as well as their experiences of 'getting a diagnosis'. In the final message posting shown here, a member expresses frustration at waiting for a diagnosis. Calling upon narratives resources that value the education and experience of medical professionals, the member personally draws on other narratives resources; in this case literary, taken from a children's story to describe her experience with some sarcasm and humour[1]. The importance of a timely diagnosis also evidenced by the reference made to a friend's brother's experience with a diagnosis of Parkinson's. Being diagnosed provides credibility to members' stories giving them a sense of permission to begin restorying themselves as someone with MS. As this member awaits a diagnosis, there is uncertainty with regard to symptoms and identity.

Diagnosis as someone with MS becomes a way of presenting an authentic identity that meets the local culture of the group. It positions a member within the group by defining their experiences in terms of the available narrative resources provided by medical discourse. Certainly, the process of diagnosis and the experiences of being diagnosed are different for all members of the group but being able to name the outcome of those experiences in one way – multiple sclerosis – is an important step in accomplishing identity.

Symptoms

MS is most commonly described as a disease where the symptoms are different for everyone; however, medical discourse provides common symptom terminology for MS. Members in the group were skilled at talking about symptoms in medical terms and integrating these terms into personal narratives. The online support group provided a place to discover if a member's symptoms were representative of having MS. In message postings about symptoms, members often asked others for clarification about symptoms they were experiencing.

As the sample indicates, members creatively develop and share a special terminology for certain symptoms that are specific to MS. In requesting information about a "tightness and numbing feeling in the upper body", a member discovers that not only is this symptom a common one but it has been given special names by those who experience it -- "MS Hug" or "the girdle effect". This provides a local narrative resource that helps members define themselves as someone who has MS. In this way, identity is actively constructed as members position their experiences in terms of personal narrative resources provided by others.

[1] "Tweedle Dumb and Tweedle Dumber" refers to two dimwitted characters (Tweedledum and Tweedledee) in the classic tale, Alice's Adventures in Wonderland by Lewis Carroll (1865).

Members responding to the initial request often confirm a similar experience making this a symptom that members may call upon to identify with having MS.

Symptoms

Does anyone have a problem with tightness and numbing in there upper body.It not painful just annoying. 

Yes! Honey!
It's called the "MS Hug" and can stay with you for a while but WILL go away!
I thought it was my bra or tight clothes or just plain fat!
However, once you know what the cause is, the problem seems less stressful.
Hope all goes OK with you! LOL!

I've heard it called "the girdle" effect. I get it all the time from one side of my stomache to the other. I also have the "tightness" around my chest too, but that could be from other things... or just plain getting old and shrinking! LOL

Treatments

Medical research into treatments for MS are abundant and learning about treatment availability, side effects, and treatment efficacy were popular topics of discussion in the online group studied here.[2] Although Internet sites for pharmaceutical companies and other medical or health sites provide volumes of information about MS treatments, membership in the online group offers an experiential and individual perspective. Members learn the medical terminology of treatments and then take up this language to restory their experiences in personal ways when talking with others. Identifying oneself as knowledgeable and experienced with certain treatments further solidifies group membership and identity as someone with MS. As medical research continues to offer up new and improved versions of numerous pharmaceutical treatments for MS, members create their own local jargon for talking about treatment options often abbreviating the most predominant treatment choices by referring to them as the ABCRs (Avonex, Betaseron, Copaxone, Rebif).

In this message sample, members work diligently to share their experiences with the "ABCRs" and in doing so draw on a number of narrative resources to story their identities. Messages include references to significant social relationships, career, and physical and psychological experiences (for example, mom, spouse, employee, informed consumer, depression).

[2] Message postings regarding medical and pharmaceutical treatments were significantly more common although in a few cases members briefly discussed complementary and alternative treatments (e.g. massage, tai chi).

Treatments

Hi everyone! I need a little help making up my mind. I went back to the neuro and he felt that it was time for me to choose one of the ABC's. I have narrowed it down to Copaxone or Avonex. I have gone to the individual drug websites, looked in some drug books to get information about them. Now I thought it might be good to ask those of you who are on or have been on either one of these your thoughts. I know that results/experiences may vary. I am a young mom with two kids… I work part time… my spouse is not always home to help out… I have alot of depressing coplications… …I didn't list my life elements not to whine, but to maybe help you to give your point of view and advise. …

I have been on Copaxone for just over a year now. Things have got better and the daily jab is so small it's not worth worrying about. I was told it takes 6 months to start working and I would go along with that. People say the jab does nothing to you but I feel it has and would recommend it to anyone. Good luck with your choice Be as well as you can be

Do you have a problem with Interferons? I do. So I have to take Copaxone. When you are first starting out on the ABCR's you just make your best educated guess and go with it. You can always change. Of course I listened to everyone else about the flu symptoms of A for months before I decided that no drug was better than being sick with the flu ALL the time. I was on C for X years and progressed downward, so I tried B for X weeks and had a major set backs. So I went back to C. Yes you do need to take a drug because there is nothing else to offer at this point but trial and error is the only method that works in picking which one.

I was on Betasaron for X yrs. Had a major attack, lost my job and my insurance and Beta would not work with me for financial help. I had the flu like symptoms for the first X months.

I was on nothing for X months until Avonex approved to help. I love the once a week injection verses the every other day with Beta. …I have had no side effects from Avonex at all. Personally, I don't want to inject myself daily, as you would with Cop, but each person has diff needs and you will have to decide what works best for you.

Members identify themselves by stating which treatment they are on or have tried and why. And members present themselves as educated about the treatments from an experiential and individual standpoint. This leads to a restorying of self in terms of treatment experiences. Identity is accomplished with reference to treatment names and options chosen – "I chose Avonex" or "I have been on Copaxone". As well, the self is storied in light of personal experience – "things have got better" or "I had flu-like symptoms". Members encourage each other to "do what works best for you" and comment that making a choice is a "personal preference". These comments inform personal narratives that support individuality in treatment choices and yet positions identity in terms of what treatments are being used.

Social Meaning: Relationships and Roles

Whereas narrative resources provided by medical discourses contributed to how illness was storied by providing specific discursive guidelines concerning diagnosis, symptoms and treatments, it is the integration of a variety of socially meaningful narrative resources outside of medical talk that offer personal depth and meaning to illness narratives. Socially constructed through the discursive forces that prevail and predominate in our culture, social meanings of illness express more than just the physical manifestations of disease. They express the social, economic, and political realities of living with illness. How we come to talk about and *do* illness is closely intertwined with other social and cultural discourses in an artful and individual way. It is an "interpretive salvage operation" in which selves are "craft(ed) from the vast array of available resources" (Holstein and Gubrium, 2000: 153).

Invoking culturally relevant and available resources that have personal meaning, members more comfortably and successfully restory their experiences and their identity online. Many message postings contained what Holstein and Gubrium (2000: 169) call "biographical particulars". In narrating a story about the everyday going concerns of having illness, members often included socially relevant biographical particulars and effectively presented themselves in reference to their careers, marital status, and other life experiences. In doing so, members were "engaged in ordinary 'biographical work' to assemble aspects of personal history that can be used to bolster claims of and about themselves" (Holstein and Gubrium, 2000:169). The value of these claims is that they provide a wider context for the self that emerges from understood social values and narratives.

Relationships

It was evident from the majority of message postings that members do not experience illness in a socially isolated world. Relationships play a vital role in the social experience of illness giving it social and personal meaning. A powerful and long time cultural discourse in our society is one in which a person with illness is supported and aided by family members. We see in the next sample posting how group members draw on socially significant narrative resources about family and parenthood to resourcefully present the challenges that illness and social role expectations bring.

Here members draw on culturally available narrative resources about what it means to be a good parent while implicating narrative resources about taking responsibility for self. In this message, members integrate social narratives about parenthood and expectations of children and family to negotiate what it means to be a responsible parent with MS. There is a struggle to incorporate the idea that 'family should help family' in the case of illness, yet as a parent the first priority is still an expectation of caring for their children. Members share biographical particulars of parenthood to story identities first as parents and then as parents with MS. Identifying as parents they express a desire to be there for their children but in their experience with MS they draw on narratives about family helping family and that it is okay to ask for support. As one member stated, "...In all reality though it is really our family and friends that we do need to reach out to in our time of need".

Relationships

I know it was my fault I didn't take my cane

This is going to sound stupid, but I decided to walk home from my (grown child's) house. It started raining and I was getting soaked…It is not that far, but I should have know better …I fell in the door coming in. (My spouse) thought I had got a ride home. … they didn't have much gas so I didn't want to ask…

… I was just trying to save (them) from…wasting gas. …I just don't wan't to be a burden to people. That is why I didn't even want to ask for a ride....

I know where your coming from.My hubby …feels that there are no excuses for certain ways that the kids are or hwo they are.I am from the old school also but i know if it was my mom nomatter what she would have been in my car and she would not have to ask me there would have been no 2 ways about it. We should not excuse our kids for not doing because that in my opinion makes them feel that nothing else matters more then their needs.

… What i am trying to say is to you and everyone else is we do need some special help from time to time and our loved ones that we ourselves would bend over backwords for should help.When we were all in better shape i am sure that most of us did plenty … … A ride home ---- a phone call-------a trip to a store etc should not be a burden for people who we love and love us!!!!

…i know how you feel. i have X kids… … my…son is great. he helps me and dad all the time. when he gets up in the morning he asks what we need him to do today. the X-year old is very understanding, too. when we have problems doing things he always says "it's just part of living with ms." it's really cute. the others often make me feel like dad and i got ms just so we could inconvenience them. hang in there and next time on the *ride* home don't forget your cane….

…i am so sorry to hear about what happened to you how inconsiderate of your (grown child) …you need to start thinking about what you can do or cant do and speak up for your self and say NO i cant do that! … i never leave my house with out my cane even for a very short distance, i am sure that you will always be taking your cane along

Roles

Although there are many ways to think about being a productive member of society the prevalent concerns expressed by members of the online group also focused greatly on careers and employability.

Roles
… I work filltime …Since my diagnosis … Ive missed a great deal of work - …with each attack depending on the severity and symptoms as it all affects my ability to work and be productive. My employer is VERY understanding and encourages me to stay home as long as I need to get better. …but I always rush back to work (trying to be as normal as possible) only to get sick again…I am now off once again…I feel soooo guilty not being there. Is there anyone in the same boat as me or have most people out there taken time for themselves to get better 'fully' before going back to work. … If I ever lost my job Id be crushed.....Any advice or people in simliar situations? I am having guilt problems too. Though I have worked through most of my attacks… since I dont have a Definate DX, I cannot justify missing a lot of work. … THere is not a whole lot I can do, I have to work for the insurance and without a DX i cannot get the meds and without the Dx I cannot get disability. I would have to say if your empolyer encourages you to stay off work until you are better take full advantage of their encouragement. … I was not as fortunate as you, I was working …when I had my first bad attack I was off work for about X months. … Before my neurologist could even type up my diagnosis my employer terminated me …there was alot of discrimination issues, my boss had the nerve to ask me to my face "What happens if you have another attack later on down the road, are we suppose to accomidate you by letting you take off work?"

Expressions of guilt, anxiety, and concern over not being able to work are further underscored by social realities that have not yet created space for alternative working lifestyles such as those that may be required in the case of chronic illness. Here members story their identity in terms of their employment experiences indicating just how prevalent and powerful this social narrative resource is as an indicator of identity.

Personal Expression

The ability to communicate online can be both liberating and limited. For those who have found this virtual space to share support and stories, it is a haven for expressing doubts, fears, and concerns about having a chronic illness. It is also a place to commiserate and celebrate with others who share similar experiences. Online support lacks the usual visual cues that expressions of support entail (such as eye contact, gestures, touch, tone of voice). With no "scenic presence" (Holstein and Gubrium, 2000: 190), online members do not share social spaces nor see or hear each other in person so there is more reliance on textual and visual cues to relate personal expressions and in essence personality and identity.

In the message samples reviewed in this study, it was pleasantly evident that there was more to posting a message than just the text. Members used different fonts and colours, and included emotional signifiers (emoticons), pictures, special online names, and positive sign-offs ("Be as well as you can be"), thereby, presenting a unique identity online. Holstein and Gubrium (2000, p. 187) draw our attention to these "material mediations" for storying the self, suggesting that the stories we construct are mediated by our material environment, social settings and the physical cues around us. The online support group is a unique example of this.

The addition of a smiley face  or a sad face  within the messages expressed the emotions of the person, or indicated their view on a discussion providing insight about a member's opinions and beliefs. Pictures used in messages provided metaphoric social and cultural resources that communicated information about identity (like lone wolf). By adding visual characterisations, members include a sense of individuality and emotion in their messages. Even in the simplest textual messages presented online, we gain a sense of who a person is by how they construct and present their messages. Restricted by the material mediations online, members endeavoured to assemble available materials in their own unique ways adding personal expression and identity cues to their messages.

The sample box below displays some of the visual resources (emoticons, pictures) used by members in their message postings. Other unique characteristics that members used to convey personal expressions included different styles and colours of text. Special care was taken to preserve the message samples throughout these results as they appeared online. However, to preserve confidentiality, special online names and sign-off messages have been omitted from the message samples.

Personal Expression

Emoticons

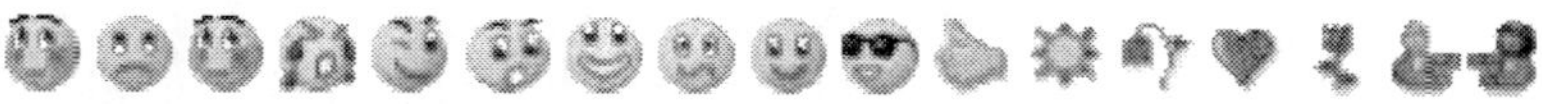

Pictures

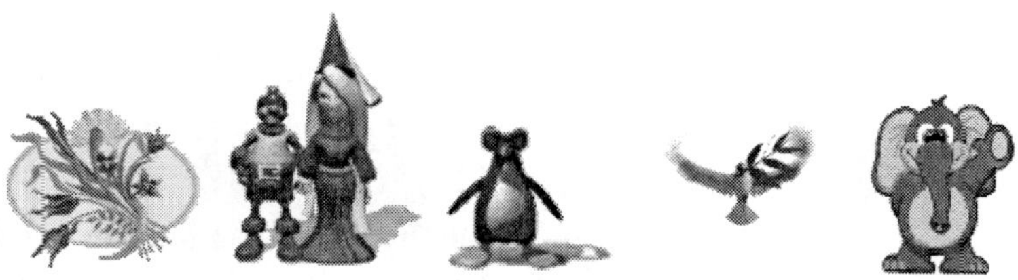

STORYING THE EXPERIENCE OF MS : SUPPORTING OTHERS, BEING POSITIVE

"People tell stories not just to work out their own changing identities, but also to guide others who will follow them" (Frank, 1995: 17). In a final analysis of the message postings, it was evident that members in the group were routinely generous with encouragement, appreciation, and support. Referencing their personal experiences with MS, members acknowledged difficulties but did so in a positive and supportive manner. There was little talk of "why me?" and more talk about facing adversity and being "as well as you can be". Members used humour and enthusiasm in their messages. Message postings that were seen as rude, negative, or of a commercial nature were quickly deleted. Local group "conventions and constraints" evidently required members to remain positive, supportive and on topic (Holstein and Gubrium, 2000: 182).

Two predominant local narratives for storying the experience of MS emerged from the data -- supporting others and being positive. These two ways of storying the experience of MS are characteristic of almost every message posted during the study. The prevalence of this way of talking about illness experiences indicates the power and significance of this narrative resource for storying experiences and identity as someone with MS.

Supporting Others

Group members regularly identified themselves as supportive and productive members in their online and real life MS communities. Taking up this supportive role indicated an authentic position as someone with MS. It was a key signifier of acceptance into a community and identity as someone with MS. The founder of the online group expresses the value and importance she placed on helping others.

Supporting Others
What made me start this site is that I realized that is that I knew that I was not alone in dealing with MS. I would start a site and even if only 1 person joined, that made it worth it. Did I expect to get over 400 ? Not in my Dreams Also, I have always worked and I needed something to do.
In response to a message of distress, online members provided the following messages of support… I know (from your post) that you are going through a hard time, but things will be looking up! If it's prayer you want, prayer you will get! There are many members here that are close to God and I'm sure we'll all put in a prayer for you. Even those that aren't religious will probably have some nice thoughts and well wishes. If you ever need a shoulder to lean on I am here. If you would like you can e-mail me at… I realize that in this situation there is so much stress and that alone is bad for the MS. … …Just to let you know you arent the only person out there dealing with these same problems. I think if you could share with us a little more detail about your situation you would find that some of us are going through the same things that you are and we

might actually be able to help each other out. Be strong things will work out. This is the best place to come for comfort and support and just to vent….
We all understand how you feel as we are all fighting daily battles, fears, and doubts. This is the best place to come where we can share our joys and sadness and others can relate to. … Remember we are all here to help each other… you have our positive thoughts and we all wish you the strength to face each day knowing you are not alone.

Members continually posted messages of support for others that worked to confirm their authentic position in the group via their own personal understandings of having MS. In the sample above members draw on a number of socially meaningful narrative resources and local group narratives thereby accomplishing their identity online (such as religion, spiritually, strength by virtue of group membership and similar life experiences, value of sharing emotional distress).

Being Positive

Being positive and hopeful are key narratives for storying identity as someone with MS. From brief words of encouragement, i.e. “good luck”, “be well”, to longer messages of support and guidance, members of the group actively and continuously storied their experiences in terms of being positive. The “be positive” narrative appeared in some form in almost every message posted during the study. The final message samples were taken from a variety of available message postings. The samples indicate the sincerity and value that this group placed on this local narrative resource and suggest just how important this way of storying the experience of MS is for accomplishing identity in the group.

Being Positive
… Our physical difficulties are circumstances that we cannot control but our mental circumstances are a choice for most of us. We can choose to be depressed and sad or we can choose to make the best of it and do the best that we can. When we are truly doing the best that we can, we cannot do more than that. If one thinks about that for a minute it should give some peace. When one is at point such as this the only acceptable choice is to make the best of it. Don't ask "why me" because there is no answer. It is frustrating to ask a question that has no answer so don't bother with the question. This may sound simple and that is because it is simple. It is a simple choice, your choice.
MS… i always remind myself i definatly could be worse (will I is Question that I can't answer and try never to harp on at all). I do not resent that I have MS because I am a person who feels instead of why me? ,I say to myself why NOT me.Why someone else and not me. …we have to go on and make the best of each day we can. …I though am extreamly grateful for days that I feel good .

> ... the human spirit that is in all of us can overcome any obstacle... MS is a problem for sure but it isn't anything that we can't handle. Since being diagnosed one of the most rewarding experiences of my life is helping others with ms. Never in my wildest dreams did I ever expect this to be the case but it is. MS has not been a negative influence on my life. I guess it was in the beginning but for the past X yrs. or so it has been like a good teacher. Some of the lessons are hard but you really learn things that otherwise might have passed you by. ...

As the sample excerpts indicate, narrative resources for doing chronic illness guide members to “do the best you can”, “find alternatives”, “don’t ask why me”. These gentle directives inform members of the importance of staying positive and persevering. And because they appear so often, they become a guide for the group and for others to recognise that living with chronic illness takes strength, character and a positive attitude. Just as medical discourse provides certain narrative resources, i.e. diagnosis, symptoms, for talking about chronic illness which help to define identity (e.g. I have MS); the way that members talk about personal experiences of illness (“we have a choice”, “do the best you can”) guides others to story the self in locally appropriate ways (i.e. positive, persevering).

A Narrative Map for Chronic Illness

This study takes up a central position between narrative resources and narrative practices -- one providing the building blocks for constructing identity and the other providing an active and discursive space for assembling and practicing how the self is storied everyday. At this theoretical intersection, we have examined the characteristic options that are available for people with chronic illness to accomplish identity. Attending to how members narratively construct and negotiate messages online affords us the ability to discern what the most prevalent narrative options for storying the self might be.

The analysis of the study suggests that there is a pattern for how members of the online support group draw on narrative resources to story their experiences and accomplish their identity online. The prevalence with which some narrative resources are drawn upon by members of the online group suggests that there is a “narrative map” that frames and guides how to talk about chronic illness, in this case multiple sclerosis (Frank, 1995; Pollner and Stein, 1996). This narrative map is not a formal template. It is an informal guide for members of the group to negotiate, draw upon, and contribute to as they come to accomplish identity as someone with chronic illness.

New members come to the group seeking ways to story their experiences when the general ways of talking about their physical discomforts and limited abilities no longer fit. Members of the online group studied here framed and expressed their experiences online in terms of medical talk about diagnosis, symptoms and treatments. These became the pervasive ways of talking about both experiences of MS and the self. Learning the narrative languages of other discourse communities (such as medical) members integrated this language into their own narratives of illness. Members also incorporated socially meaningful narrative resources to story their identity using biographical particulars (that is being a parent, employment). They incorporated the changes that illness brings into other socially meaningful ways of talking about experiences and self. The great number of references to social relationships indicates that this is a significant element of the narrative map for chronic illness.

Over time members became increasingly knowledgeable about the specific discursive frameworks for storying the illness experiences that characterise MS (that is being positive, supporting others). Members of the group drew on social and medical narrative resources and were actively engaged in practicing and producing their own personal narrative resources, guiding others about how to talk about MS. Through this active dialogue and interaction with others the narrative resources were reified, challenged, embraced and made richer from the addition of member's personal experiences. They were refined and developed as they were resourcefully practiced and shared by members of the group. All of the narrative resources became part of a dynamic online repertoire for talking about the experience of MS.

CONCLUSION: A RESOURCEFULLY PRACTICED SELF

The work of restorying the self is a complex and exhausting process. To hold down and essentialise the self in terms of personality traits or inherently individual characteristics loses sight of the active, variable, and continuous possibilities for discursively accomplishing identity. Faced with an excess of possible narrative resources and a multitude of sites for narrative practice, members of online support groups for chronic illness frame their experiences and identity in terms of the narrative resources accessible to them in everyday interactions. Online support groups offer people with chronic illness an opportunity to actively engage in restorying the self by drawing on personal and social narrative resources. Group members are guided by these narrative resources and map out an authentic and acceptable identity for others and for themselves. The self is resourcefully practised.

In this chapter, we considered how drawing from a shared pool of available narrative resources (for example, medical, social, personal), members of the online group actively work to interpret and express themselves in light of their personal experience. A negotiation and translation of sorts occurs as members share personal experiences with others using different styles, characteristics and choices of expression (that is emoticons, special names, attitudes, beliefs). As Holstein and Gubrium (2000: 11) suggest, "self-interpretation involves social input to be sure, but it's also a matter of interpretive practice, of putting forth the effort and engaging in the everyday work of orienting to each other as selves". In the sample messages, personal experience is seen to work as both a resource and a filter for engagement with available narrative resources. By expressing and interpreting available resources in individual ways a self is presented that is at once "practical, variegated, and artfully and deliberately built up in various shapes and dimensions for dealing with the circumstances in which it is located" (Holstein and Gubrium, 2000: 10).

Attending to illness narratives opens up discursive space for exploring the narrative resources that are drawn upon to story the experience of chronic illness. In online message postings, the illness experience is textually crafted into something uniquely individual and yet it holds to socially accepted narrative structures and those essentialised by local group narratives. Taken as a whole, the online messages indicate patterns or narrative maps for how to do illness. Reflecting on how these narrative maps are practiced and shared in everyday interactions, we gain a more nuanced understanding of the experience of chronic illness and the discursive moves that are implicated as members share stories and support to accomplish identity online.

ACKNOWLEDGEMENTS

Special thanks to the members of the MS online support group whose stories appear in this chapter.

REFERENCES

[1] Bakardjieva, M. and Feenberg, A., 2001, 'Involving the Virtual Subject: Conceptual, Methodological and Ethical Dimensions' *Journal of Ethics and Information Technology*, vol. 2, no. 4, pp. 233-240.

[2] Braithwaite, D. O., Waldron, V. R. and Finn, J, 1999, 'Communication of Social Support in Computer-Mediated Groups for People With Disabilities', *Health Communication*, vol. 11, no. 2, pp. 123-151.

[3] Charmaz, K., 1983, 'Loss of Self: A Fundamental Form of Suffering in the Chronically Ill', *Sociology of Health & Illness*, Vol. 5, no. 2, pp. 168-195.

[4] Conrad, P., 1990, 'Qualitative Research on Chronic Illness: A Commentary on Method and Conceptual Development', *Social Science & Medicine*, vol. 30, no. 11, pp. 1257-1263.

[5] Eysenbach, G. and Till, J. E., 2001, 'Information in Practice: Ethical Issues in Qualitative Research on Internet Communities', *British Medical Journal. <http://bmj. bmjjournals.com/cgi/content/full/323/7321/1103>*

[6] Frank, A. W., 1995, *The Wounded Storyteller: Body, Illness, and Ethics*, The University of Chicago Press, Chicago.

[7] Holstein, J. A. and Gubrium, J. F., 2000, *The Self We Live By: Narrative Identity in a Postmodern World*, Oxford University Press, New York.

[8] Hunt, L. M., 2000, 'Strategic Suffering: Illness Narratives as Social Empowerment Among Mexican Cancer Patients', in C. Mattingly and L. C. Garro (eds.), *Narrative and the Cultural Construction of Illness and Healing*, pp. 88-107, University of California Press, Berkeley.

[9] Hyden, L.C., 1997, 'Illness and Narrative', *Sociology of Health & Illness*, vol. 19, no. 1, pp. 48-69.

[10] Pollner, M. and Stein, J., 1996, 'Narrative Mapping of Social Worlds: The Voice of Experience in Alcoholics Anonymous', *Symbolic Interaction*, vol. 19, no. 3, pp. 203-233.

[11] Radley, A., 1994, *Making Sense of Illness*, Sage Publications, London.

[12] Reissman, C. K.,1990, 'Strategic Uses of Narrative in the Presentation of Self and Illness: A Research Note', *Social Science & Medicine*, vol. 30, no. 11, pp. 1195-1200.

[13] Scheerhorn, D, 1997, 'Creating Illness-Related Communities in Cyberspace', in J. Richard, L. Street, W. R. Gold and T. Manning (eds.), *Health Promotion and Interactive*

Technology: Theoretical Applications and Future Directions, pp. 171-185, Lawrence Erlbaum Associates Publishers, Mahwah, New Jersey.

[14] Statistics Canada, 2004, 'Household Internet Use Survey. Science, Innovation and Electronic Information Division'.<*http://www.statcan.ca/Daily/English/040708/d040708a.htm*>

[15] Williams, S. J., 2000, 'Chronic Illness as Biographical Disruption or Biographical Disruption as Chronic Illness? Reflections on a Core Concept', *Sociology of Health & Illness*, vol. 22, no. 1, pp. 40-67.

In: Health Research in Cyberspace
Editor: Pranee Liamputtong, pp. 229-241
ISBN 1-59454-819-6

Chapter 14

RESEARCHING THE DIGITAL NARRATIVES OF HEALTH, ILLNESS AND THE BODY

Michael Hardey

INTRODUCTION

This chapter focuses on accounts that individuals write about their health and illness, which are created through and published on the Internet. Enter a phase like 'the story of my illness' into any search engine and a vast number of potential experiential accounts of health and illness will be revealed. This influx of writing about the self is not simply accounted for by new technology. We live in times that have lost the certainties and restrictions of previously prescribed roles, whether resulting from the means of production, gender roles or belief systems that have involved a process of individualisation (Heelas et al., 1996). The consequent detrationalised and uncertain postindustrial culture confronts us with new risks while at the same time opening up new opportunities (Beck, 1992). Information is central to our ability to monitor, manage and make sense of our experiences and make choices that are continually presented to us. As Giddens (1991) suggests, our thoughts and actions are shaped by a process of casting back over previous experiences and idea in a reflexive. It can be said that individuals 'make themselves' through the choices that constitute a lifestyle. For Giddens (1991, 1994), choices include decisions about consumption, the body and personal relationships, all which equate with 'good' health. Health (or lack of it) has become central to self-identity in a culture that values thinness and fitness and views lack of health as a problem calling for a cure. Consequently, accounts of illness are spread across the popular media and stories about how individuals have 'reformed' apparently fat or unfit bodies or addicted lifestyles form the subject for whole television series and features in magazines. Not surprisingly, the Internet as a portal to information is now central to many of our consumer choices and our understanding of risk (Hardey 2004a). As this book demonstrates, the Internet has also opened up many new spaces where ideas about health and illness are created, exchanged and negotiated.

The narratives I want to consider here stem from a long tradition of auto/biographical writing but have taken on new forms as people take advantage of the potential of new digital media. In this chapter, I will look at how we may identify health related narratives published on web pages and blogs. I will then consider the matter of ethics and how we can analysis digital narratives. Before we proceed, we must first attempt to understand the roots of digital narratives and their relationship to the new technologies of the Internet.

The Internet and the Structuring of the Mediated World

In the late 1960s, the scientific community had developed various systems that linked together computers so that users could exchange digital information. Taken up by the military in the mid 1970s, what we now recognise as the Internet did not emerge from academic circles until the early 1980s. Berners-Lee (200: 133), who designed the World Wide Web as a network of connections between various forms of content, noted that "the web is more a social creation than a technical one. I designed it for social effect...". The University I worked in the 1980s used Apple Macs that were driven by the now ubiquitous graphical user interface. Thus, while others struggled with 'command lines' and other mysteries of DOS, I enjoyed the first popular 'point and click' environment. The downside is that I never plumed the depths of computer code or can lay claim to any great technical expertise (other than that where to place a paperclip when confronted with a 'sad Mac icon'). Like most Internet users, it is through the integrated graphical browser that I engage with the digital world. This user focused technology remains central to the continued expansion of the Internet that has generated "an information revolution of unprecedented magnitude" (Jadad and Gagliardi, 1998: 61). Indeed, the consequent global interactive web of information has been seen to provide the 'material basis' for the 'pervasive expansion' of 'the networking form of organisation' across all social structures (Castells, 1996: 468). In Castells comprehensive vision the 'information age' the amalgamation of text, audio and other formats into interactive digital media is regarded as having as much an impact as the spread of the alphabet in the reshaping of power relationships through information flows. This 'runaway world' (Giddens, 1991) formed around the new is media characterised by flows and liquidity (Bauman, 2003), a place where interactivity is inherent and all participants have similar opportunities to create and publish content. Rheingold's (1993) well know description of his experiences as a participant in the Whole Earth Lectronic Link (WELL) captures something of the excitement experienced by those fortunate enough to have access to the Internet in its early days. This enthusiasm was driven by the ability to write, publish and engage with others more or less instantly. For Rheingold, this recaptured a sense of community and produced a 'living encyclopaedia' constructed out of the freely given reciprocal advice by 'netizens'. The Internet is now a different place and occupied by far more users than the relatively privileged minority of the 1990s. It constitutes a space "neither private nor public . . . where private problems meet in a meaningful way . . . where ideas may be born and take shape as the "public good"" Bauman (1999: 3). The ability of anyone with access to a networked computer to write and publish content as well as engage with others remains the most revolutionary aspect of the Internet despite increasing commercialisation and attempts to impose regulation and control.

UNWIRED AND WIRED HEALTH NARRATIVES

The way the Internet has enabled users to write about their lives has led to what I have defined as the new genre of digital life-stories. This genre can be characterised as follows (Hardey, 2004b: 186).

Format and medium	Web pages and blogs that are inherently digital, dynamic, inclusive of text, pictures and other media.
Narrative pattern	Interweaving narratives that are loosely ordered by hyperlinks that are attached to an archive of material and other places on the Internet.
Writer and audience	Constructed and reconstructed for a global audience which read 'unique' narratives by making hyperlink choices.
Content	An individual life grounded in other people, localities and events.

Not only does the above categorisation help to identify such narratives, but it also places them in the context of a long history of writing about the self. Like digital life-stories, these past narratives were mediated in that they were read through an intervening medium (usually ink and paper) so that the experiences of the author were disembodied. Before the seventeenth century, few accounts of lives of either sex were published and those that were tended to focus on religion (Steedman, 1992). As literacy slowly spread, more people began to write about their experiences with a mind to publication or as a private diary or family journal. *The Autobiography of Mrs Alice Thornton* was written around 1696 as an account of the author's many illnesses, often associated with childbirth, and the deaths of many of her children. It was eventually published in1857 and is unusual, as it was not written by a member of the privileged classes. Significantly, while male writers were commonly concerned with often long-winded accounts of their military or political careers, it was women authors who entered into what we now recognise as a reflexive self-analysis of emotions and intimate feelings (Thomas, 1997). There is a project about the gendered nature of digital life-stories waiting to be done.

As a discipline, sociology signalled the significance of personal narratives in 1918 with the publication of *The Polish Peasant in Europe and America* (Thomas and Znaniecki, 1958) that contained letters and stories of individual lives. Freud used accounts of individual lives to establish what Giddens (1991) would recognise as an 'expert system' of the human condition. Such personal narratives may be seen to provide 'true' accounts of how people experience and live their lives through everyday 'dramas'. Autobiographies have also been associated with emancipation in that it is argued that they are "occasions for the staging of resistance" (Smith, 1993: 156). Indeed, such personal experiences described by women have a central place in feminist theory (Jackson, 2005). Within the sociology of health and illness 'lay narratives' are central to understanding the complexities of health (Lawton, 2003). Hence, what might be termed 'ordinary lives' gained wider audiences largely though the work of feminists, oral historians and other enterprises often associated with academic practice. It is important to recognise a division here between the common practice in health research to attempt to understand the intersections and discontinuities between individual experiences and expert clinical practice through qualitative interviews and auto/biographical narratives. The latter draw on the longer tradition of life-writing that may be constructed as a private project or with a potentially global audience in mind. Before we can consider these accounts further, we must first sketch in the background to the spaces they occupy on the Internet.

Writing on the Web: Convergence Around Browsers

There is a techno-determinism tendency in some research based on Information and Communication Technologies (ICTs) that treats the Internet itself as a 'black box'. However, information technology cannot be separated from its social settings which means we have contextualise the online in terms of its offline heritage. The story of evolution and role of ICTs is one of accident and often unforeseen social consequences. Perhaps, the best example is the way text messaging on mobile phones has come to be such an important mode of communication for young people. From the early days of the graphical web browser, individuals published their own personal home pages on the Internet. Initially, these tended give details of the author's employment and such pages are now often incorporated into employer's web pages where details of employee's background and projects are displayed. It required some technical skills to construct such pages using HTML language that set out the form of the material. Various 'point and click' driven software packages become available and simple versions were often to be found given away on the covers of computer magazines. Authors need a host or Internet Service Provider (ISP) so that their Web pages can be stored and accessed. Subsequently, Naughton (2003) notes that it took an individual with some technical experience seventeen minutes to create and publish a web page. Such a quickly constructed page would be likely to contain a relatively small amount of content and not include images, video and other material that can commonly be found on contemporary web pages. A study of web pages created by teenagers in the 1990s found that they typically included posters, pictures and music that were associated with their home life (Chandler and Roberts-Young, 1998). In effect, the construction of a web page was something of a project as is evident from the number of books published giving advice ranging from how to design a home page to how to attract visitors to your web site. Indeed, a whole new area of business emerged around professional web site design as the Internet commercialised and small business felt the need for a digital presence. Today, these companies utilise databases and site management technologies that require considerable skills and experience. While there are many millions of personal home pages, time and effort has to be spent to update, revise of add new content to them. This is significant because pages that are infrequently changed tend to date and fail to attract repeat visits from other users. The internet is highly dynamic and users seem to expect that web pages evolve and change so that those that remain static for extended periods begin to disappear from search engines and fall into the a grey background of neglected and infrequently visited sites. Personal homepages often include links to other sites that are annotated or included within the author's own text. This referencing of other sites is embedded in the culture of home pages, as it is through such links that sites can build up visitors and attract the attention of search engines. Lists of links to other sites that might be of interest to readers are frequently updated and in places annotations shift to become commentaries and advice in themselves. Indeed, these commentaries may include details of an individuals search for information or advice (for example about an illness or treatment) through the Internet in the form of what became called a web blog or bog (that is log of places visited on the web). Although the current form of the blog is commonly said to have emerged in the late1990s the concept can be traced to Berners-Lee's (2000) vision of a seamless web where both content can be as easily created as read. His original weblog is now archived by the World Wide Web Consortium.[11]

Until recently, most people used browsers (such as Mosaic, Explorer and so on) to view Web content and email (like Eudora and Outlook Express) to write and interact with others (see also Chapter 2 in this volume). The principle behind the development of the software that drives blogs was the desire to recapture the visions of a seamless web, make it easy for users to create a presence on the Internet and address the problem of personal web pages that were rarely revised. In effect, the blog marked a convergence of reading/viewing and authoring/publishing software through the medium of the Web browser. In other words, all the user needs in order to create a blog is access to a web browser. There is no need for a subscription to an ISP so that blogs may be created by people whose only route to the Internet is through cyber cafés or libraries. This freeing up from ISP membership and even the ownership of computers has led some to describe the blog as 'revolutionary' (Bennett, 2001) While blogs resemble web pages (in effect they are web pages but mediated through a interface that hides HTLM and other codes that both share), they generally adopt an incremental diary like approach with the contents displayed in a reverse chronology. However, a degree of caution in required here in that there is no generally accepted definition of what constitutes a blog and their form is one of the most rapidly changing areas of the Internet. It is now possible to find a 'Photoblog' that contain mostly photographs (the convergence of digital technologies manifest in digital cameras is has made a significant difference to the ease with which images may be published on the internet), a 'Moblog' that are created from a mobile phone or personal digital assistant by people as they travel and various other forms.

IDENTIFYING AND SAMPLING DIGITAL NARRATIVES

The Search

Health and illness forms a common thread in digital narratives as authors seek to make sense of their experiences. Indeed, for many it is the onset of a chronic condition or other health event that prompts them to seek information on the Internet (Hardey, 1999). The first problem that confronts the researcher is the identification of material on the Internet that is related to their substantive topic. For some, this may be defined by a medical condition such as diabetes. This diagnosed illness route is common in health research and has the advantage of being embedded in a defined set of symptoms and treatments. Like a consumer seeking information from the Internet, I have used a range of search engines and followed links on some web sites to produce an ever expanding set of potential material (Cline and Haynes,

1 http://info.cern.ch/

2001; see also Chapter 16 in this volume). The more defined the search is the less time will be taken up with viewing irrelevant material (Mann and Stewart, 2000). The adage 'more is less' is applicable to Internet research. This indicates that time spent devising clear inclusion and exclusion criteria is well used.

Search engines have their own limitations and priorities that may be more or less hidden to the user. Companies engaged in health related commercial activities have quickly extended their activities onto the Internet and their web pages tend to be prioritised by search engines (Goldsmiths, 2002). This manipulation of search engines came to the fore in 2002 with 'Google Bombing'. Bloggers found that Google favoured material with many links and updated content so that combined with careful use of keywords a blog could quickly force a path to the top of any search. In response, Google now has a distinct search engine devoted to blogs. Such manipulation means that a degree of tenacity and skill is required to tease out web pages and blogs related to health. In my view, any researched based on material from the Internet must use several search engines and researchers should have a familiarity with the way they track and compile material. It should also be noted that some search engines report meta sites like the BBC that will contain health information while other may ignore them. Remember that it is possible at this stage to confine searches to particular domains, languages or locations. Whatever strategy is employed it will quickly report a great many potential web pages and blogs. Many of these can be quickly examined by reading the brief notes attached to the universal resource location (url) displayed by the results of the search. Webrings (a group of Internet sites that are linked by subject and monitored by a 'ringmaster') organised around particular conditions may also be revealed and these can provide a useful additional source of web pages and blogs. It is also worth exploring newsgroups such as those found within Yahoo and elsewhere often have groups devoted to health diaries using blogs. Those accessing the Internet through university or other organisations should examine any codes of practice and where relevant discuss their research with the head of computing services. This is particularly important for those researching for material that may in some way be sexually or politically related. For example, a study of HIV risk behaviour related to people who are introduced via e-dating sites many require visiting web pages that in fact seek to sell sexual services or distribute pornographic material. A similar dilemma may confront other health researchers in that the body has been colonised by both medicine and the pornography industry (for example, a search for 'breast cancer' will reveal more than the naïve internet researcher might imagine).

The Internet is highly dynamic and so there may be a need to revisit searchers several times during the life of a project. Much of the content like radio or television is ephemeral so that web pages and blogs are always emergent but unlike newsgroups lack an assessable back store of previous material. The chronological form of many blogs may give access to past material however authors may also remove or modify their past posts. The act of changing a web site can regularly destroy its predecessor as each previous version is erased when a new version is produced. Therefore, researchers need to have a way of storing material. Fortunately, it is not difficult to 'save' material from the Internet through the 'file' menu on most browsers. For some purposes simple text files will be sufficient while other research, may demand the acquisition of the whole or part of a web site or blog. Whatever the case this material constitutes the 'data' of a research project. Should the archiving of Internet material not be viable researchers can employ a form on online tracking by which the content of sites are recoded on pre-formatted report sheets. Such an exercise can be repeated for the same sites to track change over time. Finally, I have to echo that old computer warning that the researcher should always frequently back up their work and keep at least one copy at another location than the one where they regularly work.

Representation and Sampling

In survey and positivistic social research, sampling theory is the cornerstone of validity (see also Chapter 7 in this volume). However, we need to know the nature of a population before we can think about sampling and in the dynamic world of the Internet this is a problem. There is no identifiable 'population' of narratives about health or any particular illness or experience. In my work, no 'representative' samples have been used. Rather, I have used a combination of the search strategies outlined above and a 'snowball' approach that involves following links from one narrative to others. Examining the initial narratives gave a great deal of information, as did the next and the one after that. By around the sixtieth, I had begun to understand how illness related to the writer's life and experiences on and offline. After examining another thirty accounts, I was able to situate the accounts in previous research on health narratives and auto/biography and felt that a clear picture of the reflexive nature of digital life-stories and health had began to emerge. Reading more narratives added nuances but otherwise largely confirmed what had already been understood. In other words, I had engaged in a process whereby knowledge is saturated. This is a different level of representation from the positive tradition in that rather than the simple description of a survey it taps into sociological and other knowledge that generates an understanding. To be clear, if we want to know how young people may vote in an election a representative survey will provide the most valid and useful information. Should we want to understand why some choose not to vote we need to engage with a methodology that will produce a more nuanced account. I am not trying to argue that one approach is superior, but that both have a place and should be used in accordance with the intentions of the research project.

Ethics

At this point, it is necessary to consider the question of ethics. There are two broad approaches to Internet ethics. The first follows conventional offline practice whereby researchers make clear their aims and ask permission to use material, even if the 'real' identity of the author of the material is uncertain (Waskom and Douglas, 1997). The second approach argues that anonymity and uncertain identities obliterates the need to obtain permission or informed consent. The assumption is that if subjects are not identifiable "'there is no risk to subjects, and therefore the protection of rights and interests no longer applies'" (Jones, 1994:33). Web pages and blogs are in one sense public documents in that they are published through a global medium. A similar argument can be applied to newsgroups where people post comments for others to read (Sharf, 1999). Thus, researchers can take the role of 'lurkers' who are simply reading material available to all (Sharf, 1997; see also Chapters 1 and 8 in this volume). Besides, as Jones (1994) suggests, we are all anonymous in cyberspace so what can be the harm of such covert research? What should concern us is the sense of privacy, reciprocity and community that participants of many venues on the Internet feel (Burrows et al., 2000; see also Chapter 1 in this volume). Moreover, as networks increasingly rotate around digital media, an individual's identity on the Internet is likely to come closer to their offline selves. To turn material into 'data' without any acknowledgement, warning or agreement has overtones of a surveillance society and potentially undermines trust in all forms of Internet research. While I acknowledge the public nature of web documents, I also want to stress the way the health narratives are reflexively engaged with people's lives (Hardey, 2002a; see also Chapters 13, 15, 16, 17, 18, 19 in this volume). They are public and private, intimate and objective, and as such we should respect them as personal documents. I have applied the principle of informed consent in relation to digital life-stories. Authors invariably have an email address visible on the Internet material they create. Details of any research can be sent to them so that they can give permission for the material to be used for research purposes. Finally, it should be noted that the copyright of material published on the Internet is uncertain and it may be wise to include a note in a research protocol related to the potential publication of extracts from web resources. Cyberspace is an anonymous medium and individuals may hide their offline identify behind any number of email addresses. However, it behoves researchers to always respect those whose experiences contribute to our understanding of the social world.

Email Interactions

I noted above that email is central when we need to gain consent to participation in research. It may also be the used as a conduit for asynchronous interviews or questionnaires (for example Hardey 2002). These can be used to systematically collect information that may not be evident within all digital narratives (Gillett, 2003; see also Chapters 6, 9, 11 in this volume). Exchanges between researchers and participants may be relatively short or extend beyond the life of an individual research project (Mann and Stewart, 2000). Like face-to-face interviews, a relationship of trust can be built up and participants may enter into an extended correspondence (Bampton and Cowton, 2002; see also Crouch and Liamputtong in this volume). It is important to draw some boundaries here. Researchers should remember that the research relationship should be defined by a research protocol and ethics that all parties are working with and should not be tempted to for example act as an advocate or offer expert advice. They should also be clear about the end of the research project and when they are acting as a researcher as opposed to a member of the online community. In other words, researchers must be aware of the boundaries of their work and the potential transitions to other forms of relationship. Such dilemmas are common fodder in any social research course, but the seamless nature of the Internet makes it easy to slip across the researcher/researched divide. I am not attempting to highlight this boundary out of some belief in the superiority of academic research, but rather out of a belief that clear boundaries or roles protect both the researcher (for example from unwanted emails or spam) and participants (such as unscrupulous attempts to sell products or recruit individuals through apparent research projects).

A Matter of Interpretation

I am sometimes struck when 'reading' digital narratives how subtle and deep what academic experts have, in another context, labelled 'lay' narratives can be. Like narratives mediated through print digital accounts can embrace a range of literary and other devices. Frank's (1991) well known account of his illness includes poems and other literary devices that help situate the reader in his experiences. There are links with the arts and especially literature here where illness is on occasions romanticised (Sontag, 1978). Indeed, illness narratives may resemble dramatic forms including tragedies, thrillers, comedies and romantic sagas. They have their own logic that is informed by the author's own lifeworld and involve a particular representation of the self (Williams, 1984). Without the guiding hand of an interviewer, authors draw on their knowledge of other stories when they create their digital narratives. This raises the question of authenticity. The problem of 'reality' has from the beginning been a key component of the debate about the possibilities of using material from then Internet for research. There is a whole area of the Internet devoted to discussing and publishing fictional stories that authors may previously have attempted to offer to publishers. As we noted early, digital life-stories exclude such fictional accounts so it is important that any research project differentiates between fantasy and embodied experiences. One strategy is to 'take back' fieldwork to participants for verification and comment. Willis (1977), in his now classic study of the 'lads' who were 'learning to labour' in Hammertown, gave the results of analysis back to the lads. While they recognised their experiences in Willis's vignettes, they dismissed his interpretation and theoretical concerns. This dismissal of sociological expertise is not surprising as in everyday life we do not normally need (or desire) an expert commentary to make our social actions more intelligible. Email makes it easy for participants and researches to exchange material, but as researchers, should we expect participants to be interested and engage with our analysis?

By 'reading', I want to indicate that analysis will often involve more than just text. As we have seen web pages and blogs inevitably contain links to other places on the Internet, often display images and increasingly include sound and/or video material. I have found web pages on which the author has included video clips of his last operation and blogs that have videos of 'out baby's birth'. Images of the author's own body parts that display relevant symptoms or similar graphics taken from other web sites or scanned from medical books are rather more common. These images form part of the account and often serve to allow the reader to compare their symptoms with that of the author. Before and after images are also used to show the outcome of a particular treatment. For example, a woman who has experienced poor results following breast enhancement surgery may use images to reinforce her concern to warn others of the dangers of certain implants, treatments or surgeons. The structure of the material (in what sequence it is displayed on web pages in particular, how it is laid out and so on) should not be ignored. Links are important as they situate the author within the Internet and communities of users (Schnieder and Foot, 2004). For example, a person who has sought to address symptoms through homeopathic means may reinforce their experiences with links to others who share symptoms, sites that provide particular services and note critically sites that reject homeopathy. We are not, as Grafinkel (1967) notes, 'cultural dopes' and it is evident that authors create their Internet narratives based on a mass of experience and information. The result is a complex marriage of the personal and the social, expert scientific knowledge and information about non-biomedical approaches to health. As Shaw (2003) notes, scientific ideas and language percolate common-sense accounts of illness. Indeed, the framework and language used in digital narratives may be set in modes of expression that resonance with what Rose (1989) has associated with the spread of 'psy' ideas within popular culture. As individuals struggle with ideas about health and illness their narratives may take such a confessional and therapeutic turn. This reflects the complexity of information and choices that can be made about health. The increase in use of alternative and complementary health strategies echoes the use of the Internet for information and the wide array of individual experiences that are available through it (Eisenberg et al., 1998).

At a practical level, it is possible to simply drop text from digital narratives into a computer assisted qualitative data analysis software such as Ethnograph or QSR NVivo and to proceed to follow some conventional form of narrative analysis. For some purposes, this strategy will yield reliable results. However, a few general factors should be born in mind when beginning to analyse the accounts discussed in this chapter. Digital life-stories should be treated as layered accounts that unfold to achieve meaning, both in terms of the embodied author and as an actor within the story. This recognises that the author is an actor in his/her own experiential account and so will engage in the complex business of creating a story full of contextual nuances. This is important because illness or health is not a neutral scientific category but full of meaning. Cornwell's (1984) well know study of families in East London shows how people may view their health as 'good' when they suffer from various clinically recognised conditions. However, these accounts were initiated by academic researchers and, as Atkinson (1997) notes, interviews should be viewed as a social encounter where sets of norms are negotiated. The creation of narratives on the Internet is a more individual act usually confined to the author and computer screen. However, we can move beyond this and conceptualise the Internet material as the result of an ongoing interaction between the originator of the material and those who through email and other resources interact and ccontribute to it. A note of caution is needed here to ensure that we do not 'over' interpret digital narratives. It is important to acknowledge that the software the narratives are constructed from shapes their form to a greater or lesser degree. The Internet is a system like any other systems, as Foucault (1979) reminds us, might offer greater freedoms while at the same time hiding the way they control activities, possibilities and experiences. We must, therefore, resist the temptation to over analysis some aspects of digital narratives. For example, the chronological ordering of a narrative in which the author tells the story of his/her illness may simply reflect the way the software encourages users to display their material.

In the analysis of Internet material, we must also be aware of the social context of such narratives. Indeed, it is common for people to explain why they have created their web page of blog as part of the narrative they construct (Hardey, 2002b). Researchers may be interested in following up such explanations with the author through email. In any event, these explanations are often central to the story that is being told. For example, a person who has an undiagnosed or clinically controversial condition may be keen to gain medical legitimacy and use the Internet as part of a larger campaign for recognition. Others, while experiencing ill health, may also be actively selling advice or products through their web page or indirectly via an ebay 'store'. This points to the problem of how an interpretive understanding of the material may be achieved and integrated within a final analysis. As researchers, we collect and extract material that is then reconstituted so that experiences are repositioned and situated within a more or less theoretical framework. Like ethnographers, there is sometimes a desire to establish the validity of an analysis through claims as to the 'authenticity' of participants' voices. Indeed, like others I have implicitly underscored this by providing extracts from participants material published on the internet to illustrate or support a particular point made in a paper.

CONCLUSION

Rethinking the Self, Narrative and the Internet

Had Foucault (1978) been able to observe the proliferation of digital life-stories, he may have seen them as a reflection of some aspects of what he considered characterised a confession culture. For some, it may be tempting to dismiss these narratives as digital detritus that are poor echoes of talk shows and reality television where participants seek a moment of fame or simply a chance to access support services that may be unaffordable where public health services are minimal. However, as I have sketched out in this chapter, digital accounts of health and illness have a deeper heritage in auto/biographical writing and are embed in sociological approaches to health and illness. The analysis of these narratives reveal how they are part of the development of 'self making' whereby the processes of individualism, confessional culture and lived lives are reflexively shaped into a coherent experiential account (Skeggs, 2004). The publication of these narratives on the Internet also marks the culmination of a process whereby subjective and often mundane experience is no longer marginalised in the public sphere. I hope that this chapter has pointed to the significance of digital accounts of health and illness in shaping our understanding of health and illness. As C W Mills (1970: 34) put it: "no social study that does not come back to the problem of biography, of history, and of their intersections within a society, has completed its intellectual journey". It seems to me that these intersections have never become more evident than in a society where social actions of all kinds are increasingly mediated though the new digital media.

REFERENCES

[1] Atkinson, P., 1997, *The Ethnographic Imagination: Textual Constructions of Society*, Routledge, London.

[2] Bampton, R. and Cowton, C. J., 2002, 'The e-interview', *FQS Forum: Qualitative Social Research*, vol. 3, no. 2. *<http://www.qualitative-research.net/fqs-texte/2-02/2-02 bamptoncowton-e.pdf>*.

[3] Bauman, Z., 1999, *In Search of Politics*, Polity Press, Cambridge.

[4] Bauman, Z., 2003, *Liquid Modernity*, Polity Press, Cambridge.

[5] Beck, U., 1992, *Risk Society: Towards a New Modernity*, Sage Publications, London.

[6] Bennet, J. C., 2001, 'Angloshpere: The New Reformation?', *United Press International* December 29 *<www. Upi.com/view.cfm?StoryID=28122001-050733-7164r>*

[7] Berners-Lee, T., 2000, *Weaving the Web: the Original Design and Ultimate Destiny of the World Wide Web*, Harper Collins, New York.

[8] Burrows, R., Nettleton, S., Pleace, N., Loader, B., and Muncer, C., 2000, 'Virtual Community Care? Social Policy and the Emergence of Computer Mediated Social Support', *Information, Communication and Society*, vol. 3, no. 1, pp. 95–121.

[9] Castells, M., 1996, The Rise of the Network Society, Blackwell, Oxford.

[10] Chandler. D., and Roberts-Young, D., 1998, *The Construction of Identity in the Personal Homepages of Adolescents <http://www.aber.ac.uk/media/Documents/short/strasbourg.html>*

[11] Cline, R.J.W., and Haynes, K.M., 2001, 'Consumer Health Information Seeking on the Internet: The State of the Art', *Health Education Research* vol. 16, pp. 671-92.

[12] Cornwell, J., 1984, *Hard Earned Lives: Accounts of Health and Illness from East London*, Tavistock, London.

[13] Couser, G. T., 1997, *Recovering Bodies: Illness, Disability and Life Writing*, University of Wisconsin Press, Madison.

[14] Eisenberg, D.M., Davis, R.B., Ettner, S.L., Appel, S., Wilkey, S., van Rompay, M. and Kessler, R.C., 1998, 'Trends in Alternative Medicine use in the United States, 1990–1997', *New England Journal of Medicine*, vol.280, pp.1569–75.

[15] Foucault, M., 1979, *Discipline and Punish: The Birth of the Prison*, Penguin, London.

[16] Foucault, M., 1978, *The History of Sexuality Volume One*, Random House, New York.

[17] Frank, A. W., 1991, *At the Will of the Body: Reflections on Illness*, Houghton Miffa, Boston.

[18] Garfikel, H., 1967, *Studies in Ethnography*, Prentice-Hall, Englewood Cliffs.

[19] Giddens, A., 1990, *The Consequences of Modernity*, Polity Press. CambridgeGiddens, A., 1991, *Modernity and Self-Identity: Self and Society in the Late Modern Age*, Polity Press, Cambridge.

[20] Giddens, A., 1994, 'Livinging a Post-Traditional Society', in U. Beck, A. Giddens, and S. Lash, (eds.), *Reflexive Modernization*, pp. 56–109, Polity Press, Cambridge.

[21] Gillett, J., 2003, 'Media Activism and Internet Use by People with HIV/AIDS', *Sociology of Health and Illness*, vol. 25 no. 6, pp. 608–624.

[22] Goldsmith, J., 2002, 'How will the Internet Change our Health System?', *Health Affairs*, vol. 191, pp.148-156

[23] Hardey, M., 1999, 'Doctor in the House: The Internet as a Source of Lay Health Knowledge and the Challenge to Expertise, *Sociology of Health and Illness*, vol.21, no. 4 , pp. 820–835.

[24] Hardey, M.,2002, 'Life Beyond the Screen: Embodiment and Identity Through the Internet', *Sociological Review*. Vol. 50, no. 4, pp. 571-585.

[25] Hardey, M., 2002a, 'E-health: The Internet and the Transformation of Patients into Consumers and Producers of Health Knowledge', *Information, Communication and Society*, vol. 4, no. 3, pp.388–405.

[26] Hardey, M., 2002b, 'The Story of My Illness': Personal Accounts of Illness on the Internet', *Health*, vol. 6, no.1, pp. 31-46.

[27] Hardey, M., 2004a, 'Digital Life-stories: Auto/biography in the Information Age', *Auto/biography*, vol.1, no.3, pp. 183-200.

[28] Hardey, M., 2004b, 'Internet et Société: Reconfigurations du Patient et de al Médecine? *Sciences Sociales and Santé*, vol. 22, no. 1, pp. 21-42.

[29] Heelas, P., Lash, S., and Morris, P., 1996, *Detraditionalization*, Blackwell, Oxford.

[30] Jackson, S., 2005, 'Rethinking the Self: Constructions of Gender and Sexuality in Late Modernity', in M. Kimmel, (ed.), The Sexual Self: The Construction of Sexual Scripts, pp. 152-173, University Press, Vanderbilt.
[31] Jadad, A. R., and Gagliardi, A., 1998, 'Rating Health Information on the Internet: Navigating to Knowledge or Babel?', *Journal of the American Medical Association*, vol.. 2798, pp. 611-614.
[32] Jones R. A., 1994, 'The Ethics of Research in Cyberspace', *Internet Research*, vol. 4, no. 3, pp.30-5.
[33] Lawton, J., 2003, 'Lay Experiences of Health and Illness: Past Research and Future Agendas', *Sociology of Health and Illness*, vol. 25, Silver Anniversary Issue, pp.23–40.
[34] Mann, C., and Stewart, F., 2000, *Internet Communication and Qualitative Research*, Sage Publications, London.
[35] Mills, C.W., 1970, *The Sociological Imagination*, Penguin, London.
[36] Naughton, J., 2003, *A Brief History of the Future. The Origins of the Internet*, Phoenix, London.
[37] Rheingold, H., 1993, *The Virtual Community: Homesteading on the Electronic Frontier*, Addisons-Wesly, Reading MA.
[38] Rose, N., 1989, *Governing the Soul*, Routledge, London.
[39] Schnieder, S. M, and Foot, K. A., 2004, 'The Web as an Object of Study', *New Media and Society*, vol. 6, pp, 114-122
[40] Sharf, B.F., 1999, 'Beyond Netiquette. The Ethics of Doing Naturalistic Discourse Research on the Internet', in S. Jones, (ed.), *Doing Internet Research*, pp.243-56, Sage Publications, London.
[41] Sharf, B.F., 1997, 'Communicating Breast Cancer On-Line: Support and Empowerment on the Internet', *Women and Health*, vol. 26, no. 1, pp.65-84.
[42] Shaw, I., 2003, 'How Lay are Lay Beliefs?', *Health*, vol. 6, no. 3 pp.287–300.
[43] Skeggs, B., 2004, *Class, Self, Culture*, Routledge, London.
[44] Smith, S., 1993, *Subjectivity, Identity and the Body: Women's Autobiographical Practices in the Twentieth Century*, Indiana University Press, Bloomington.
[45] Steedman, C., 1992, *Past Tenses. Essays on Writing, Autobiography and History*, Rivers Oram Press, London.
[46] Sontag, S., 1978, *Illness as Metaphor*, Farr, Straus and Giroux, New York.
[47] Thomas, W. I. and Znaniecki, F., 1958, The Polish Peasant in Europe and America, Dover Press, New York.
[48] Thomas, R., 1997, *Text and Narrative,* Howarth Press. London
[49] Waskom, I. and Douglas, R., 1997, '*Researching the Net': Health Information on the Internet', Royal Society of Medicine Press* vol. 5, pp. 1-3.
[50] Williams, G., 1984, 'The Genesis of Chronic Illness: Narrative Reconstruction', *Sociology of Health and Illness*, vol. 6, no. 2, pp.175–200.
[51] Willis, P., 1977, *Learning to Labour*, Saxson House.

In: Health Research in Cyberspace
Editor: Pranee Liamputtong, pp. 243-256

ISBN 1-59454-819-6

Chapter 15

INTERNET NEWSGROUPS AS A SOURCE OF DATA FOR QUALITATIVE HEALTHCARE RESEARCH: ISSUES, CHALLENGES AND THE PRACTICALITIES OF EXPLORING YOUNG PEOPLE'S MENTAL HEALTH ACCOUNTS

Stephen K. Bradley and Bernie Carter

BACKGROUND

In this chapter, we provide an account of a research project, conducted from the UK, which sought to address the paucity of empirical research that investigates young people's perspectives on child and adolescent mental health (CAMH) issues and experiences. We tell the story of this qualitative inquiry project because, in seeking to access young people's accounts of mental health experiences, we investigated the Internet as a promising source of appropriate material. This led us to focus particularly on exploring the potential of Internet newsgroups as a rich resource for healthcare researchers of, largely untapped, data. We share lessons from the project so as to indicate some of the issues that researchers need to consider, the sources we found helpful in addressing these issues and some of the solutions that we arrived at. We concentrate particularly on conceptual and methodological issues, but also include *some* of the outcomes of the project as indication of the potential of such research.[1] Our hope is that this chapter might encourage others to consider investigating Internet newsgroup materials in their own healthcare research.

The mental health of children and particularly adolescents is a growing cause for concern in most Western countries. In the UK, the Government estimate that 20% of children suffer from mental health problems at some time before reaching adulthood (Audit Commission, 1999). In response, provision for CAMH is firmly on the political agenda. The UK Government has recently published its Children's National Service Framework that seeks, for

[1] For those interested in a more detailed account of the findings, please contact the first author.

the first time, to integrate CAMH concerns within overall National Health Service (NHS) health and social care service improvement targets for children (DOH, 2004). Along with increased interest and some increased Government expenditure has come a focus on 'customer satisfaction' within healthcare provision; specifically, on hearing the views of clients, relatives and carers (DOH, 2001, 2002). More generally, taking into consideration the views of children and young people regarding issues that affect them has been spurred by the United Nations Convention on the Rights of the Child (UN, 1989).

Against this background, the recent CAMH academic/professional literature provides a rich dialogue concerning the problems with existing *services*, how to improve them and, thus it is assumed, the mental health outlook for young people. Discussion centres around the need for increased priority (Geanellos, 1999), more and better facilities (Polnay, 2000), more effective outreach services (Stein et al., 1991), more flexible and innovative services (Allison et al. 2000), early intervention (Walker, 2001), increased development of preventative education and parenting training (Scott 1999), better integration of services (Kraemer, 1995) and so on. However, what is singularly lacking from this expansionist, service focussed, literature is any consistent place for listening to the voices of young people themselves.

Recently commenced high-profile studies that claim to be doing so (NCB, 2001; Young Minds 2002), remain resolutely service driven. The approach of such studies remains 'managerialist/consumerist', aimed primarily at the development and improvement of existing provision. There appears little place within such studies for a 'democratic/empowerment' approach (Beresford 2002),developing a critical exploration of the experience of CAMH informed by young people's expressed perspectives. Such studies have yet to be developed (James, 2002; Parker, 2002). Traditionally, lack of interest in client's views regarding mental health services (Parker et al., 1995), and the views of children as having something valuable to contribute in their own right (Taylor, 2000) played a major part in this deficit. It may now be viewed in some quarters as more desirable to research young people's perspectives and to view their experiences and cultures as worthy of study in their own right (France et al., 2000); rather than to continue to hear only the predominant voices of the 'professional ventriloquists' (Carter, 2002). However, conceptual, ethical and practical difficulties remain.

Moving Towards Internet Newsgroup Research

The initial problem facing this project arose from these difficulties. How can an ethically defensible methodological approach that 'hears the voices' of young people as clearly as possible, concerning their experiences of such a sensitive area of life as CAMH, be developed? Addressing this problem was compounded by the lack of an existing developed corpus of appropriate work within CAMH to draw upon for inspiration. Therefore, finding a way forward inspired by the literature in other associated fields was necessary. Harris (2000) had faced comparable difficulties in seeking to research the experiences and perspectives of women who self-injure. Her decision to avoid face to face interviewing and to design a correspondence study to gain access to sensitive personal accounts pointed to a possible way forward. Hardey (2002), in researching personal accounts of ill health as detailed on the pages of personal Internet websites, also indicats a potentially promising avenue for conducting research into sensitive areas of human experience. Taken together, these two studies made a major contribution towards stimulating the methodological thinking that informed this project.

Before going on to detail the methodological approach that was developed, it is necessary to briefly identify two issues of a conceptual nature that underpinned the project; namely, a commitment to understanding the world in terms of its 'social construction' and an emphasis on the key role of 'narrative'. The intention is not to present a detailed discussion of these issues, but merely to highlight key ideas that informed the methodological approach taken.

Constructionism stands opposed to traditional conceptions of language which see words as purely descriptive (Gergen, 1999). The primary insight is to draw attention to the 'work' that words do; that language produces meaning and creates social reality (Richardson, 2000). Furthermore, by attending to the constitutive, social and interactive, constructionists problematise the assumption of the existence of stable, separable, individually and internally sited psychological entities and processes (Stenner and Eccleston, 1994). From a constructionist position, it is vital to consider the social and cultural dimensions to any human activity; an insight which is also argued to be foundational to 'new' or 'interpretive paradigm' research (Denzin and Lincoln, 2000).

Following on in this project from a commitment to constructionist understanding, the key point to highlight regarding narrative is the contention that research with the stories that people tell to make sense of their lives/experiences must be fundamental to any understanding in human inquiry. Stories are viewed as fundamental building blocks of social life, allowing us to speak of our lives, whilst at the same time establishing many of the limits to those very lives that we describe and share with others (Kotre, 1984; Bruner, 1987; Rosenwald and Ochberg,1992; Riessman, 1993; Frank, 1995; Bochner, 2001). To ignore the impact of the storied nature of the human condition is to weaken any study that purports to research that condition (Sarbin, 1986). The intention here is to signal that the focus of this project was to consider the power and impact of stories, specifically of child and adolescent mental ill health; paying particular attention to the stories that *are told*, the stories that are *not told*, and the stories that *could be told* (Dreyfus and Rabinow, 1982; Prior, 1997; Howells, 1999; Kendall and Wickham, 1999). The key research question pursued was: 'what are the stories informing thinking about CAMH?'

So, as indicated, the initial challenge facing this project was how to develop an ethically defensible methodological approach that would allow access to 'hear the voices' of young people, as clearly as possible, concerning their experiences of such a sensitive area of life as CAMH. Whilst not impossible to allay, ethical concerns regarding potential psychological harm to 'vulnerable' minors arising from asking them to relive possible traumatic events for the benefit of postgraduate research were highlighted during the process of developing an appropriate project. Also worth noting is that this project was developed at a time in the UK (Autumn 2001) when research, particularly on/with children, was being especially rigorously scrutinised; in the wake of high profile 'scandals' in Bristol and Liverpool. Harris's work (2000, 2002) had pointed towards the benefits of avoiding face to face methods when researching sensitive issues. Hardey's paper (2002) had highlighted the largely untapped documentary resource for research in the human sciences that the Internet potentially represents (see also Hardey in this volume). However, since Hardey's article was published concerns have begun to be raised as to the intellectual property rights of personal web pages (Riessman, 2002). Therefore, the research reported here accessed only pre-existing archived materials, voluntarily contributed ('posted') to Internet newsgroups (also known as Usenet discussion groups). Ethical thinking, current with the development of this project, was that such contributions could be safely viewed as a secondary source, like any other archive material. The nature of Internet newsgroups is such that contributors can expect that their posts will be read and commented upon by others. By contributing in the first place, they may be taken to have consented to this (Robinson, 2001). However, such consent must be 'implied', rather than being 'informed consent' in the traditionally accepted sense within healthcare research. Whilst we were happy to go forward with this research, based on implied consent to access materials within the public domain, we accepted the potential of being considered 'spooks'; secretly spying on the Internet newsgroups that we investigated.

Hence, by accessing pre-existing archived material, it was possible to access young people's accounts without having any contact with them; so allaying any ethical concerns regarding potential harm. However, the cost of this innovative solution was that we grappled with other equally complex problems. Firstly, the research protocol that we developed, so as to minimise the concerns of the ethics committee that we should not access interactive 'chat rooms' (another ethico-political 'hot potato' at the time), expressly forbade any interactive activity. Therefore, this project was necessarily serendipitous. It was only possible to access whatever material could be found. Also, newsgroup contributor's claims had to be taken at face value as it was not permissible to contact a contributor to ask questions of clarification, or to find out 'what happened next' if that information was not forthcoming in a later post. Coming from constructionist understanding with an interest in investigating accounts, questions such as 'how do you know that when someone claims to be fifteen that they are telling the truth' were not of great concern to us. Our concern was whether the other contributors to the newsgroup accepted an account as plausible. If it was an acceptable account to them, then it was of interest to us. However, we lost count of the number of times that we were asked just such questions after workshop/conference presentations and during academic scrutiny from colleagues. Researchers coming from more realist orientations, for example, would obviously have more problems with such questions and would need to arrive at other answers were they to pursue Internet newsgroup research; possibly by developing research protocols which allowed them to 'follow up' interactively.

Whilst the Internet is by no means the sole preserve of the young, demographic surveys of its users consistently indicate that it has become a popular medium for children and teenagers (Kennedy, 2000). The world's largest newsgroup archive is held at 'Google Groups', which claims to contain over 850 million posts (April 2005). This archive was, therefore, likely to be a potentially promising resource for this project; to allow non-interactive collecting and collating of young peoples' pre-existing accounts of CAMH experiences for investigation. Initial exploration of the archive confirmed this proposition; hence the development of our research aims:

1. To survey the internationally recognised integrated Internet newsgroup archive held at 'Google Groups' (http://groups.google.com), identifying and downloading a corpus of first-person accounts of CAMH experiences for further investigation;
2. To develop a critical examination of these accounts, consistent with the approaches described as being concerned with "contexts and consequences" within Mishler's typology of Narrative Analysis (Mishler, 1995); approaches concerned with how storied understandings work in impacting 'lived experience'.

THE PRACTICALITIES OF GETTING STARTED

The 'Google Groups' search facility was used to identify accounts of mental ill health experiences contributed to Internet newsgroups by young people (see also Chapter 14 in this volume). Given the international nature of the Internet and the variability of definitions in different countries, 'young people' was pragmatically defined at the outset as legal minority in the country of origin of the researchers (that is less than 18 years in the UK). Given the overall aims and focus of the project, the question of 'sampling' does not apply to the demographics of the authors of the newsgroup contributions. Rather, the sampling applies to the accounts themselves. It is these that are of interest. Therefore, the sampling was purposive when applied to the collection and collation of data from the 'Google Groups' archive. At the outset of the data gathering phase, accounts had to meet the following criteria for inclusion:

- Author's age at time of events detailed in account must be claimed to be less than 18 years;
- Account must identify personal experience of a mental ill health condition accepted within an internationally recognised classificatory system (DSM-IV or ICD-10);
- Account must meet Chatman's (1978) definition of 'narrative' (that is contain identifiable characters, events, narrative form);
- Accounts must be sufficiently detailed so as to contribute worthwhile data to the study.

As will be seen later, these apparently reasonable initial criteria were to present some difficulties in practice and needed to be slightly revised.

The first searches of 'Google Groups' Internet newsgroup archive used combinations of search terms, such as 'teens', 'teenagers', 'child', 'children', 'mental health', 'depression', 'eating disorders' and so on to establish where within the archive appropriate posts were likely to be found. Results from these initial searches suggested any number of possible newsgroups that might contain contributions from young people regarding mental health. Given the size of the archive and the focus of the project, it was decided to search for a newsgroup that was specific to young people and mental health, arriving at an appropriate group[2] which at the time of the commencement of the project ran to some 22000 archived 'threads'[3] on the 'Google Groups' archive.

The rationale for further investigating this specific group was threefold. Firstly, by its very constitution the group claims to be a forum for 'teens' and so might reasonably be expected to attract contributions from the age group of interest to this project. Secondly, the

---

[2] We have not included specific details of the groups considered. This omission is not an oversight, but after lengthy consideration is taken motivated by our concern that any readers, not sensitive to the ethical nuances of this research, might cause unwitting psychological distress to contributors to the newsgroup were we to make the newsgroup details known. Readers with a legitimate reason for wishing to explore such specific details further are again invited to contact the first author.

[3] A newsgroup 'thread' comprises all the individual contributions (posts) made to that particular topic for discussion. A thread can be as short as one contribution, to which no one else replied; or could comprise say 20, 30 or more contributions (theoretically infinite) to an ongoing dialogue. Usually a thread comes to a natural conclusion as the subject is finished with, or perhaps 'peters out' as other (more interesting?) threads attract contributors' interest. A post can be one sentence or many pages long. 'Worthwhile' posts for the purposes of this project were ones which develop a detailed account or discussion.

group focuses on 'depression'. It can be argued that 'depression' has become the most commonly occurring, and thus effectively, de-stigmatised of conditions generally accepted to be within the purview of mental health (Behar, 1996). Thus, a newsgroup concerning 'depression' might be expected to be more frequently visited and so provide a rich source of data. Thirdly, the stated intent of the group is to be concerned with 'support'. Therefore, it might reasonably be expected to be a place where the sharing of personal experiences might be found. It is difficult to conceive of too many circumstances in which those asking for support would be able to do so without sharing something of the reasons why; in effect, to tell something of their personal story. Taken together, this specific newsgroup appeared to be a highly promising source.

This one newsgroup was then investigated further, following Hardey's suggested search strategy (2002), using the term 'my story' as the most likely to yield appropriate data, given that the interest was in accessing personal stories. The 'my story' search yielded some 717 posts. Of these, the most recent 100 were followed up by working backwards chronologically, using the above stated inclusion criteria. This exploration yielded some eight qualifying personal narrative accounts for further analysis. Given this small number, the next 100 results were scrutinised, yielding a further nine qualifying accounts. An inclusion rate of only 8.5% (17 from 200) was of sufficient concern to prompt review of the inclusion criteria.

Three factors were identified as to why over 90% of posts were being excluded using the initial criteria. Firstly, a strict interpretation of the age criteria was excluding many accounts. Unless a post included a phrase that identified a specific age less than 18 years, the contribution was excluded. The second factor leading to a large number of exclusions was the narrative construction criterion, which reflected the *a priori* narrative commitment of the project. Whilst believed to be a fairly wide definition, when applied in practice it proved to be an unexpectedly tough inclusion criterion to meet. Whilst many posts told personal stories that met this definition of narrative, many other posts did not. There appeared to be diversity amongst the posts on this newsgroup that was in danger of being overlooked by applying a strictly narrative approach from the outset. Thirdly, this apparent diversity of posts also highlighted a problem with the mental health definition criterion. Reappraisal of the excluded contributions identified that a significant number evidenced understanding of the experience of mental ill health without necessarily explicitly identifying 'personal experience'. To exclude these contributions *en masse* without further investigatory work appeared unwise. Conversely, the deliberately wide and inclusive nature of the definition of mental ill health was problematic when applied in practice. The ubiquity of the term 'depression', and its derivatives, presented a problem. The spectrum of usage appeared to go from 'I'm feeling a little off colour today' through to what a psychiatrist might recognise as a severe problem in need of urgent treatment. As used on the studied newsgroup, it proved to be a problematic term to rely on as evidence of 'personal experience of a mental ill health condition'. Whilst self-identification of depression would technically meet this criterion, it was found in practice to be too vague. For example, several accounts that met the above three criteria of age, mental ill health experience and narrative form needed to be excluded on further consideration because the 'depression' being claimed amounted to effectively 'I feel bad because of a relationship problem'. Such contributions may have been more appropriately posted to a more general advice group, rather than to a group seeking to offer support to those experiencing 'depression'.[4]

Taken together, a reappraisal of the criteria seemed justified. Persevering with these criteria in this form ran the risk of missing the fullness of what could be learned from the contributions to this newsgroup. This initial exploration had in effect acted somewhat analogously to a 'pilot study'. Hence, a revised approach to the identified data was instituted that sought to identify and categorize the contributions to this newsgroup; to be more data driven, and to 'map the terrain', so to speak. The data set was increased in size to the maximum allowed by 'Google Groups' search facility. This allowed some 350 of the 717 threads identified by the 'my story' search to be followed up. These 350 posts were reviewed with the following revised criteria:

- author's age at time of writing, or at time of events detailed in account, to be reasonably believed to have been less than the legal age of majority pertaining to their particular geographical/political setting;
- account discusses a mental ill health condition accepted within an internationally recognised classificatory system (DSM-IV, ICD-10), describing appropriate symptoms in addition to any diagnostic title;
- account contains sufficient detail so as to contribute worthwhile data to the study.

Given this revised approach, some 172 posts were identified for further investigation from the 350 search results allowed at the time by the 'Google Groups' search facility. The majority of exclusions were made due to one of three factors. Firstly, that there was no way of establishing the age of the contributor from the material that they had provided in their posting, or that they positively identified themselves as outside of the age parameter. Secondly, that the posting was a very short note or comment in response to a larger post. Thirdly, posts that claimed 'depression', for example, without mentioning any other symptoms were excluded. So, a post that talked only of depression related to a recent relationship break-up was excluded. However, such a post that made mention of, say, prolonged sleep disturbance, significant interruption of daily routine and functioning, or a self-injury attempt would be included.

The 172 posts for further investigation were downloaded from 'Google Groups' archive into 'ATLAS.ti 4.2', a qualitative data analysis computer software package. Although this package allows for automatic coding by key word or phrase, and for 'theory building', its use in this project was solely to enhance data management and manual coding. Reading, re-reading and coding of the texts allowed key issues, themes and categories to emerge from critical engagement with the data rather than being derived from preconceived groupings. The informed critical analytic reading that developed through the process of repeated reading, coding and then category development bears comparison with the approach described as 'content analysis' (Plummer, 1995; Plummer, 1983); being concerned to identify occurrences of discrete categories within textual material (Bryman, 1988). However, such an approach is generally taken to be primarily concerned with quantification; identifying the number of times

[4] This is not to say that mental ill health problems and relationship difficulties do not bear on each other, but rather that some of these posts appeared to be inappropriate. When in doubt over a particular posting, a good 'rule of thumb' that developed was to look at the quantity and quality of the replies that were posted, particularly by 'regulars' to the newsgroup. If they took the posting as appropriate, then it seemed reasonable for us to do so as well.

that a particular pre-determined category appears in the text being analysed (Silverman, 2000). Hence, whilst being informed by the concerns of content analysis, the critical reading of textual material presented here differs from the classical form of that method in two important respects. Firstly, the coding approach employed did not search for instances of pre-determined categories. Rather, an iterative process of category development from within the coded data, filtered by the researchers' reflexively positioned understanding, was adopted. This is an eclectic approach informed as much by the concerns of grounded theory methodology (Glaser and Strauss, 1967; Glaser, 1992; Charmaz, 1995), ethnographic work in relation to documentary sources (Atkinson and Coffey, 1997; Tierney, 2000), discourse and narrative analysis (Burman and Parker, 1993; Riessman, 1993; Mishler, 1995; Potter and Wetherell, 1987, 1995;), as by those of content analysis. Secondly, coding in terms of counting the number of occurrences within each post of a word, phrase or concept was not integral to the analysis. The aim of this project was hermeneutic, not nomothetic. The key question asked of the data at this stage was 'what is happening here in terms of the types of post being made?'

Following this initial phase of data analysis, a second dimension to the 'what is happening' question also then needed pursuing: 'what is happening here in terms of the subjects being discussed?' This second investigatory phase was able to consider an enlarged data set of some 287 posts. This enlarged set was made possible by re-visiting the source archive held at 'Google Groups' to update the data set with any appropriate new posts made since the initial data collection. Whilst some such new posts were identified, the increase from 172 to 287 posts, found by repeating a computerised search for posts containing the words 'my story', was largely accounted for by a technical change in the functioning of the 'Google Groups' search facility. This change allowed for a larger number of search results to be accessed than had been the case earlier.

'Emerging' Themes and Issues

Table 1: 'Emerging' Themes and Issues – Types of Posts/Topics of Interest

'Emerging' Themes and Issues – Types of Posts
Personal Material - Narrative accounts/stories - Statements - Expressive material - Appeals - Farewells
Help Response - Personal - Impersonal - General
Discussion Contribution

Table 1: 'Emerging' Themes and Issues – Types of Posts/Topics of Interest (cont.)

'Emerging' Themes and Issues – 'Mental Health' Topics of Interest to Contributors
Self-injury
Experiences of professional help (psychiatry/therapy)
Prescription drugs
Experiences of depression
Panic attacks/anxiety
Eating Disorders
Suicide: ideation; attempts
Fears and phobias

Analysis of the contributions to the newsgroup under study suggested that three distinct *types* of contribution were being made: 'personal material', 'help response' and 'discussion contribution' (see Table 1).

As might be expected, the category 'personal material' included a preponderance of the personal stories initially sought after, but it was not limited to accounts that tell only something of a person's life history. As well as such narrative accounts (stories), other 'personal material' placed in this category were 'statements' (personal material without narrative form); 'expressive material' (such as original poems); 'appeals' (for personal help/advice); and, 'farewells' (either to the group or as a 'virtual suicide note'). The key feature in this category of contributions was the personal nature of the material. The contributor spoke of events that had happened to them, or about occurrences that were relevant to them in some way. Secondly, a strong sense of drive to put the material 'out there' (i.e. to relatively anonymous 'others') was common to this category.

The definition of the category 'help response' is self-explanatory in broad terms. Most 'help responses', but not all, are prompted by a specific personal material posting. The apparent intent of the 'help response' is synonymous with the intention of the group more generally; to offer 'support'. Again, sub-categories of 'help response' can be identified: 'personal help responses' (includes the introduction of 'personal material' in a reply); 'impersonal help responses' (absence of any personal material in the reply); and, 'general help responses' (not posted in reply to a specific posting, but spontaneously proffering help on an issue of the author's choosing).

The final category, 'discussion contribution', is the only one which by definition does not contain personal material. Discussion contributions are, as the name suggests, posts that are focussed on the exchange of 'factual' information pursuant to discussing and debating an issue. Reading such discussion contributions may, of course, be personally helpful to the reader. However, that is not a necessary condition for definition of a 'discussion contribution'.

The second phase of investigation of the data set (now enlarged to 287 posts) was to approach the 'what is happening here' question in terms of the topics of interest being discussed by the contributors to the newsgroup. The process of repeated reading, coding for topics being written about, and then subsuming the generated codes into broader categories being discussed, resulted in the identification of 27 'topic categories'. Of these, 19 topic categories could be described as discussing 'general issues'; for example, 'difficulties with parents', 'romantic difficulties', 'bullying', and 'illegal drugs'. The remaining eight topic categories were identifiable as 'mental health issues'. Given that our interest was primarily to investigate 'the stories informing thinking about CAMH', it was these eight topic categories that were pursued in more depth. Many of the posts within these mental health topic categories were unremarkable, or conversely remarkable because of their relative scarcity. For example, posts concerning 'panic attacks/anxiety', 'eating disorders', 'fears and phobias' were found less frequently than might be expected; most likely due to the existence of newsgroups more specifically focussed on such issues. However, a number of striking issues/themes were particularly identified.

'Following The Data'

Having identified the types of post being contributed and the topics of interest to the contributors to the studied newsgroup, we decided to 'follow the data'; in the sense of pursuing those issues that appeared highly important to the young people. What was particularly noticeable during investigation of the 'what is going on' questions were the high number of posts that discussed self-injury and suicide. Approximately 24% of posts studied discussed self-injury (69 out of 289), whilst 13% (37 out of 289) discussed suicide attempts and/or ideation. Given that some, but not all, posts discussed both issues approximately 30% of posts studied discussed self-injury and/or suicide; to us, a surprisingly high percentage. These are also issues of national and international concern (NCB, 2001).

Focussing particularly on self-injury, the received wisdom in the academic/professional literature suggests two broad categories of self injury behaviour. Firstly, there is self-injury that is deemed to be of 'serious' suicidal intent and thus, when not successful, is viewed as a failed suicide attempt. Secondly, there is 'parasuicide'; a self-injury attempt with low likelihood of fatal outcome, which is frequently viewed as a 'cry for help' or to 'attract attention'(Shaffer and Gutstein 2002; Sharman 1997). As indicated, the studied newsgroup contains a significant literature of it's own on self-injury (particularly by 'cutting') which appears to describe a more diverse and complex picture. Scrutiny of the 'cutting' posts suggests a number of sub-categories of self-injury behaviour that did not appear to be being pursued by the current academic/professional literature (see Table 2).

Furthermore, our investigation suggested that some contributors were describing self-injury attempts that had no suicidal intent whatsoever. This possibility does not appear to be adequately discussed in the existing professional/academic literature. Even the recent creative qualitative correspondence study conducted by Harris (2000), within which she identified a type of self-injury attempt as a 'management strategy' that allowed her participants to cope with stressful times without resorting to potentially lethal actions, still apparently maintains the traditional conceptual link between self-injury and suicide that our investigations question.

Table 2: Newsgroup Posts – Self-injury Sub-categories (with indicative examples)[5]

Newsgroup – Sub-categories of Self-injury
'Compulsive Self-injury' - being driven to cut: "when i was 14-16 i had an odd habit, every friday night i'd cut my wrist, my throat, my finger, anything until finally all i had was scars and blood all over me... well, to make a long story short, i ended up hurting my self in more ways than one--->drugs, alcohol, smacking a hammer to my head.
'Reinforced Self-injury' - repeat cutting encouraged by some sort of benefit: "the thing is, i wasn't depressed i was happy, and when i cut my self i became happier"
'Recreational Self-injury'- self-injury in concert with others: "I've been cutting since I was about 17... My roommate knows about it. She even tried it once to see what I got out of it... Two of the guys did it together... I don't understand how they could sit in a room with each other and cut."
'Secretive Cutting' - which appears to directly contradict the 'attention seeking' nuances of the 'parasuicide' thesis: "thats why u should stick to one arm... i needed a blood test... but i only rolled up one (my 'good' arm) hehe and everything was fine... my mom later saw my cuts but i told her i fell and whatever".

CONCLUSION

In this chapter, we have provided a primarily methodological account of a research project that accessed young people's accounts of CAMH posted on Internet newsgroups. In so doing, we have indicated and critiqued some of the key pragmatic aspects of this type of research in conceptual and methodological terms including some of the outcomes of the project as indication of the potential of such research. Whilst using posted accounts is not without challenges, our hope is that this chapter has encouraged others to consider investigating Internet newsgroup materials in their own healthcare research.

[5] The examples included in this table are chosen because they highlight the category succinctly. Original format, grammar, spelling, and so on are retained as far as possible so as to allow readers a 'feel' for the posts.

REFERENCES

[1] Allison, S., Roeger, L., Dadds, V. and Martin, G., 2000, 'Brief Therapy for Children's Mental Health Problems: Outcomes in a Rural Setting', *Australian Journal of Rural Health*, vol. 8, pp. 161-166.

[2] Atkinson, P. and Coffey, A., 1997, 'Analysing Documentary Realities', in D. Silverman (ed.), *Qualitative research: Theory, method and practice*, pp.45-62, Sage Publications, London.

[3] Audit Commission, 2002, *Children in Mind: Child and Adolescent Mental Health Services*. *<http://www.audit-commission.gov.uk/publications/brcamhs.shtml>*

[4] Behar, R., 1996, *The Vulnerable Observer: Anthropology that Breaks Your Heart.* Beacon Press, Boston.

[5] Beresford, P., 2002, '*User involvement in research*'. Paper presented at Qualitative Research in Health and Social Care Conference, Bournemouth, UK.

[6] Bochner, A. P., 2001, 'Narrative's Virtues', *Qualitative Inquiry*, vol. 7, pp.131-157.

[7] Bruner, J., 1987, 'Life as Narrative', *Social Research*,. vol. 54, pp. 11-32.

[8] Bryman, A., 1988, Quantity and Quality in Social Research, Unwin Hyman, London.

[9] Burman, E. and Parker, I. E., 1993, *Discourse analytic research: Repertoires and readings of texts in action*, Routledge, London.

[10] Carter, B., 2002, 'Chronic Pain in Childhood and the Medical Encounter: Professional Ventriloquism and Hidden Voice', *Qualitative Health Research*, vol. 12, pp. 28-41.

[11] Charmaz, K., 1995, 'Grounded Theory', in J.A. Smith, R. Harré and L. Van Langenhove (eds.), Rethinking Methods in Psychology, pp.27-49, Sage Publications, London.

[12] Chatman, S., 1978, *Story and Discourse: Narrative Structure in Fiction and Film*, Cornell University Press, New York.

[13] Denzin, N. K. and Lincoln, Y. S., 2000, 'Introduction: The Discipline and Practice of Qualitative Research', in N.K. Denzin and Y.S. Lincoln (eds.), *Handbook of Qualitative Research*, pp.1-29, Sage Publications, Thousand Oaks, CA.

[14] Department Of Health, 2001, *Essence of Care*, Department of Health, London.

[15] Department Of Health, 2002, *Children's Taskforce: An Introduction*, Department of Health, London.

[16] Department Of Health, 2004, *National Service Framework for Children, Young People and Maternity Services*, Department of Health, London.

[17] Dreyfus, H. L. and Rabinow, P., 1982, *Michel Foucault: Beyond Structuralism and Hermeneutics*, Harvester Wheatsheaf, Hemel Hempstead.

[18] France, A., Bendelow, G. and Williams, S., 2000,'A 'Risky' Business: Researching the Health Beliefs of Children and Young People', in A. Lewis and G. Lindsay (eds.), *Researching Children's Perspectives*, pp.150-162, Open University Press, Buckingham.

[19] Frank, A. W., 1995, *The Wounded Storyteller: Body, Illness, and Ethics*, University of Chicago Press, Chicago.

[20] Geanellos, R., 1999, 'A Review of the Sociopolitical Context of Adolescent Mental Health and Adolescent Mental Health Nursing in Australia', *Australian and New Zealand Journal of Mental Health Nursing*, vol. 8, pp. 134-142.

[21] Gergen, K. J., 1999, *An Invitation to Social Construction*, Sage, London.

[22] Glaser, B. G., 1992, *Emergence vs Forcing: Basics of Grounded Theory Analysis*, Sociology Press, Mill Valley, CA.

[23] Glaser, B. G. and Strauss, A. L., 1967, *The Discovery of Grounded Theory*, Aldine, Chicago.

[24] Hardey, M., 2002, "The Story of My Illness': Personal Accounts of Illness on the Internet', Healt, vol. 6, pp. 31-46.

[25] Harris, J., 2000, 'Self-Harm: Cutting the Bad out of Me', *Qualitative Health Research*, vol. 10, pp. 164-173.

[26] Harris, J., 2002, 'The Correspondence Method as a Data-gathering Technique in Qualitative Enquiry', *International Journal of Qualitative Method*, vol. 1, no. 4. *<http:// www.ualberta.ca/~ijqm/ 2002>.*

[27] Howells, C., 1999, *Derrida: Deconstruction from Phenomenology to Ethics*, Polity Press, Cambridge.

[28] James, A., 2002, Critical Work on CAMH in Childhood Studies? Personal Communication.

[29] Kendall, G. and Wickham, G., 1999, *Using Foucault's Methods*, Sage, London.

[30] Kennedy, A. J., 2000, *The Internet: The Rough Guide 2000*, Rough Guides, London.

[31] Kotre, J., 1984, *Outliving the self: Generativity and theInterpretation of Lives*, John Hopkins University Press, Baltimore, MD.

[32] Kraemer, S, 1995, 'The Liason Model: A Guide to Mental Health Services for Children and Adolescents', *Psychiatric Bulletin*, vol. 19, pp. 138-142.

[33] Mishler, E. G., 1995, 'Models of Narrative Analysis: A Typology',. *Journal of Narrative and Life History*, vol. 5, pp. 87-123.

[34] NCB, 2001, *Child and Adolescent Self-harm in Europe (CASE Study). <http://www.ncb. org.uk/projects/pmain.asp?projno=145>*

[35] Parker, I., 2002, Critical work on CAMH?, Personal Communication.

[36] Parker, I., Georgaca, E., Harper, D., McLaughlin, T. and Stowell-Smith, M., 1995, Deconstructing Psychopathology, Sage Publications, London .

[37] Plummer, K., 1983, *Documents of Life*, Allen and Unwin, London.

[38] Plummer, K.,1995, 'Life Story Research', in J.A. Smith, R. Harré and L. Van Langenhove (eds.), *Rethinking Methods in Psychology*, pp.50-63, Sag Publications, London.

[39] Polnay, L., 2000, 'Continuity of Behaviour Problems from Infancy to Early Adulthood'. *<http://tap.ccta.gov.uk/doh/refr_web.nsf/Switch+Body/916FC8272B57AD1200256951>*

[40] Potter, J. and Wetherell, M.,1987,Discourse and Social Psychology: Beyond Attitudes and Behaviour, Sage Publications, London.

[41] Potter, J. and Wetherell, M., 1995, 'Discourse Analysis', in J.A. Smith, R.Harré and L. Van Langenhove (eds.), *Rethinking Methods in Psychology*, pp.80-92, Sage Publications, London.

[42] Prior, L., 1997, 'Following in Foucault's Footsteps: Text and Context in Qualitative Research', in D. Silverman (ed.), *Qualitative Research: Theory, Method and Practice*, pp. 63-79, Sage Publications, London.

[43] Richardson, L., 2000, 'Writing: A Method of Inquiry', in N.K. Denzin and Y.S. Lincoln (eds.), *Handbook of Qualitative Research*, pp.923-948, Sage Publications, Thousand Oaks, CA.

[44] Riessman, C. K., 1993, Narrative Analysis, Sage Publications, Newbury Park, CA.

[45] Riessman, C. K, 2002, Narrative Analysis Workshop. Held at Qualitative Research in Health and Social Care Conference, Bournemouth, UK.

[46] Robinson, K. M., 2001, 'Unsolicited Narratives from the Internet: A Rich Source of Qualitative Data', *Qualitative Health Research*, vol. 11, pp. 706-714.

[47] Rosenwald, G. C. and Ochberg, R. L. , 1992, 'Introduction: Life Stories, Cultural Politics, and Self-Understanding', in G.C. Rosenwald and R.L. Ochberg (eds.), *Storied Lives: The cultural politics of self-understanding*, pp.1-18, Yale University Press, New Haven.

[48] Sarbin, T. R., 1986, 'The Narrative as a Root Metaphor for Psychology', in T.R. Sarbin (ed.), *Narrative Psychology: The Storied Nature of Human Conduct*, pp.3-21, Praeger, Westport, CT.

[49] Scott, S., 2002, 'Parent Training Groups for Childhood Conduct Disorders'. *<http://www.iop.kcl.ac.uk>*

[50] Shaffer, D. and Gutstein, J., 2002, 'Suicide and Attempted Suicide',in M.Rutter and E. Taylor (eds.), *Child and Adolescent Psychiatry*, pp.529-554, Blackwell, Oxford.

[51] Sharman, W., 1997, *Children and Adolescents with Mental Health Problems*, Bailliere Tindall, London.

[52] Silverman, D., 2000, *Doing Qualitative Research: A Practical Handbook*, Sage Publications, London.

[53] Stein, M. B., Hyde, K. L. and Monopolis, S. J., 1991, 'Child and Family Outreach Sevices as an Adjunct to Child and Adolescent Mental Health Treatment', *International Journal of Partial Hospitalization*, vol. 7, pp. 69-75.

[54] Stenner, P. and Eccleston, C., 1994, 'On the Textuality of Being: Towards an Invigorated Social Constructionism', *Theory and Psychology*, vol. 4, pp. 85-103.

[55] Taylor, A. S., 2000, 'The UN Convention on the Rights of the Child: Giving Children a Voice', in A. Lewis and G. Lindsay (eds.), *Researching Children's Perspectives*, pp.21-3, Open University Press, Buckingham.

[56] Tierney, W. G., 2000, 'Undaunted Courage: Life History and the Postmodern Challenge', in N.K. Denzin and Y.S. Lincoln (eds.), *Handbook of Qualitative Research*, pp.537-554, Sage Publications, Thousand Oaks, CA.

[57] United Nation, 1989, *UN Convention on the Rights of the Child.* New York, United Nations.

[58] Walker, S., 2001, 'Developing Child and Adolescent Mental Health Services', *Journal of Child Health Care*, vol. 5, pp. 71-76.

[59] Young Minds, 2002, 'Towards a New Adolescent Mental Health Service'. *<http://www.youngminds.org.uk/professionals/research/research.html>*

In: Health Research in Cyberspace
Editor: Pranee Liamputtong, pp. 257-272
ISBN 1-59454-819-6

Chapter 16

HEALTHCARE-RELATED WEB FORUMS IN SAUDI ARABIA: UNDERSTANDING THEIR USE THROUGH SILENT OBSERVATION AND THEMATIC CONTENT ANALYSIS

Yeslam Al-Saggaf and Radwan Kharabsheh

INTRODUCTION

Silent observation and thematic content analysis have long been used to research offline environments in qualitative, and even in some quantitative, research. This is because of the ability of the first in gaining rich and in-depth experiential accounts from research participants and the ability of the second in offering numeric values that allows reflective inferences of the major themes about a certain topic to be made. The Internet offers yet another medium through which silent observation and thematic content analysis can be carried out. The Internet has made possible the conduct of research in settings that were previously difficult to access. It is now possible for researchers to study conservative societies, such as the Saudi, and groups of people, such as females in the Saudi gender-segregated society who are otherwise inaccessible[1], without moving from their chairs.

This chapter focuses on the use of online forums for healthcare-related purposes in Saudi Arabia. Both of us (the first is a Saudi Arabian resident, the second is a Jordanian) are well versed in the customs, religion and traditions of the Saudi society and are frequent users of online forums. Our interest goes back to when the Saudi Arabian government introduced the Internet to the public in early 1999 and online forums began. Today, the number of Internet users in the country has reached nearly two million which is about 10% of the total population (Al-Watan, 2004). Of these, according to JeddahNews.net (2005), 50% participate in online forums.

---

[1] To male researchers.

Online forums have not been subjected to the strict regulations applied to other components of the Internet in the country. Anyone with a computer, a modem and a telephone line can join them, which is one of the things that made them popular among people. In addition to the thousands web forums from which people learn about healthcare risks and options from each other, specialised healthcare-related websites have also mushroomed in recent days in Saudi Arabia with more than 480 websites offering advice to people in all sorts of medical practices. The absence of free health care cover in Saudi Arabia and the high cost of health care services in the country, appear to have made healthcare-related forums significant in people's lives.

Lack of studies on healthcare-related online forums in Saudi Arabia inspired our research. It was further encouraged by the apparent lack of studies on online forums in general being conducted in the Arabian Gulf countries and the other Arab countries as Western researchers have noted (Ess, 1998). Moreover, with the exception of the first author's studies on social and political online forums (Al-Saggaf, 2004; Al-Saggaf and Weckert, 2005), there is a paucity of research on online forums. This chapter takes a step in the direction of addressing this paucity. Its emphasis is on the philosophical underpinnings of the study and two key components of the study's qualitative method, namely silent observation and thematic content analysis that were used to gather data for this study.

Philosophical Underpinnings

The study took an interpretivist (or interpretive) approach, which is associated with qualitative research methods. Interpretivists believe that the social world is interpreted or constructed by people and is, therefore, different from the physical world. They emphasise natural settings and seek to gain deep understanding of the meanings of the actors involved in the social phenomenon under study (Glesne, 1999; Sudeweeks and Simoff, 1999; Williamson, 2002). Given that the purpose of our study was to understand how people in Saudi Arabia use healthcare-related online forums from within their social and cultural contexts, qualitative research methods emerging from an interpretivist framework seemed to be most appropriate.

The constructivist paradigm, coming as it does under the interpretivist umbrella, was chosen. This paradigm assumes a relativist ontology (multiple realities), a subjectivist epistemology (investigator and respondent co-create understandings), and a naturalistic (in the natural world) set of methodological procedures (Denzin and Lincoln, 2000: 21). Constructivists believe that there is no single objective reality 'out there'; instead, there are multiple constructed realities about the phenomenon under study. They accept that they themselves influence the research process and for this reason they reflect on their own roles when writing the report (Marshall and Rossman, 1999). They also believe that they should study the phenomenon in the field where it occurs, because they recognise the importance of understanding the meanings and cultural practices of the people from within the everyday settings in which they take place. Schwandt (1994: 128) believes that research carried out within a constructivist paradigm is very similar to naturalistic inquiry as outlined in Lincoln and Guba (1985).

There are principally two kinds of constructivist theories. Kelly's (1963) personal construct theory which focuses on how individuals interpret their world, and Berger and Luckmann's (1967) social construct theory which emphasises the influence of society, culture, and social environment on individual reality. Personal constructivists claim that, associated with a particular social phenomenon are multiple, constructed realities that exist in the minds of individuals who are involved in the phenomenon (Charmaz, 2000; Denzin and Lincoln, 2000; Schwandt, 2000). In other words, reality for each individual is determined by each individual's perceptions (Lincoln and Guba, 1985) and each individual's perceptions of what is real may differ from that of others (Kelly, 1991; Hammersley, 1995; Saule, 2000). This means that, while in the constructed view, events, persons, objects are tangible entities, the meanings derived from them in order to make sense of, or organize, them are constructed realities (Lincoln and Guba; 1985: 84).

Social constructionists argue that meaning is developed through the interactions of social processes involving people, language and religion (Berger and Luckmann, 1967). Williamson (2002: 30) says that social constructionists see people as developing meanings for their activities together, that is, they socially construct reality. Schwandt (1994: 127) adds that the focus of social construct theory "is not in the meaning-making activity of the individual mind, but on the collective generation of meaning as shaped by conventions of language and other social processes". Additionally, social constructionists recognise the impact of society, culture, and social environment on the way people behave and make meanings in that society (Berger and Luckmann, 1967).

In line with the literature in which both points of view are represented (Markham, 1998; Costigan, 1999; Fernback, 1999; Dodge and Kitchin, 2001; Manaszewicz et al., 2002), ours is influenced by both constructivist theories. Jones (1998: 5), for example, argues that the online community is "constituted in conversation and interaction". Building on Berger and Luckmann's (1967) theory on the social construction of reality, he argues that "the social construction of reality is not constituted *by* the networks of Computer-Mediated Communication users utilise, it is constituted *in* the networks" (Jones, 1998: 5), suggesting that it is not the computer screens, and physical networks but the people and the interactions between them that create social reality.

On the other hand, Fernback (1999), who takes a personal constructivist view, thinks that the reality about online environments is personally constructed, because these realities exist mainly in the minds of the participants. Markham (1998) agrees, believing that through the exchanges of text, individuals construct their individual accounts and their individual experiences about their online environments, implying that the reality about online environments is multiple (Markham, 1998; Costigan, 1999).

Both of the above theories are useful for understanding healthcare-related online forums in Saudi Arabia. Personal construct theory can be used to understand how participants individually develop their sense of place and their perception of the value of these forums. Social construct theory can be used to understand how individuals develop shared meanings about their online experience together and how their culture and the online forums affect their participation online. The fact that religion and culture in Saudi Arabia not only shape people's attitudes, practices and behaviours, but also the way they see and do things and perceive their lives, makes social construct theory particularly appropriate for understanding online forums in that society.

From Philosophy to Method

Ethnography, one of the methods favoured by constructivists, was chosen for the study. One of the important aspects of ethnography is that it allows multiple interpretations of realities and alternative interpretations of data to be presented (Fetterman, 1989), which fits well with the purpose of constructivism. Ethnography is closely linked with participant observation (Liamputtong and Ezzy, 2005). For example, Saule (2000: 160) describes ethnographers as "studying people in their everyday contexts" and Minichiello et al. (1990:18) describe participant observation as "studying people by participating in social interactions with them in order to observe and understand them". Modern ethnography or participant observation uses a range of techniques such as interviewing, focus groups, observation and questionnaires (Liamputtong and Ezzy, 2005) and "also has the flexibility to emphasise some techniques over others, and to leave some techniques out altogether" (Bow 2000: 249).

Data were collected and analysed for this study using two techniques[2]. These were silent observation of a popular healthcare-related online forum and thematic content analysis of another similar healthcare-related online forum. Findings obtained through these techniques were triangulated to assist in establishing the trustworthiness of this research (Lincoln and Guba, 1987; Maxwell, 1996; Bow, 2000). This triangulation of data will also give the reader the opportunity to critique the truthfulness of the results.

As silent observers in the first forum, we avoided disturbing the normal flow of events in that forum and were able to observe the natural behaviour of participants (Angrosino and Mays de Perez, 2000; Locke et al., 2000). We also avoided confusion over our roles and becoming emotionally close to the participants, which could have caused some distortions to the research findings (Paccagnella, 1997; Glesne, 1999). Without the need to participate, we were able to concentrate on our observation. As pointed out in the literature, being an observer and a participant at the same time involves two distinct roles, which the researchers may not often accomplish successfully (Lincoln and Guba, 1987; North, 1994; Tedlock, 2000).

On the other hand, we also gained enormously from doing thematic content analysis of another similar healthcare-related online forum. Doing thematic content analysis in this forum offered us numeric values that allowed reflective inferences about the themes contained in topics to be made. Conducting content analysis in this way allowed the themes and patterns related to the studied online forums to emerge from the text and the final result was hopefully an accurate picture of the characteristics of the studied forums. Using content analysis in this way (that is emerging from an interpretivist framework) seemed to be most appropriate because the benefit sought from using this technique is to also understand how healthcare-related web forums are being used by people in Saudi Arabia. This approach is also consistent with how content analysis is used in the literature and is often followed in descriptive studies such as the present study (see for example, Neuman, 1994; Aronson, 1994; Neuendorf, 2002; Cammaerts and Audenhove, 2003).

---

[2] The first researcher takes the position of distinguishing between the terms 'technique' and 'method'. The former should mean the specific procedures that are used to collect or analyse data. The latter should mean the general rules that govern the implementation of these procedures.

THE SILENT OBSERVATION – SETTING AND PROCESS

The silent observation began first and was carried out over a four-week period, from March 1 2005, until March 31, 2005. The healthcare-related online forum selected as the research site for conducting silent observation is called Al-Saha[3] Al-Tubiah[4] and is located at www.alsaha.com. The Al-Saha forums which are asynchronous public discussion web forums, are by far the most widely spread forums in Saudi Arabia (Al Arabiya, 2004). The observed forum has a design similar to that found in most forums in the country. At the time of observation, the main page in the forum contained links to newly posted topics or messages only. Older topics resided in other pages that could be accessed through small links that were found on the main page.

While entry to the forum is open to anyone with a computer and Internet connection and subscription was free of charge and involved only the provision of a nickname and a password, because of the popularity of this forum registration has been closed down since five years ago. To observe the forum silently, also called lurking (Jones, 1997; see also Chapter 1 in this volume), we did not need to subscribe, gain permission from a gatekeeper, seek permission to conduct observations from the participants in the forum, or seek their permission to use some of what they said in the forum. Rigorous checking of the ethical issues involved, revealed that conversations in publicly accessible discussion forums are public acts deliberately intended for public consumption. Recording, analysing and reporting of such content, where individuals' identities are shielded, is in line with the ethics of doing research on online environments (King, 1996; Paccagnella, 1997; Frankel, 1999; Glesne, 1999; Eysenbach and Till, 2001; Ess, C. and AoIR Ethics Working Committee, 2002; see also Chapter 1 in this volume).

During the four-week period, the process of observation and the recording of field notes in a journal, in which date and time were also entered, took three to four hours daily, depending on the volume of new topics. The process went in two stages with the first stage, lasting one week (first), being unstructured. In this stage, we entered the setting with a broad view, which involved looking at activities and characteristics that were salient. This stage assisted us in becoming familiar with the atmosphere of the online forum and the nature of the topics. In the field notes, the second author identified the key features of participation and made a brief checklist of observational categories for use in the second stage. It should be noted while both of us did the silent observation individually, only the second author took field notes. He then, on a regular basis, discussed his notes with the first author. This process tackled issues of subjectivity that could arise if only a single observer was present.

In the second stage, field notes focused on these categories were made daily. Messages and information related to the topics discussed were recorded and the key features of participation accordingly categorised. The second author also wrote his own reactions, reflections and interpretations about his observations. Quotes that contained interesting statements or insights into behaviour, or that seemed illuminating of the purpose of the study, were copied and translated immediately in the same journal, in a different font to distinguish them from other data. When translating the Arabic expressions, the second author regularly consulted with the first and sought his opinion.

---

[3] Al-Saha, and also Al-Muntada, in Arabic means a forum

[4] In English this word means medical or healthcare

Analysis of Data from Silent Observation

Data from silent observation were analysed as they were collected. The daily observational field notes were recorded in MS Word and saved as RTF documents, with a single document covering one week of field notes. At the end of each week, this RTF document was imported into NVIVO (a Software package for managing qualitative data) for analysis, meaning that the analysis of field notes was performed on a weekly basis. This is not to say, however, that the process of analysis was not iterative as the field notes were re-analysed as more data were collected.

The document passages from the observational and participation field notes were arranged under headings, based on time and date of recording, to form sections. After editing the documents in the NVIVO editor, they were read more than once so that a feel for the data was gained. Keywords were identified after careful studying of each word and each line in the document passages. Themes were then developed based on these keywords and the NVIVO Coder was used to assign nodes representing those themes. Next, the node browser in NVIVO was invoked to view all segments of text, from all the weekly documents, for the purpose of printing them out. Very importantly, the nodes stored all the data related to a particular theme from all the weekly documents. That is, these nodes became buckets or baskets into which segments of text, from all the weekly documents, related to a particular theme were placed.

The printed segments of text pertaining to a particular node were carefully read to make sure that the themes developed were appropriate. For the purpose of ensuring their appropriateness also, each was defined and evaluated. The process of evaluation involved ensuring that certain phrases (or similar to them) were found in the data. The evaluation process was followed by two important steps. First, items of data from all documents that had been assigned to a particular node were compared and contrasted to ensure that they were assigned to the appropriate node. Second, all nodes were further structured or organised into groups based on the general concepts of the research they addressed. Finally, for the purpose of producing a summary of the data, statements that encompassed the developed nodes (themes) were written. These statements were combined to form paragraphs that formulated the results some of which are presented below.

Thematic Content Analysis

The thematic content analysis of the other healthcare-related online forum, with considerable efforts being made to ensure it was similar to the first one, began about one week later, and involved analysing four weeks worth of posts from April 7, 2005 until May 5, 2005. The unit of analysis was each individual post. While many traditional (statistical) approaches to content analysis rely on fixed or stable units of analysis, for example, word counts, the focus in this study was on the occurrence of selected themes within each topic. The broader nature and purpose of each topic posted was also taken into consideration during the process of analysis. The decisions of assigning selected themes to topics were made after gaining an idea about the context or contexts each topic fitted.

Assigning selected themes to topics based on judgments about their context can no doubt be somewhat subjective (although we did this component of the research also together). To limit this subjectivity and enhance the reliability and validity of the findings, we triangulated the findings from content analysis with findings obtained through silent observation. In order also to enhance the reliability and validity of the findings, we will explain the process of coding and analysis of data in great detail so as to make this study replicable as much as possible (Neuendorf, 2002).

THE PROCESS OF CODING

While most posts were coded with only one category (see Figure 1 below), in a few cases topics were coded with an additional one or two categories. In thematic content analysis, it is acceptable that items are coded with more than one category at the same time (see for example, Frankos, 2000). This is because the basis for categorisation is the context of the topic which makes it likely that a topic will belong to more than one category or a theme at the same time. Having said that, however, assigning a topic to more than one category occurred very seldom as in the majority of cases only a single theme was found to be representative of the topic. This is shown in Table 1 below.

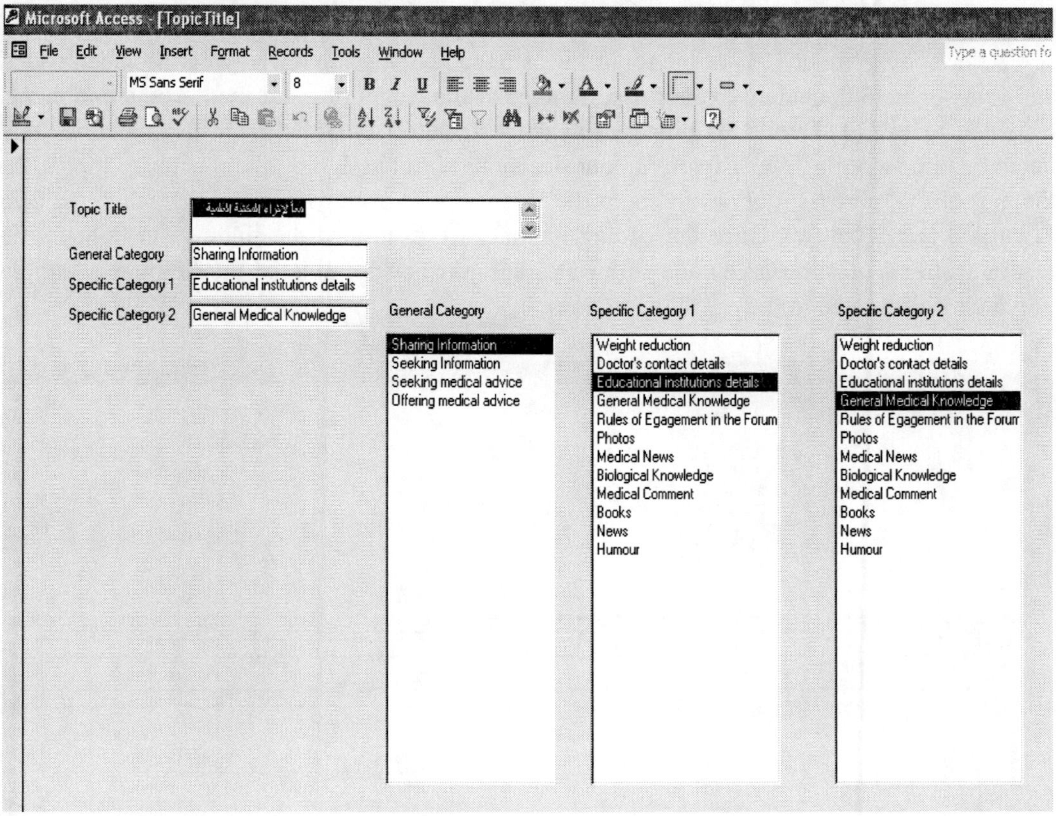

Figure 1. The process of categorisation

First, topic's titles in the form of clickable hyperlinks were copied and pasted into a Microsoft Excel sheet. The clickable hyperlinks titles, which represented links to topics, were copied in groups as they were located on one page on the forum. Next, and after titles were arranged in Excel, they were imported to Microsoft Access as a single table. In Microsoft Access, three fields were added to that table and named category 1 to 3. The three added categories represented the three possible themes a topic could be assigned. In Microsoft Access also another table with a number of pre-determined categories was created. (See Figure 1 above for a list of the categories.) The source of the pre-determined categories was the information obtained from the four weeks of silent observation of the first forum. It is important to note that additional categories were added as the analysis progressed. This meant that the study relied on both predefined and interactive categories. This introduced a level of coding flexibility as it allowed new and important material that could have significant bearings on the findings to be incorporated into the coding process.

To code data, the topic in Excel was first clicked and read (by both of us) from its location on the Internet. In many cases, the replies to a topic were also read to be sure about the context the topic fitted. Second, the topic was assigned a category from a Microsoft Access System screen in which the first author developed. The form consisted of a textbox that contained the topic title, three empty textboxes to accept the assigning of categories, and three list boxes which had copies of the categories developed earlier (see Figure 1 above). When a topic was selected (after it was read) and upon selecting a category from one of the list boxes, the corresponding empty textbox was automatically filled with the selected category. This process of coding was carried out for all the topics in the main table.

After coding about 10% of the topics, we stopped coding, reviewed what has been coded and in a separate document explained a number of the categories and made some comments on when to assign them. This process (Neuendorf, 2002) provided us with guidelines that helped us in becoming consistent with our decisions about assigning the themes to topics. At the end of this process, queries to count the frequency of each category were generated (see Figures 2 and 3 below). Once the coding is done, we examined the findings in light of the results from silent observation and formed paragraphs that formulated the findings a sample of which is presented in the next few sections.

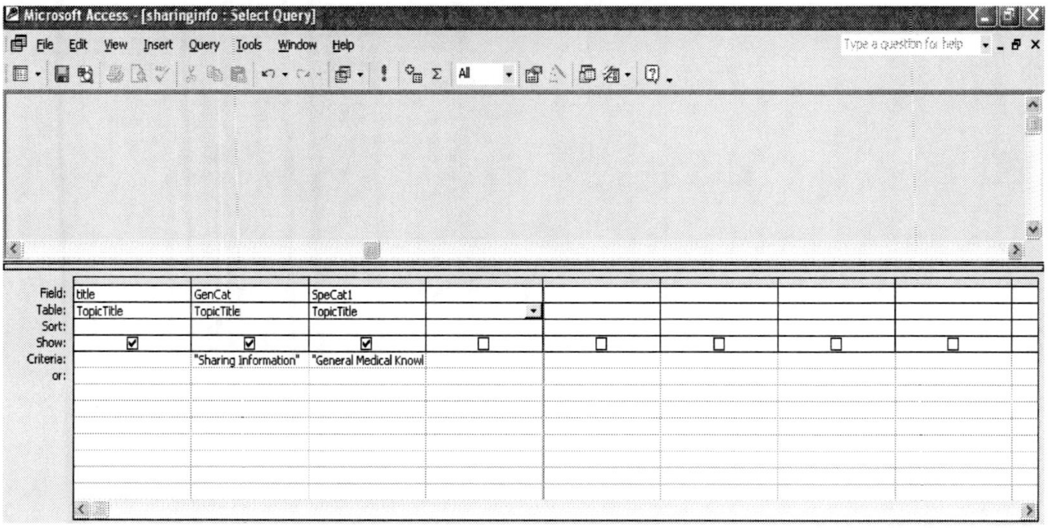

Figure 2. The generation of queries

Microsoft Access - [sharinginfo : Select Query]

File Edit View Insert Format Records Tools Window Help

title	GenCat	SpeCat1
نصائح لعينيك	Sharing Information	General Medical Knowledge
اضرار فرقعة الاظافر والرقبة..	Sharing Information	General Medical Knowledge
سيء السمعة	Sharing Information	General Medical Knowledge
الجاثوم ..	Sharing Information	General Medical Knowledge
فصائل الدم ؟؟؟	Sharing Information	General Medical Knowledge
من يستوعب الديسلكسيا	Sharing Information	General Medical Knowledge
النانو تكنولوجي والطب	Sharing Information	General Medical Knowledge
العلاج بالألوان	Sharing Information	General Medical Knowledge
[align=left]"USE IT OR LOSE IT" wanna know whats t	Sharing Information	General Medical Knowledge
الحبة السوداء	Sharing Information	General Medical Knowledge
فوائد التمر..	Sharing Information	General Medical Knowledge
أفضل طريقة للتخلص من البكتيريا والجراثيم	Sharing Information	General Medical Knowledge
خطر نفخ البالون	Sharing Information	General Medical Knowledge
بدون عنوان	Sharing Information	General Medical Knowledge
عندما تتحدث عيناك!!	Sharing Information	General Medical Knowledge
سلاح البروكولي والطماطم معاً في وجه السرطان	Sharing Information	General Medical Knowledge
الأطفال الأذكياء أقل إصابة بأمراض الشيخوخة	Sharing Information	General Medical Knowledge
الشيكولاته	Sharing Information	General Medical Knowledge
اكتشف باحثون أن الاكتئاب قد يزيد من مخاطر الإصابة بأمراض الق	Sharing Information	General Medical Knowledge
التدخين يقصر عمر المرأة	Sharing Information	General Medical Knowledge
أول مشاركة وأول طلب هام للأطباء وطلاب كلية الطب	Sharing Information	General Medical Knowledge
بعد عشر سنوات لن نحتاج الادويه ولن نرى انسان عاجز((اكتشاف طب	Sharing Information	General Medical Knowledge
المناعة كنز لا يفنى	Sharing Information	General Medical Knowledge
مهم جدا	Sharing Information	General Medical Knowledge
بكتيريا قاتلة تحيّر العلماء	Sharing Information	General Medical Knowledge
هـــل تصـــــــــدق... الشمس تعالج الأرق	Sharing Information	General Medical Knowledge
رائحة الزهور تخفف الاكتئاب وكذلك الصداقة..	Sharing Information	General Medical Knowledge
لحماية القلب واظب بتنظيف اسنانك!	Sharing Information	General Medical Knowledge
ما هو الطب النفسي بإيجاز ؟	Sharing Information	General Medical Knowledge
الطب الحديث يكشف المزيد من أسرار السواك	Sharing Information	General Medical Knowledge
الحاسة السادسة حقيقة وليست وهم	Sharing Information	General Medical Knowledge
طبيب عربي يتوصل إلى نظرية جديدة لعلاج أمراض العيون	Sharing Information	General Medical Knowledge
بدقّة يمكن أن يشخّص اختبار الدّم السّكتة القلبيّة في مرضى ال	Sharing Information	General Medical Knowledge

Figure 3. An example of the result of a query

Sample of the Findings

In this section, we provide a sample of the findings relating to the main themes that characterised healthcare-related web forums in Saudi Arabia. The findings presented in this section have been obtained using both silent observation and thematic content analysis. The section also presents some interpretations of these findings from within the social and cultural contexts of Saudi society.

SHARING INFORMATION

Information sharing was by far the most common theme that characterised Saudi healthcare-related web forums. This observation accords well with the findings obtained through thematic content analysis. 87% of all the topics posted to the second forum were for the purpose of sharing information. Of course there were all different types of information that was shared. Participants regularly posted topics to update others about developments in medicine (17% of all topics) and medical research or new cures or procedures in which they learned about through the media. They used their forums to share with others their general medical knowledge (71% of all topics) about, for example, weight reduction, diabetes, bones or joints diseases. They also provided others with doctor's and medical institution's contact details (3% of all topics); although some members had reservations about this type of sharing of information from fear that some might think that they were using the forum as an advertising tool for their own or favourite medical doctors, products or medical institutions. Members also shared their personal stories and experiences particularly in relation to an illness they were having or had in the past. Patients or concerned members in the families benefited from these personal stories and experiences. The shared stories and experiences assisted existing patients in reducing tension and anxiety that stemmed from their own illness.

The diversity of the backgrounds of the participants was reflected through their contributions to the forums. The observed forum, for example, included members who appeared to be medical doctors, specialists and university medicine students. The observed forum also contained members who seemed to be interested and well-read in medicine as they frequently provided news extracts from newspapers and online media sources. The forum also included the regular type of members many of whom were past/present patients with personal stories or experiences to tell, and knowledge of doctors and medical institutions to share.

It was very clear that one of the main aims of healthcare-related web forums is providing medical advice and consultations to those who sought them (although only 3% of all topics revolved around that issue in the second forum). Members who are medical doctors or specialists visited the observed forum regularly for the purpose of offering those who sought medical advice on their medical problems their diagnosis or expert opinions. Occasionally, the specialists were observed asking patients (members) for more information or the results of their medical reports. In some cases, patients, in an attempt to help specialists make an informed opinion, provided their medical history or the results of their medical examinations online as an attachment to the forum.

Some of the patients (members), and their familles, used the observed healthcare-related web forum to seek medical doctors' help with verifying the diagnosis made by their personal doctors especially when the medicine prescribed by their doctors did not cure the problem or the symptoms. A good example of this was when a member inquired about a hearing aid for his brother. The member's brother, who was using a hearing aid for a long time prescribed by a German hospital in Riyadh, started to loose his hearing ability to the extent that he could only hear the very loud voices. Some members in the forum offered him the contact details of the top specialists in this area in the country. A specialist (forum member), however, asked that person for more information about the case and for all the tests that had been conducted on the patient. After the member provided a case history and attached a pdf file which contained a copy of the results of all the tests conducted on his brother, the specialist replied to him with a new consultation for his brother.

WOMEN

Although it was difficult to identify the gender of the participants in the observed online forum, by continuously observing the members and their interactions and closely examining the topics they posted, it was possible in many cases to guess their gender. Moreover, results from studies by the first author (Al-Saggaf, 2004) did not suggest that members deliberately disguised their gender. On the contrary, these results showed that because members operated in these online forums for very long periods of time, many even chose to reveal their real life names. Unmarried young females in the observed forum, however, appeared to be very reluctant about revealing their true genders and their real life names. Older married females, on the other hand, felt comfortable revealing their true genders and occasionally even their real life names. This could be because either older married females felt less threatened by the presence of males (that is males might not see them as having the potential for entering into a relationship with them and thus they would not target them) or could be the result of their marriage experience which could have made them lees inhibited towards males and more experienced in dealing with them.

The anonymity, lack of public self-awareness, and the medium's lack of oral and non-verbal cues which, according to Joinson (1998) and Mar (2000), cause abandonment of social inhibitions, apparently fostered a liberating effect on the members in general and on females specifically. Females seemed to be more liberated, uninhibited and more willing to participate and be open about their personal opinions and experiences in a way that is unusual to their attitude in the real life. This was especially true when debating topics that were considered to be sensitive or taboo in the Saudi society. One example of this was during a debate that revolved around the effect of masturbation on Saudi males/females. This topic, which even males in Saudi Arabia would feel embarrassed to discuss with their friends, due to its sensitivity and to the conservative nature of the Saudi society, attracted some female members. During the debate, female members participated in the discussion of this topic and did not hesitate from giving their opinions and thoughts on it.

Gender itself had an effect on member's participation in healthcare-related web forums. Female members received more attention than regular male members. This was evident in the amount of responses females received compared to what males would normally receive in the forum. Males were also observed to make fun of females less (compared to what they do to males), replied to female messages quicker and complimented them on their contributions generously. This reflects the eagerness of Saudi males to interact with females which makes sense given that in the real life, the long-established traditions prevent them from having a casual conversation with females. This means that these forums have allowed males and females in this gender-segregated society to communicate in ways not previously possible (see also Chapter 1 in this volume).

Political Jokes and Political Comments

One of the interesting observations was the members' use of their forum to post political jokes and political comments (3% of all topics). The members' use of their forum in this way reflects the importance of internal politics in their lives. It also supports findings from an earlier study (see Al-Saggaf and Weckert, 2005) that suggests that because freedom of expression in general in Saudi Arabia is somewhat limited, people turned to online forums to express themselves and present their ideas and views to others in their forums. Given that in the real life these people can not express their opinions openly, any medium that could enable them to do so they would use. For example, when a concerned parent of a child, who swallowed a coin, sought members' advice on what to do, one of the funny comments he received was

> You are worried about a poor little child who swallowed just one coin! What about the millions of dollars which people swallow everyday and no one says anything about them [Silent observation, Week 1, 7 March 2005]

The above quote hints towards the financial corruption of some of the politicians and businessmen in the country. Another funny comment the father of the child received was from one asking him to be careful when carrying the chid through the security gates in airports. The man said with the coin inside the child's stomach, if the metal detector detected the coin it would set the alarm and the child would be treated as a young terrorist! This, again, carries an implicit indication regarding the phobia of being a terror suspect that some Saudis experience when travelling overseas particularly after September 11, 2001.

It appears that political comments were made within healthcare-related topics in the observed forum whenever the context of the topic allowed. Different topics of course tackled different issues, mainly un-talked about publicly in the real life, such as nepotism in hiring and firing, financial corruption, and politics. In this sense, even healthcare-related online forums were used by people to communicate their ideas and opinions to others, let their voices heard, and get their messages across to others.

Conclusion

Silent observation and thematic content analysis have proven to be successful in researching healthcare-related online forums in Saudi Arabia and combining these approaches brought the benefits of each to the study. In addition to their low cost, speed of return, and ease of access to a wider geographical area (that is, members in the studied forums came from all over the country), they enabled the researchers to conduct their research from the comfort of their chairs. It was also clear from the findings of the study that silent observation was effective in providing in-depth and rich descriptions of the main characteristics of the forum and its use. It offered the researchers thick descriptions about the people (that is, women) in their own context in a way that could not be done using thematic content analysis. On the other hand, thematic content analysis facilitated comparisons of data and provided the researchers with numeric values that allowed reflective inferences about the themes in this study to be made. The triangulation of data from the two techniques gave the researchers some reassurance about the results that emerged from this research and enabled the establishment of their trustworthiness.

The choice of the constructivist paradigm to study online environments in Saudi Arabia enabled this deep exploration of the online forums in their cultural context to be undertaken. The lens of personal and social construct theories have proven to be useful for the understanding of these forums. The theory of personal construct was useful for understanding the ways members individually constructed their realties about these forums; that is some used these forums for sharing information while others used it for making political statements. Social construct theory was useful for understanding how the members, for example males towards females, collectively behaved online and how they developed together the meanings about their online experiences. This theory was particularly useful for understanding the ways in which the offline culture and the web-forum technology affected members' behaviour online and in many cases caused changes in attitudes online to occur.

The interpretive-qualitative research methodology used in the study also proved to be appropriate. Conducting ethnography from within a constructivist paradigm enabled the use of silent observation and thematic content analysis, which produced findings that are deep, indicative and rich in nature. Had a quantitative research method been used, the findings could only have been broad and superficial. The use of a quantitative content analysis or a survey by self-administered questionnaires, for example, for this study could not have provided the rich data revealed by observation.

REFERENCES

[1] Al Arabiya, 2004, 'The owner of Al-Saha is in the "Cage of Accusation"'. *<http://www. alarabiya.net/>*

[2] Al-Saggaf, Y. and Weckert, J., 2005, 'Political Online Communities (POCs) in Saudi Arabia', in S. Marshall, W. Taylor and X. Yu (eds.), *Encyclopaedia of Developing Regional Communities with ICT*, Idea Group Reference, London (in print).

[3] Al-Saggaf, Y., 2004, 'The Effect of Online Community on Offline Community in Saudi Arabia', *Electronic Journal of Information Systems in Developing Countries EJISDC*, vol. 16, no. 2, pp.1-16. *<http://www.ejisdc.org>*

[4] Al-Watan, 2004, 'To Improve Services for Subscribes and Promote Research'. *<http:// www.alwatan.com.sa>*

[5] Angrosino, M. and Mays de Perez, K., 2000, 'Rethinking Observation: From Method to Context', in N. K. Denzin and Y. S. Lincoln (eds.), *Handbook of Qualitative Research*, 2nd edition, pp. 673-702, Sage Publications, Thousand Oaks, CA.

[6] Aronson, J., 1994, 'A Pragmatic View of Thematic Analysis', *The Qualitative Report*, vol. 2, no. 1. *<http://www.nova.edu/ssss/QR/BackIssues/QR2-1/aronson.html>*.

[7] Berger, P.L. and Luckmann, T., 1967, *The Social Construction of Reality: A Treatise in the Sociology of Knowledge*, Anchor Press, New York.

[8] Bow, A., 2000, 'Ethnographic Techniques', in K. Williamson (ed.), *Research Methods for Students and Professionals: Information Management and Systems*, 2nd edition, pp. 247-262, Centre for Information Studies, CSU. Wagga Wagga.

[9] Cammaerts, B. and Audenhove, L.V., 2003, *ICT-Usage among Transnational Social Movements in the Networked Society: To Organise, to Mediate & to Influence*, unpublished report, ASCoR, Amsterdam Free University, Amsterdam.

[10] Charmaz, K., 2000, 'Grounded Theory: Objectivist and Constructivist Methods', in N. K. Denzin and Y. S. Lincoln (eds.), *Handbook of Qualitative Research*, 2nd edition, pp. 509-535, Sage, Thousand Oaks, CA.

[11] Costigan, J. T., 1999, 'Introduction: Forests, trees, and Internet research', in S. G. Jones (ed.), *Doing Internet research: Critical issues and methods for examining the Net*, pp. xvii-xxiv, Sage Publications, Thousand Oaks, CA.

[12] Denzin, N.K. and Lincoln, Y.S., 2000, 'Introduction: the Discipline and Practice of Qualitative Research', in Denzin, N.K. & Lincoln, Y.S. (eds.), *Handbook of Qualitative Research*, 2nd edition, pp. 1-29, Sage Publications, Thousand Oaks, CA.

[13] Dodge, M. and Kitchin, R., 2001, *Mapping Cyberspace*, Routledge, London.

[14] Ess, C., 1998, 'First Looks: CATaC'98', in C. Ess and F. Sudweeks (eds.), *Proceedings of Cultural Attitudes Towards Communication and Technology*, Uni of Sydney,Australia

[15] Ess, C. and AoIR Ethics Working Committee, 2002, 'Ethical Decision-Making and Internet Research: Recommendations from the Aoir Ethics Committee'. *<http://www. aoir.org/reports/ethics.pdf>*

[16] Eysenbach, G. and Till, J. E., 2001, 'Ethical Issues in Qualitative Research on Internet Communities', *British Medical Journal*, vol. 323, no. 7321, pp. 1103-1105.

[17] Fernback, J., 1999, 'There Is a Their There: notes Toward a Definition of Cybercommunity', in S. G. Jones (ed.), *Doing Internet research: Critical issues and methods for examining the Net*, pp. 203-220, Sage Publications, Thousand Oaks, CA.

[18] Fetterman, D.M., 1989, *Ethnography: Step by Step*, Sage Publications, Thousand Oaks, CA.

[19] Fetterman, D. M., 1998, 'Ethnography', in L. Bickman and D. J. Rog (eds.), *Handbook of Applied Social Research Methods*, pp. 473-504, Sage Publications, Thousand Oaks, CA.

[20] Frankel, M.S., 1999, 'Ethical and Legal Aspects of Human Subjects Research on The Internet'. *<http://www.aaas.org/spp/dspp/sfrl/projects/intres/report.pdf>*

[21] Frankos, C. E., 2000, *Interactivity and Community: Social Interaction in An Online Community*, Unpublished MA thesis, UMI. California State University, Ann Arbor, Michigan.

[22] Glesne, C., 1999, *Becoming Qualitative Researcher: An Introduction*, 2nd edition,: Longman, New York.

[23] Hammersley, M., 1995, *The Politics of Social Research*, Sage Publications, London

[24] JeddahNews.net, 2005, 'Where Do You Spend Most of Your Time Over the Internet?' *<http://www.jeddahnews.net>*

[25] Joinson, A. 1998, 'Causes and Implications of Disinhibited Behaviour on the Internet', in J. Gackenbach (ed.), *Psychology and the Internet*, pp. 43-59, Academic Press, San Diego.

[26] Jones, S. G., 1997, 'The Internet and its Social Landscape', in S. G. Jones (ed.), *Virtual Culture: Identity and Communication in Cybersociety*, pp. 7-35, Sage Publications, London.

[27] Jones, S. G., 1998, 'Information, Internet, and community: Notes toward an understanding of community in the information age', in S. G. Jones (ed.), *CyberSociety*

2.0: Revisiting Computer-Mediated Communication and Community, pp. 1-35, Sage Publications, Thousand Oaks, CA

[28] Jones, S.G. and Kucker, S., 2001,'Computers, the Internet, and Virtual Cultures', in J. Lull (ed.), *Culture in the Communication Age*, pp. 212-225, Routledge, London.

[29] Kelly, G. A., 1963, *A Theory of Personality: The Psychology of Personal Constructs*, W.W. Norton & Company, New York.

[30] Kelly, G. A., 1991, *The Psychology of Personal Constructs*, Routledge, London.

[31] King, S. A., 1996, 'Researching Internet communities: Proposed ethical guidelines for the reporting of results', *The Information Society*, vol. 12, no. 2, pp. 119-128.

[32] Liamputtong, P. and Ezzy, D., 2005, *Qualitative Research Methods*, 2nd edition, Oxford University Press, Melbourne.

[33] Lincoln, Y. S. and Guba, E. G., 1985, *Naturalistic Inquiry*, Sage Publications, Newbury Park, CA.

[34] Lincoln, Y. S. and Guba, E. G., 1987, *Effective Evaluation*, Jossey-Bass, San Francisco.

[35] Locke, L. F., Spirduso, W. W. and Silverman, S. J., 2000, *Proposals That Work*, 4th edition, Sage, Thousand Oaks.

[36] Manaszewicz, R., Williamson, K. and Mckemmish, S., 2002, 'Breast Cancer Knowledge Online: Towards Meeting The Diverse Information Needs of The Breast Cancer Community', Proceedings of Electronic Networking 2002 Building Community Conference, 3-7 July. Melbourne, Australia.

[37] Mar, J. 2000, 'Online On time: The Language of Internet Relay Chat', in D. Gibbs and K.-L. Krause (eds), *Cyberlines: Languages and Cultures of the Internet*, pp. 151-174, James Nicholas Publishers, Albert Park, Melbourne.

[38] Markham, A. N., 1998, *Life Online: Researching Real Experience in Virtual Space*, AltaMira, Walnut Creek, CA.

[39] Marshall, C. and Rossman, G. B., 1999, *Designing Qualitative Research*, 3rd edition, Sage Publications, Thousand Oaks, CA.

[40] Minichiello, V., Aroni, R., Timwell, E. and Alexander, L., 1990, *In-depth Interviewing: Researching People*, Longman Cheshire, Melbourne.

[41] Maxwell Joseph A., 1996, *Qualitative Research Design: An Interactive Approach*, Sage Publications, Thousand Oaks, CA.

[42] Neuendorf, K. A.., 2002, *The Content Analysis Guidebook*, Sage Publications, Thousand Oaks.

[43] Neuman, L., 1994, *Social Research Methods: Qualitative and Quantitative Approaches*, Simon and Schuster, Massachusetts.

[44] North, T., 1994, 'The Internet and Usenet Global Computer Networks: An Investigation of Their Culture and Its Effects on New Users', Unpublished MA thesis, Curtin University of Technology, Perth, Australia. <http://www.scribe.com.au/timn/thesis/>

[45] Paccagnella, L., 1997, 'Getting the Seats of Your Pants Dirty: Strategies for Ethnographic Research on Virtual Communities', *JCMC*, vol. 3, no. 1. *<http://jcmc. indiana.edu>*

[46] Saule, S., 2000, 'Ethnography', In K. Williamson (ed.), *Research Methods for Students and Professionals: Information Management and Systems*, 2nd edition, pp. 159-176, Centre for Information Studies, CSU, Wagga Wagga.

[47] Schwandt, T. A., 2000, 'Three Epistemological Stances for Qualitative Inquiry: Interpretivism, Hermeneutics, and Social Constructionist', in N. K. Denzin and Y. S.

Lincoln (eds.), *Handbook of Qualitative Research*, 2nd edition, pp. 189-214, Sage Publications, Thousand Oaks, CA.

[48] Schwandt, T.A., 1994, 'Constuctivist, Interpretivist Approaches in Qualitative Research', in N. Denzin and Y. Lincoln (eds.) *Handbook of Qualitative Research*, pp. 118-137, Sage Publications, Thousand Oaks.

[49] Kollock, P. and Smith, M., 1999, 'Communities in Cyberspace', in M. Smith and P. Kollock (eds.), *Communities in Cyberspace*, pp. 3-25, Routledge, London.

[50] Sudweeks, F. and Simoff, S. J., 1999, 'Complementary Explorative Data Analysis: The Reconciliation of Quantitative and Qualitative Principles', in S. G. Jones (ed.), *Doing Internet research: Critical issues and methods for examining the Ne*t, pp. 29-56, Sage Publications, Thousand Oaks, CA.

[51] Tedlock, B., 2000, 'Ethnography and Ethnographic Representation', in N. K. Denzin and Y. S. Lincoln (eds.), *Handbook of qualitative research*, 2nd edition, pp. 455-486, Sage Publications, Thousand Oaks, CA.

[52] Williamson, K., 2000, *Research Methods for Students and Professionals: Information Management and Systems*, Centre for Information Studies, CSU, Wagga Wagga.

In: Health Research in Cyberspace
Editor: Pranee Liamputtong, pp. 273-284
ISBN 1-59454-819-6

Chapter 17

GENTLE HUGS: RESEARCHING ONLINE SUPPORT SYSTEMS FOR WOMEN WITH LUPUS

Cindy Mendelson

INTRODUCTION

Internet listservs and bulletin boards are an important source of support for women living with systemic lupus erythematosus and are venues from which participants can be recruited for qualitative research conducted via electronic communication. In this chapter I will discuss the Internet component of an ethnographic study of women with lupus (Mendelson, 2003, in press). In the course of this discussion I will present methodological and ethical challenges facing researchers pursing this type of research.

Lupus is a chronic systemic autoimmune illness of poorly understood etiology that affects women nine times more frequently than men and disproportionately affects women of color (Rus and Hochberg, 2002). Despite being the second most common autoimmune disease affecting women during their childbearing years (Bongu et al., 2002), lupus is not well understood. In the United States, the prevalence of lupus is estimated to be between 15 and 122 cases per 100,000 individuals (Rus and Hochberg, 2002). The Lupus Foundation of America suggests a conservative estimate of 5 million people diagnosed worldwide and an annual incidence of 100,000 new cases (Centers for Disease Control and Prevention, 2005). The wide range of numbers, in part, is reflective of the difficulty of diagnosing the illness. The manifestations of lupus are varied and can mimic many other illnesses (Kuper and Failla, 2000). The initial symptoms, such as fatigue, sun sensitivity, rashes, arthralgia, and weight loss, which are ubiquitous and often fleeting, are frequently disregarded or unrecognized, making diagnosis difficult. Because the manifestations of lupus vary from person to person and often evolve over time, definitive diagnosis may be difficult and often takes years (Wallace, 2002).

Lupus tends to wax and wane, with individuals experiencing unpredictable periods of flare and remission. The manifestations of lupus vary from person to person; some are minimally affected, with symptoms limited to inflammation of the joints and skin, whereas others may have life-threatening involvement of major organs (Kuper and Failla, 2000).

Although there are a variety of symptoms and experiences common to lupus, each person's illness experience is not only unique, but frequently varies over time (Grossman and Kalunian, 2002). Consequently, women with lupus must learn to live with a variety of unpredictable symptoms, making a consistent source of support and information a key component of day-to-day illness management. For many women, the Internet fills this need.

Online support for those with chronic illness is a logical outgrowth of the increasing availability of the Internet and popularity of Internet communities. According to Nua Internet Surveys (n.d.), there are over 605.6 million online users worldwide. The Pew Internet and American Life Project reports that 60 million Americans have sought health-related information on the Internet (Rainie and Packel, n.d.), and 4 million Americans have indicated that the Internet helped them "cope with their own struggle with a major illness in the past two years". (Kommers and Rainie, n.d.: 2). As increasing numbers of people turn to Internet sites, such as listservs, bulletin boards, and homepages to seek information and support and to connect with others in similar situations, researchers have become increasingly interested in understanding the nature of support and communication offered on these sites (Klemm et al., 1998; Ward, 1999; Dickerson et al., 2000; White and Dorman, 2000; Hardy, 2002; Mendelson 2003; see also Chapters 8, 13, 14, 16 in this volume). Researchers are also increasingly turning to the Internet as a venue for recruitment (Fleitas, 1998; Barry, 2001; Mendelson, 2005) and a location for delivering health care intervention (Bliss et al., 1998; Cudney and Weinart, 2000; Weinert, 2000; see also Chapter 3 in this volume).

THE STUDY

The genesis of this study was my own experience of being diagnosed with a connective tissue disease. I was symptomatic for several years prior to diagnosis, and I found it difficult to find accurate information and to get reasonable explanations for my symptoms. I also found it isolating because I had not met others in a similar situation. Although my family was supportive and believed that I had "something," there was little that they could do in the face of mystery symptoms and no diagnosis. After receiving a tentative diagnosis, I attempted to research the illness. I moved through the lay resources quickly and turned to the nursing literature for insight into living with lupus. A review of the core nursing journals in the CINAHL data base, which is the primary data base of nursing literature, returned 85 articles on multiple sclerosis, 41 on rheumatoid arthritis, 12 on fibromyalgia, and only 5 on lupus, despite statistics that suggest that lupus is more common than multiple sclerosis. Despite a well-established role in nursing to supporting daily management of individuals with chronic illness, it became apparent that the voices of people living with lupus were missing not only from the nursing literature but also from the medical discourse in general.

Consequently, in 2002, I conducted an ethnographic study to identify predominant themes in women's experiences of living with lupus. The study included three face-to-face interviews with 7 women with lupus recruited from the local community and an Internet component designed to evaluate the effectiveness of using the Internet to recruit participants for narrative-type research, to solicit first-person narratives on living with lupus, and to evaluate the nature of support available on lupus-focused listservs. This chapter will focus on the Internet component of the study.

The Internet was used to recruit participants willing to submit a single narrative describing their experiences with lupus and to identify and describe the nature of online support available on Internet listservs. Participants for the narrative component were recruited into the study by posting a study announcement on Internet listservs and bulletin boards that serve the needs of people with lupus. Internet sites that focus on lupus were identified through a Google search. Nine sites with an asynchronous interactive component (two message boards and seven listservs) were initially selected to receive the study announcement. To access the listservs, I subscribed to each list. If a site moderator could be located, an e-mail was sent directly to the moderator requesting permission to post the announcement; otherwise, the request was posted directly to the site. In each message, I introduced myself as a nurse and researcher with a connective tissue disorder and said that I became interested in the topic as a result of my own diagnostic and treatment experiences. I was able to successfully post messages on six of the nine sites that I originally identified.

SOLICITING NARRATIVES FROM INTERNET PARTICIPANTS

The announcements invited women diagnosed with lupus to participate in a study exploring their experiences of living with the illness. Responses to the announcement were rapid and universally positive. A total of 53 women with lupus responded to the messages within the recruitment period. A follow-up e-mail was sent in response to each query that included an information sheet describing the study, the inclusion criteria, and study materials with directions for completing and returning the questionnaires and stories. A packet of questionnaires that included a demographic profile, medication inventory, and provider inventory for the previous 12 months was sent via e-mail attachment to each potential participant.

A total of 26 women returned packets, 23 of which were useable. Most were returned promptly. A reminder notice was sent to those with unreturned stories approximately 1 month after the original e-mail to inquire if they were still interested in participating and reminding them of the deadline to submit their stories. Several women responded to the e-mail indicating that their stories were forthcoming (although not all were received). Other women wrote to explain why they could not participate, such as being too busy, feeling too sick, or not meeting the inclusion criteria. All communication with the participants occurred through e-mail. Most of these e-mails included some form of thanks or encouragement for the study. For example, one list member who did not meet the inclusion criteria wrote, “I sure wish I could participate but I understand! Good luck with your research and THANK YOU”. Although I provided my office phone number, I only had voice contact with one participant, who called me at my office to ensure that my request was legitimate and that I was indeed associated with a university.

IDENTIFYING ELEMENTS OF SUPPORT BY OBSERVING INTERNET LISTSERVS

The second Internet component of this study was an analysis of the type of support provided by listservs. All the postings to three of the listservs that accepted recruitment posts were read for a 3-month period; the fourth list was not followed because it had very little activity. A subset of posts for each site was downloaded for analysis. Posts for analysis were collected by downloading all the posts to a single listserv for 7 consecutive days at the beginning of the month. This process was repeated for each of the three listservs such that in the course of 3 months, 7 days worth of posts were downloaded from each site. As the posts were downloaded the e-mail addresses were replaced with a participant number. A separate list was maintained throughout the period of data collection that linked the e-mail address with the participant numbers to ensure accurate tracking. This list was destroyed after data collection and analysis were complete. Any identifying information, such as the names of doctors, cities, and family members were removed from the posts. Additionally, signature tags were removed and reference lines that contained identifying information were altered to ensure anonymity. The sample consisted of 1,187 discrete posts to three Internet listservs made by 90 participants, as identified by e-mail addresses. There is no way of knowing if the sample represents 90 different individuals or fewer individuals posting under a variety of e-mail addresses (see also Mustanski in this volume). There was no attempt to further identify individuals according to age, diagnosis, or other type of demographic information because this would be speculative. It was clear, however, that the vast majority of the participants were women who had lupus or believed they had lupus.

LIVING WITH LUPUS: A VIEW FROM THE NET

The findings of this study have been reported in detail elsewhere (Mendelson, 2003, 2005) but will be summarized briefly. The demographics of the participants recruited for the narrative component are shown in Table 1.

Table 1. Demographic Characteristics of Narrative Participants

	Mean	Range
Age (years)	39	18–57
Years since diagnosis	7	2–22
Number of medications	10	3–37
Number of health care visits	23	3–149
Years to diagnosis	7	0–47

The average age was 39 years, and diagnosis took at least 2 years and as many as 22. The women took an average of 10 different medications. Medications included over-the-counter drugs, drugs prescribed by their health care providers, and alternative treatments, such as homeopathic remedies. The most commonly mentioned medications included steroids, antimalarials, and nonsteroidal anti-inflammatory medications. Many of the participants also took antidepressants, and several took narcotic pain relievers, at least on occasion, to control pain. Participants had an average of 23 health care visits in the preceding 12 months. Health care providers included primary care providers, such as physicians and nurse practitioners, physical and occupational therapists, mental health professionals, and alternative practitioners, such as chiropractors and acupuncturists.

All the stories were compelling and deeply personal glimpses into the participants' experiences of living with an unpredictable, chronic illness. Most of the participants focused on their diagnosis experiences, and many discussed the dramatic changes that the illness necessitated in their lives. Overall, the participants described their lupus as an embodied state that, over time, they came to implicitly know and understand. This embodied knowledge of how their illness manifested was often disregarded by the medical community. Living with lupus was described as *Living a Medically and Socially Complex Life,* which was manifest by the following themes: (a) *A Life of Uncertainty,* which comprised the processes of getting a diagnosis, coping with unpredictable flares and remissions, and learning to live with the unpredictable course of the illness; (b) *A Shifting Sense of Identity,* which included the role changes associated with lupus, coming to terms with an altered body image and an altered future, and managing lifestyle changes necessitated by the illness; and (c) the *Financial Burden of Illness,* which encompassed issues associated with time lost from work and treatment costs (see Mendelson, in press, for a complete discussion of these themes).

The listserv statistics are shown in Table 2. Only 3 of the 90 participants posted to more than one observed site. Each site had a core group of individuals who participated on a regular basis and a smaller group of participants who posted to the site less frequently. Additionally, each site had a large number of lurkers, or listserv members who did not actively participate in the list by posting a message to the list.

Table 2. Listserv Statistics

	Listserv 1	Listserv 2	Listserv 3
Subscribers (n)	258	351	204
Downloaded posts (n)	926	115	67
Active participants (n)	38	33	22
% of List participating	15	9	11

Five themes that characterized the posts were identified: (a) *Exchanging Advice and Information* included messages designed to share lupus-related information; (b) *Living with Illness* described posts in which participants discussed how their lives had been affected by lupus; (c) *Life Goes On* described the events in participants' lives that occur despite a diagnosis of lupus; (d) *Life in Cyberspace* referred to the mechanics of operating in an online environment; and (e) *Being There for Each Other* described support in the most traditional sense (see Mendelson, 2003, for a detailed discussion of these findings). The most striking aspect of the listservs was the unique personality of each site. The most active site was an online network of friends who supported each other through life's events and who had lupus. Although lupus was the connection they shared, the majority of the messages dealt with a broad range of life events. The content of the second site was primarily a source of social support related to living with the illness, with informational content and support for life activities a secondary function. The content of the last site was primarily informational, although participants also provided support to those living with the illness.

CONDUCTING QUALITATIVE RESEARCH USING THE INTERNET

The Pew Internet and American Life Project documents the increasing importance of the Internet for individual research on matters of health and illness (Rainie and Packel, n.d.). A quick search of Google groups attests to the numbers of people seeking information and support in virtual communities. Qualitative research approaches are especially appropriate to understanding how people form self-help communities on the Internet and how they incorporate these virtual interactions into the daily management of physical and psychological consequences of chronic illness. As an emerging venue for research, especially one in which the technology continues to change and develop, issues of access, representation, and ethics remain in a formative stage of discussion (see also Chapters 1 and 2 in this volume).

Gatekeeping

The role of gatekeepers in controlling access to sites and in censoring the activities of sites in the study became obvious immediately. To post on the listservs, I subscribed to each of the lists; however, I was only successful in posting the study announcement on four of the seven lists. The moderators of three of the listservs, one very large and established, prevented me from posting on their site because they felt that it would be an unwelcome intrusion. Those that rejected the study announcement indicated that the sites were "safe places" for the participants to post and that researchers were not welcome. To honor the request of the moderator, I immediately unsubscribed from these lists and consequently cannot report on the nature of support on these lists or cannot evaluate whether the dynamics of these lists are different from those that accepted the posts. I was surprised by the moderator's perception that my motives were dangerous or that list participants needed to be protected from opportunities to participate in legitimate research. The study announcements merely asked list members to consider volunteering to participate in research. However, a study by Hudson and Bruckman (2004), in which they evaluated the reactions of chat room participants to being studied, supported the notion that, at least in some cases, Internet participants object to being the object of research (see also Chapters 1 and 9 in this volume).

The other four lists allowed me to post directly to the site, although one moderator suggested that, instead of posting a request to the list for participants, I observe the list for a period and then individually contact members and invite them to participate in the study. This approach would have allowed me to engage in more purposive sampling; however, it also would have limited sampling to the very small percentage of list membership that posted. Of the 23 participants recruited from the Internet, several indicated that they followed the activities of the list on which they saw the announcement but rarely or never posted to the list.

Feedback from the participants on these sites was overwhelmingly positive regarding both my study and the need for research about the experiences of living with lupus. This may, however, be reflective of the specific dynamics of the list; without having the opportunity to post on a greater number of sites, it is difficult to tell if the response was typical of participants with lupus or idiosyncratic to the lists. Each list had a very distinct personality; one was mostly social, the other was mostly informational, and the third was informational but emphasized support (Mendelson, 2003), and I can imagine that certain lists may be more or less welcoming to research requests. This phenomenon may be reflective of the willingness of some of the gatekeepers to welcome the posts and others to reject them.

Regardless, the willingness of participants to not only voice support for the study but then to follow up and participate deserves further exploration. Choosing to participate involved actively engaging in the study; participants had to complete a demographic questionnaire, and two inventories, including a 12-month recall of health care appointments, and additionally had to submit a narrative. Conservatively, even the shortest narrative probably took at least 1 hour to complete, and I'm sure several participants spent several hours reconstructing their medical background and creating their narratives. The thought and consideration that went into crafting the narratives are exemplified by a woman living with lupus for over 20 years. She missed the initial deadline to submit her narrative and I wrote her to see if she was planning on participating. She wrote back, "I'm still working on it, I'm up to 1994 now… when you have had lupus for 20 years there is a lot to write about". When I followed up with her about a week later, she replied, "the bulk of it is done. I worked on it for at least six hours this weekend. I just need to add some finishing touches and include a couple of things I forgot. I should have it completed in a couple of days".

Participants often began or ended their stories with a brief statement about either why they were participating or thanks for allowing them to participate. One participant wrote, "Please feel free to contact me if you have any questions…this helps me, kind of therapeutic". Another wrote, "I am interested in sharing my story, not only from my perspective as a patient, but also as an RN". She went on to recount that nothing in nursing school had prepared her for what it was like to live with lupus. A third participant was hopeful that this was a way to communicate to the health care community the difficulty of the disease. She wrote, "Well, that's my story up to now and I only hope that eventually someone can make the medical professionals see that this is a disease to be reckoned with and that we women who have it are no hypochondriacs, but are in a lot of pain and need help. Thanks". Another participant was hopeful that in telling her story she could give hope to others: "I hope my story can help ease any fears or worries you might have. We are connected by our illness, but also by the love of God and through him all things are possible. I pray for all of us every day and I love all of you, we will be o.k".

I believe that the study tapped into a true desire of women with lupus to be heard and understood. By introducing myself to the participants and by sharing my own diagnosis, the participants were able to see me as someone who was not only interested in understanding their experiences but capable of grasping the essence of their experience. To me, the most poignant responses, and the most troubling, were from participants who were simply thankful for the opportunity to tell the story: "I hope my story is helpful to you. Thanks for letting me tell it", "Thank you for the opportunity to participate in this study", "Here is my story... let me know if you need anything else or something.... or I forgot to put something in that you want". "Thank you for including m". The need to have their experiences heard was a very powerful motivator for the participants and clearly demonstrated the extent to which this population of women has been marginalized and in some cases harmed by the attitudes of health care professionals and members of their social and professional networks.

Flaming, or hostile, aggressive communication, which is quite common on many bulletin boards, was not present on the listservs under observation and was not noted on the bulletin boards on which I placed postings but did not do intensive observations. Studies have shown that anonymity contributes to the increased likelihood of critical comments (Reinig and Mejias, 2004) and flaming (Douglas and McGarty, 2001). The typical practice on the observed sites was for new list members to introduce themselves to the list and provide an outline of their personal story. List members would acknowledge the introduction and welcome the new participants to the list (Mendelson, 2003). Although site moderators frequently posted reminders to participants not to share personally identifying information, many participants often signed their names to the their posts or revealed enough personal information that, despite using a screen name, group members interacted as if they were acquainted, reducing the perception of anonymity. Gatekeeping activities by the moderator could have also contributed to these generally tranquil environments because access to the site was limited by the moderators and posts could be vetted. Regardless, it is reasonable to question if aggressive gatekeeping in the name of "providing a safe environment" that does not distinguish recruitment for legitimate research from intrusive spam serves to further isolate women with chronic illness and to reify the notion that health care providers are not interested in understanding the dynamics of living with the illness.

Representation, Presence, and Consent in Listserv Research

The vastness and the anonymity of the Internet might be one of the greatest strengths and problems for researchers working in this environment. Because one has the ability to remain anonymous, participants may be more willing to participate in sensitive research or more fully disclose their stories than they may be in face-to-face settings or to the researcher who is also a member of a community in which they live (see also Hessler and Mustanski in this volume). On the other hand, the risk of deception is high. Within the Internet culture, taking on multiple identities is not uncommon, and the potential to encounter participants who may not be who they say they are is a real risk to the truth value of findings; reports of Munchausen syndrome by Internet have been documented on Internet discussion groups (Feldman, 2000). In the current study, I made certain assumptions about the data, which included that people were who they said they were, and their stories were representations of events that occurred in their lives that were written out for the purpose of this study. In this study, many participants signed e-mail responses to me with first and last names, and many also gave me their phone numbers if I had additional questions, which added a degree of assurance that their stories were genuine. Even more importantly, all the stories were coherent presentations of events that might occur in an illness such as lupus. Although some represented extreme examples of misdiagnosis, extensive medication usage, and maltreatment at the hands of medical professionals and family members, none were beyond the reach of plausibility.

The analogy of an iceberg is an appropriate description for listserv communication in that the number of participants who post are often only a small portion of those who actually receive list messages. Consequently, care must be taken when describing list activity to distinguish the nature of communication that occurs from the opinions or attitudes of list members, who for the most part do not actively participate in list discussion. Because only a small percentage of subscribed participants actually posted messages, the benefits derived from reading messages without posting should be considered. The lists provided a variety of potential benefits to subscribers whether or not they actually posted. The lists are populated by people who have common health concerns and are likely to have had similar experiences dealing with their illness. Face-to-face support groups, especially those for relatively uncommon illnesses or illnesses that cause disabling symptoms, are difficult to mount. Joachim (1998) found that the desire for a support group was often tempered by people's time, schedules, and perceived need for support at any given time. The flexibility of asynchronous listservs allows participants to check in at a time convenient for them. Moreover, the ability to lurk, or "listen" without participating is quite common in online groups (White and Dorman, 2001) and usually not acceptable in face-to-face groups (Dickerson et al., 2000). Weinberg and colleagues (1996) reported that the participants in a small computer-mediated breast cancer support group found reading the posted messages even more valuable than posting. In my study, list participants who described themselves as lurkers but posted on occasion frequently included a statement in their posts attesting to the benefits that they derived from following the discussions. For those who participate in the list discussions, the ability to share their experiences and provide support to others is powerful. For those who post rarely, the list represents a resource for individuals who have access to expertise should they need it and also the ability to stay informed based on the ongoing conversations

Internet research poses unique challenges in terms of consent and representation. As an emerging venue of research, many questions as to the appropriate use of Internet data remain unanswered, and the scholarly discussion into these issues is in a formative stage (Eysenbeck and Till, 2001; Sixsmith and Murray, 2001; Pittenger, 2003). These issues revolve around questions pertaining to what types of Internet research constitute research with human subjects, what components of Internet research are documentary analysis, and whether or not communication that occurs on the Internet represents public or private discourse.

The current research was reviewed by the University Institutional Review Board and deemed exempt because it represented minimal risk and all identifiers would be removed from the data. However, the differing levels of involvement with and by the participants and the differing levels of disclosure necessitated differing approaches to notifying and securing permission from participants for their involvement. Participants recruited into the narrative component were asked to share demographic information and treatment information in addition to their written story. Consequently, these participants were sent an information sheet and disclaimer with the study information explaining the study, how the information would be used, and how their privacy would be protected. By returning the study information, participants agreed to allow the information they provided to be used in the study. Although participants were only known by their screen names and e-mail addresses, even this information was separated from the documents, and participants were assigned a study name.

The issues associated with securing permission to passively observe the communication on listservs and chat rooms are complex, involving discussions about whether the lists are public or private sites and whether analysis of posts is human subject research or documentary analysis (see also Chapter 1 in this volume). I operated from the position that the research involved human subjects and, because all the listservs were available via subscription to anyone who requests them, the sites were essentially public. However, because list members may perceive their communication as private or at least sheltered, measures were taken to ensure the anonymity of the site and the participants. Because membership on Internet listservs is fluid, and participant lists are usually not accessible, securing and maintaining informed consent from each member is not possible, and it is questionable whether or not a list owner or moderator can provide consent on behalf of the list. In minimal risk research, removing all identifying information from the posts often eliminates the need for consent. However, this precaution may not adequately protect the anonymity of listserv participants if direct quotes from the posts are used because Internet search engines can link very small strings of words back to the original post, thereby potentially revealing the identity of the participant. To protect the identity of the participants, all identifying information was immediately removed from the posts, the process of observation was passive (Eysenback and Till, 2001), and I did not post to the list nor did I announce my presence on the list beyond the original study announcement. Additionally, the findings are reported in summary and do not include direct quotes because consent to use quotes was not secured from the list participants. Although this approach is consistent with published literature, the reader is not able to share in the richness of the findings. To further ensure the anonymity of listserv participants, the sites are reported as lupus listserv (LLS) 1, LLS 2, and LLS 3, and their Web locations and affiliations are not disclosed (Eysenback and Till, 2001; Klemm et al., 1998; Sixsmith and Murray, 2001). Further research and debate into the ethical issues of Internet research will help clarify these issues and provide direction to researchers working with listserv data.

Final Thoughts

Very little is known about the daily experiences of women living with lupus. The study discussed in this chapter documents the experiences of women with lupus from symptom recognition through diagnosis to the management of daily life in the presence of chronicity. The Internet component of this study provided insight into the frustrations of living with the illness that were not well developed in the face-to-face component of the study. Participants in the Internet component appeared to find support that was otherwise unavailable to them and was elusive to some of the participants who participated in face-to-face interviews. The Internet also provided access to a wider participant base than would ordinarily be available for a relatively small qualitative study and accessed the voices of women who, because of the isolation of the disease and fatigue, might not ordinarily participate in research. Although Internet ethnography is certainly in a nascent stage, the phenomena of online self-help communities coupled with increasing accessibility of the Internet provide compelling support for developing strategies to explore the role of virtual communities in the conduct of chronic illness management.

NOTE

This research was supported by a Dean's Research Award from the College of Nursing at the University of New Mexico, USA. Portions of this chapter have been published previously as: Mendelson, C., 2003, Gentle hugs: Listservs as sources of support for women with Lupus. *Advances in Nursing Science,* vol. 26, no. 4, pp. 299–306, and are used with the permission of the publisher.

REFERENCES

[1] Barry, D. T., 2001, 'Assessing Culture via the Internet: Methods and Techniques for Psychological Research', *CyberPsychology and Behavior*, vol. 4, no.1, pp. 17-21.

[2] Bliss J., Allibone C., Bontempo B., Flynn T. and Valvano N. E., 1998, 'Creating a Website for On-Line Social Support, Melanocyte', *Computers in Nursing,* vol. 16, no. 4, pp. 203–207.

[3] Bongu, A., Chang, E. and Ramsey-Goldman, R., 2002, 'Can Morbidity and Mortality of SLE Be Improved?', *Best Practices and Research in Clinical Rheumatology*, vol. 16, no. 2, pp. 313–332.

[4] Centers for Disease Control and Prevention, Office of Minority Health, 2005, 'Eliminate Health Disparities in Lupus'. *<http://www.cdc.gov/omh/AMH/factsheets/lupus.htm>*

[5] Cudney, S. A. and Weinert, C., 2000, 'Computer-Based Support Groups: Nursing in Cyberspace', *Computers in Nursing,* vol. 18, no. 1, pp. 35–43.

[6] Dickerson, S. S., Flaig, D. and Kennedy, M. C., 2000, 'Therapeutic Connection: Help Seeking on the Internet for Persons With Implantable Cardioverter Defibrillators', *Heart Lung,* vol. 2, no. 4, pp. 248–255.

[7] Douglas, K. M. and McGarty, C., 2001, 'Identifiability and Self-presentation: Computer-Mediated Communication and Intergroup Interaction', *British Journal of Social Psychology*, vol. 40, pp. 399–416.

[8] Eysenback, G. and Till, J. E., 2001, 'Ethical Issues in Qualitative Research on Internet Communities', *British Medical Journal,* vol. 323, no. 7321, pp.1103–1105.

[9] Feldman, M. C., 2000, 'Munchausen by Internet: Detecting Factitious Illness and Crisis on the Internet', *Southern Medical Journal,* vol. 93 no. 7, pp.669–672.

[10] Fleitas, J., 1998, 'Spinning Tales From the World Wide Web: Qualitative Research in an Electronic Environment', *Qualitative Health Research,* vol. 8, no. 2, pp. 283–292.

[11] Grossman, J. M. and Kalunian, K. C., 2002, 'Definition, Classification, Activity and Damage Indices', in D. J. Wallace and B. H. Hahn (eds.), *Dubois' Lupus Erythematosus, 6th edition,* pp. 19–31, Lippincott Williams and Wilkins, Philadelphia.

[12] Hardy, M., 2002, '"The Story of My Illness": Personal Accounts of Illness on the Internet', *Health: An Interdisciplinary Journal for the Social Study of Health Illness and Medicine,* vol. 6, no.1, pp. 31–46.

[13] Hudson, J. M. and Bruckman, A., 2004, '"Go Away": Participant Objections to Being Studied and the Ethics of Chatroom Research', *The Information Society* vol. 20, pp. 127–139.

[14] Joachim, G., 1998, 'The Birth and Dissolution of an Inflammatory Bowel Disease Support Group: Lessons in Providing Support', *Gastroenterology Nurse,* vol 21, no. 3, pp. 119–124.

[15] Klemm, P., Reppert, K., and Visich, L., 1998, 'A Nontraditional Cancer Support Group on the Internet', *Computers in Nursing*, vol. 16, no.1, pp. 31–36.

[16] Kommers, N. and Rainie, L., n.d., Use of the Internet at Major Life Moments, The Pew Internet and American Life Project Web site. *<http://www.pewinternet.org/pdfs/PIP_Major_Moments_Report.pdf>*

[17] Kuper, B. C. and Failla, S., 2000, 'Systemic Lupus Erythematosus: A Multisystem Autoimmune Disorder', *Nursing Clinics of North America,* vol. 35, no. 1, pp. 253–265.

[18] Mendelson, C., 2003, 'Gentle Hugs: Listservs as Sources of Support for Women With Lupus', *Advances in Nursing Science,* vol. 26, no. 4, pp.299–306.

[19] Mendelson, C., in press, 'Living Medically and Socially Complex Life: Women Living With Lupus', *Qualitative Health Research.*

[20] Nua, n.d., 'How many online?' Nua Internet Surveys. *<http://www.nua.ie/surveys/how_many_online/index.html>*

[21] Pittenger, D. J., 2003, 'Internet Research: An Opportunity to Revisit Classic Ethical Problems in Behavioral Research', *Ethics and Behavior,* vol. 13, no. 1, pp. 45–60.

[22] Rainie, L. and Packel, D. n.d., 'More online, doing more'. The Pew Internet and American Life Project Web site. *<http://www.pewinternet.org/reports/toc.asp?Reports=30>*

[23] Reinig, B. A. and Mejias, R. J., 2004, 'The Effects Of National Culture And Anonymity On Flaming And Criticalness In GSS-Supported Discussions', *Small Group Research,* vol. 35, no.6, pp. 698–723.

[24] Rus V. and Hochberg, M. C., 2002, 'The Epidemiology of Systemic Lupus Erythematosus', in D. J. Wallace and B. H. Hahn (eds.), *Dubois' Lupus Erythematosus, 6th edition,* pp. 65–83, Lippincott Williams and Wilkins, Philadelphia

[25] Sixsmith, J., and Murray, C. D., 2001, 'Ethical Issues in the Documentary Data Analysis of Internet Posts and Archives', *Qualitative Health Research,* vol. 11, no. 3, pp. 423–432.

[26] Wallace D. J., 2002, The Clinical Presentation of Systemic Lupus Erythematosus', in D. J. Wallace D. J. and B. H. Hahn (eds.), *Dubois' Lupus Erythematosus, 6th edition,* pp. 621–628, Lippincott Williams and Wilkins, Philadelphia.

[27] Ward, K. J., 1999, 'Cyber-Ethnography and the Emergence of the Virtually New Community', *Journal of Information Technology*, vol. 14, pp. 95–105

[28] Weinberg, N., Schmale, J., Uken, J. and Wessel, K., 1996, 'Online Help: Cancer Patients Participate in a Computer-Mediated Support Group', *Health and Social Work,* vol. 21, no. 1, pp. 24–29.

[29] Weinert, C., 2000, 'Social support in cyberspace for women with chronic illness', *Rehabilitation Nursing,* vol. 254, pp. 129–135.

[30] White, M. H. and Dorman, S. M., 2000, 'Online Support for Caregivers: Analysis of an Internet Alzheimer Mail Group', *Computers in Nursing*, vol. 18, no. 4,, pp.168–179.

[31] White, M. and Dorman, S. M., 2001, 'Receiving Social Support Online: Implications for Health Education', *Health Education Research,* vol. 16, no. 6, pp. 693–707.

In: Health Research in Cyberspace
Editor: Pranee Liamputtong, pp. 285-296

ISBN 1-59454-819-6

Chapter 18

BREAST CANCER CYBERSPACE: A HITCHHIKER'S GUIDE

Barbara Thomas

INTRODUCTION

Receiving the diagnosis of breast cancer can be likened to the initial premise in the *Hitchhiker's Guide to the Galaxy* (Adams, 1979). As the novel opens, the main character, Arthur Dent, is having a very bad day. He awakens to discover bulldozers ready to tear down his house, Planet Earth is about to be demolished to build a hyperspace freeway and his best friend turns out to be an alien. He goes out and lies down in front of the bulldozers. His best friend comes by Arthur's house and offers him his only chance for survival, to hitch a quick ride on a passing spacecraft.

For people searching for information in the galaxy of breast cancer resources, the Internet may be just the spacecraft they need. It is increasingly used by the public to locate health-related information and the demand is unlikely to diminish. The Internet information may be targeted to different audiences such as patients or healthcare professionals. It may be scientific or anecdotal so it can be difficult to find information that matches an individual's specific needs. As the fastest growing health information source, the Internet has become an important tool for patients, their families, health care providers and researchers. Web sites on the broad topic of breast cancer are among those most frequently visited. However, in order to make sense of the galaxy of breast cancer topics addressed in these websites, a guide may be useful.

Using breast cancer as the example, this chapter examines various usages of this evolving medium including researching online. The Internet provides a multifaceted resource for hitchhikers searching for medical information and support, two of its more important uses (Mayer and Till, 1996). The plethora of websites available may be overwhelming for someone seeking information and support for a recent breast cancer diagnosis.

GUIDE TO INFORMATION

While not everyone chooses information gathering as a priority when they are faced with cancer, the availability of Internet information enables those who do, to have more information and to help evaluate the possible treatments. The information they obtain may influence the treatment course originally suggested by their physician.

In recent years, many Internet breast cancer resources have appeared, including online breast cancer journals like The Breast, the Breast Cancer Research and Treatment and cancer registries like the Physician Data Query (PDQ). The PDQ is an online database developed and maintained by the National Cancer Institute (2003). This guide is designed to provide health professionals and the public with the most current, credible, and accurate cancer information available. Peer-reviewed summaries on cancer treatment, screening, prevention, complementary and alternative medicine, and supportive care are provided. As well, a registry of clinical trials for cancer from international centers and directories of physicians, professionals, and organizations that provide cancer care are available (National Cancer Institute, 2003). There are also websites of non-profit breast cancer organizations, medical associations and institutions that provide users with clinical guidelines, schedules of international breast cancer events, and news and abstracts from breast cancer conferences.

When seeking information on breast cancer, there are a number of criteria to consider. These include the quality and reliability of the information provided. The National Cancer Institute maintains a website that provides questions and answers on how to evaluate health information on the Internet (Table 1).

Table 1. Key Points in Evaluating Health Information on the Internet (adapted from the National Cancer Institute, 2003)

Who runs the website?	Organization or person responsible should be clearly identified, noted on home page and every major page.
Who pays for website?	Source of funding can influence the content, how it is presented, what owners want to achieve with site.
Purpose of website	Purpose is related to who runs site; helps users evaluate trustworthiness of information.
Original source of information	Original source should be clearly identified; If person or organization in charge of site did not write material, original source should be clearly cited.
Documentation and selection of website information	Medical facts, statistics should be referenced; Credentials of reviewers/editorial boards should be identified; Opinions should be separate from "evidence-based" information.
How current is website?	Should be updated regularly; Clearly post date of most recent review.
What information about users does website collect?	If personal information is requested, users should read and understand privacy policies and not sign up for anything they do not fully understand.

Hoffman-Goetz and Clarke (2000) found that most websites in their study lacked critical information that could enable consumers to make informed decisions about site quality. For example, sources of information for the content on the website were provided in only 30% of sites studied and owner's credentials were cited in 31%. Shon and Musen (1999) revealed similar results with basic publishing elements such as authorship, attribution and currency in low frequency. They suggest the design of metadata-based system to evaluate the quality of medical information on the World Wide Web to improve quality assurance. Santoro (2003) suggests that it is fairly easy to find high quality breast cancer websites if appropriate indexes such as Cancerlit or MedlinePlus are used. However, when suddenly faced with the need to obtain breast cancer information, the automatic response my not be to use sophisticated indices.

In a study of women's preferences about receiving online breast cancer information, Unruh et al. (2004) found that trust in the content provider as well as in the organization collecting personal data was important. They concluded that personal searching assistance was helpful. As well, they suggested that disclosures of content sources and a privacy policy that explains how personal data is handled should be provided.

Satterlund, McCaul and Sandgren (2003) studied where women found medical information about their illness and tracked changes over time when they moved from active treatment to survivor status. They found that more years of formal education and younger ages were significant predictors of Internet usage. Stage of disease was not a significant predictor. Although they found that the percentage of women using the Internet 16 months after diagnosis dropped slightly, their use of other major sources of information like books and videos, dropped off sharply.

In a study of the information needs of people with breast and prostate cancer, (Rozmovits and Ziebland, 2004), respondents indicated that their information needs were complex and changed over time. They valued practical information and appreciated experiential suggestions. Participants were not only aware of Internet information limitations but also had developed strategies to deal with them. They identified being cautious of commercial health sites and questioned stories from individual patients. Involvement in organizations that promote active treatment such as surgery over less interventionist approaches, may strongly influence the way people perceive their own information needs both currently and retrospectively. There are thousands of websites that provide information on breast and prostate cancer. For people experiencing diseases that are more rare and less well known, they are likely to have very different information needs as less information and support may be available.

Teo and colleagues (2005) incorporated a voluntary online questionnaire into their website. Women responded that they were interested in obtaining research-related and technical information on benign and malignant breast diseases. They also wanted an online consultation facility and a directory of local breast clinics. Using the feedback from the questionnaire, they were able to refine the site content to more closely reflect the requirements of their users.

In summary, the Internet provides a vehicle that may be very helpful when attempting to maneuver through the vast galaxy of breast cancer of information.

GUIDE TO SUPPORT

Evaluations of community-based cancer support groups, including both face-to-face groups and Internet groups, suggest that they provide a number of benefits. It is more reasonable to expect that such interventions will have greater impact on psychosocial functioning and /or health-related quality of life than on survival (Till, 2003).

Fogel et al. (2002) found that the use of the Internet for information was associated with greater social support and less loneliness in women with breast cancer. Although participants indicated they did not benefit from tangible social support, they may use the information to give them a sense of control. They also found that only about one third of the Internet users for breast health issues chose e-mail as a helpful resource for their breast health while 91% used e-mail for general use. Listservs, news groups and Internet self-help groups were also underused by this group. Although many physicians refer their cancer patients to various support services, patient use of these services is quite low, ranging from 2% to 8% (Eakin and Strycker, 2001). However, more knowledge is needed about the quality of the web sites used, the types of information sought and whether patients or physicians believe that there are potential clinical benefits of the social support available from the Internet.

Some users find the option that the Internet can be used interactively to communicate with individuals and groups in geographically diverse areas while allowing for anonymity to be very helpful. For topics such as personal concerns or problematic side effects that are difficult to discuss in person, the Internet can provide a special bond.

Winzelberg et al. (2003) noted that web-based breast cancer support groups are widely used although little is known about their effectiveness. They studied a group of 72 women with primary breast cancer, who were randomly assigned to a web-based social support group (Bosom Buddies), and moderated by a health care professional. They found that the program was effective in reducing participants' scores on depression, perceived stress and cancer-related trauma measures. They concluded that the web-based social support group offers many advantages but that ethical issues in this medium need to be addressed. The ethical issues they identified included how the participants understand the role of the moderator since it was a psychoeducational support group, and not a form of psychotherapy. Group members offered each other advice, but the group moderator did not.

Another ethical issue considered was the privacy of the participants. The website used in their study was password-protected. Participants could read personal stories from survivors, share their relevant experiences, and keep a web-based personal journal. The latter was not open to other group members. They were also instructed not to disclose any information that they learned about group members to others and not to allow family members or friends to access the website. Limits to the confidentiality of any web-based intervention were discussed because no internet-connected system can be completely secure from experienced computer hackers. It was noted that all participants in support groups should be reminded regularly of the limits of confidentiality when using the Internet for personal matters. They should treat their postings as potentially public documents.

Since some forms of breast cancer are being viewed as a chronic illness, there is a need to address the ongoing concerns of people living with breast cancer and other members of their social support networks. As a guide to the galaxy of popular online support groups, many are peer-moderated, rather than professionally-moderated. In an evaluation of online support groups, different models of the role of the guide or navigator need to be taken into account. Some conceptual models are outlined for the evaluation of the navigator role in meeting the informational, decisional and educational needs of women with breast cancer.

Farber et al. (2002) carried out an environmental scan of navigator roles in meeting the needs of women with breast cancer in Canada. Key informants who would have information about the navigator role were identified, and 40% of them were interviewed. Three conceptual models were identified. According to Farber, the navigator is actively involved in helping affected individuals to navigate a way through the care system in the Active Coordination Model. The navigator provides information, support and encouragement in the Facilitating Navigator Model. The Shared or Tacit Model involves several people providing navigation, either tacitly, or intentionally. For an unmoderated support group, experienced or long time members may assume the role of a tacit peer navigator.

Since the tacit peer-navigators are volunteers, the navigator role is fulfilled at no extra cost to group members. Evaluating the effectiveness of online support groups, in comparison with each other, and with more traditional face-to-face support groups seems appropriate. It is likely that the more effective the navigator role is, the more cost effective the support group will be, whether it is online or not. From this perspective, systemic evaluation outcome variables, and especially those addressing the navigator role, may be most important (Till, 2003).

Application of the concept of a navigator role to support groups in general, and to unmoderated online groups has received little attention in the research literature. The navigator role should be taken into account in outcome-oriented research on this increasingly important aspect of cancer communication.

Guide to Art and Aesthetics

Art provides the hitchhiker with another view of the galaxy of breast cancer resources. It is a form of expression and communication that can effectively convey health messages through the medium of the Internet. Although art and aesthetics have not been the traditional mode of providing health information or health promotion, they have been effectively used to give vision and voice to women experiencing breast cancer. Robb and Murray (1992) suggest that aesthetics provide opportunities for innovative approaches to learning and help us know ourselves and the world around us. The humanities, including art, incorporate knowledge of the meaning of life individually and as a collective whole (Bruderle and Valiga, 1994). Through art, one can receive another's expression of feeling and experience the same emotions and thoughts (Hoshiko, 1985; Mohr, 1995). Art conveys messages about life and health experiences and can potentially influence health practices among people.

Thomas et al. (2002a) examined websites for aesthetic quality. The criteria that resulted from this evaluation are outlined in Table 2.

Table 2. Key Points in Evaluating Aesthetic Quality of Breast Cancer Websites (adapted from Thomas, Gold/Smith, Forrest, and Marshall, 2002)

Color	Visually appealing; Appropriate color more engaging than black and white.
Layout	Font should be easily readable, character size should allow for information to be posted on one screen with minimum scrolling required.
Content	Have title, table of contents, text or body of the page on each page to avoid having to backtrack through site; Avoid lengthy text.
Use of Graphics and Images	Choose logo or symbol to complement topic of website; Maintain consistency throughout website with use of symbols/images; Images are clear, sized to fit on page.
Loading of pages	Pages load in reasonable time.

In a unique study, Thomas et al. (2004) interviewed artists after they participated in a breast health awareness project for which they created visual artworks. The artworks were exhibited in a community gallery as well as being placed on a University of Windsor (2001) website (*www.uwindsor.ca/eob*) designed especially to provide breast health information and enable viewers to take a virtual gallery tour. The interview data showed a strong personal connection to breast cancer either through themselves or a loved one. Many also indicated a perceived personal risk of breast cancer. Although the focus of the project was on breast health, over half of the interviewees approached the theme from a breast caner and medical perspective. Two-thirds of the respondents connected their work with the breast health theme through the use of symbolism. They used images, color, and different materials to represent women and breast health.

The main themes that were identified were a strong personal connection to and fear of breast cancer, a desire to promote health within the community and the uni-dimensional nature of breast health and breast cancer. This project demonstrated that visual art can be used to promote breast health to large populations through the Internet as it can communicate with a wide variety of people, regardless of age or language (see also Chapter 1 in this volume).

Guide to Quality Control and Feedback

Another useful guide to the galaxy of Internet breast cancer resources is in the area of monitoring and quality control of cancer care. The Internet provides a valuable resource that can publicly demonstrate the type of progress is being made in cancer care in a region and where improvements are needed.

For example, in Canada, the province of Ontario has developed an innovative Cancer System Quality Index (Cancer Care Ontario, 2005) that aims to demonstrate its accountability in cancer care by providing current information on the state of cancer care in the various provincial regions. This includes prevention programs, regional wait times for surgery and radiation and quality of care. This index, the first of its kind in North America, provides a broad picture of cancer services in the province and will show patients, health care providers and government the areas that need urgent action.

The website addresses five broad areas: accessibility of services to patients, efficiency of resource utilization, how people are affected by cancer and cancer risk factors, quality of treatment and the ability to understand and measure improvements.

Since many of today's cancer patients are well-educated and have often scanned the Internet for the latest data on their type of disease, this index will give patients comprehensive and current information. The Internet enables the monitoring system to report publicly on cancer system performance and to provide opportunity for feedback from the users.

GUIDE TO HOW THE INTERNET CHANGES THE EXPERIENCE OF CANCER FOR PEOPLE

The Internet offers many possibilities to people with cancer to have active participation in their own health care. Physicians may be concerned about the quality of information patients will obtain and that the patients may become victims of questionable marketing techniques. If the public views Internet information with similar caution to that which they apply when books and articles are reviewed, then there is less reason for concern. If however, the information on the Internet is used to challenge hierarchical roles and relationships between doctors and patients, it has the potential to diminish the power of the medical profession.

Ziebland (2004) used in-depth interviews to demonstrate how the Internet was used to gather information, gain support and make sense of the experience of cancer. She notes that The Internet may also influence the relationship between physicians and patients and questions how transformational the Internet may become. It provides a new source of consumer advocates in health care policies, research and management. People with cancer use the Internet to be active collaborators in their treatment plan and care. They are also using Internet support groups and may establish their own personal web pages to share their information and experiences. Blumenthal (2002) recommends that physicians develop skills as decision analysts, as specialists in health care informatics and use the Internet to enhance their work and interaction with patients.

Accessibility remains a serious limitation for many who would not search for their own information or discuss what they found with their physician. With easier access to Internet health information and a changing relationship between doctors and patients, one of the outcomes may be the feeling by patients that they have to present themselves as and expert or critical patient who can question their health care providers and learn about effective treatments themselves. Ziebland (2004: 1792) suggests that the ability of patients to access their health information on the Internet may give them "an opportunity to display a particularly modern marker of competence and social fitness".

GUIDE TO INNOVATIVE USES

The Internet has been used to develop and evaluate an interactive computer tool for teaching breast imaging to senior medical students (Roubidoux et al., 2002). Student surveys results showed that the website provided educational value, that it was more interesting than the handout provided and that it provided extra reinforcement. Students liked the accessibility of the web and most agreed that it was appropriate for other medical specialties.

Lundin and others (2004) developed an atlas of breast histopathology using web-based virtual microscopy. A website was constructed after slides were scanned at high resolution and archived on a server in a high speed university server. The virtual slide atlas is organized according the World Health Organization 2003 classification. It is anticipated that web-based virtual microscopy will become widely used in many aspects of pathology teaching.

Several authors have studied the patient information needs as reflected in websites from different countries and languages. For example, Weissenberger et al. (2004) found English and German language websites varied considerably. German websites more often addressed the topics of palliative treatment, alternative medicine and disease related information while therapy related information such as surgery details, chemotherapy, radiation therapy and stem cell transplantation were more often found on English language websites. Their intercultural results have implications for patient education.

Guide to Using the Internet as a Research Tool: Practical Issues, Difficulties and Personal Experiences

The Internet is a powerful tool for many types of quantitative and qualitative research. It is assuming an increasingly important role in health care research. Data can be collected quite expeditiously after a website has been carefully planned and mounted. Once the program is set up, large amounts of data can be managed and analyzed as they are received (see Chapter 1 in this volume).

When planning a web site to promote breast health and education using visual art and aesthetics, the researchers (Thomas, Gold/Smith, Forrest, and Marshall, 2002a) were not experts in web site design and technology. They were however, average computer users who employed this limitation to their benefit. They searched for existing websites related to their topic, as might anyone who was looking for information. Then they analyzed the web sites for accessibility and aesthetics. They utilized a web site consultant for essential expertise and assistance in the conceptualization and creation of their breast health web site. Once established, it was evaluated for possible improvements. Updates and future events were posted regularly to encourage visitors to the site to return for another visit. They noted that the hardware of the user such as modem capabilities, available memory and processor speed will influence the efficiency with which the computer will receive data. Other factors, such as the Internet service provider's method of data transference, reliability and the number of subscribers for a particular provider, will also affect the ability to download at a reasonable speed. This is particularly important when establishing a web site that is integrates photographs and graphics as essential elements of the site.

Thomas et al. (2000) also used the Internet to extend previous research in breast health education and screening from a regional population of women to a national and international population of women. Since breast health may be a very personal concern, strategies to maintain anonymity of the respondents were implemented. This meant that tracking methods such as "cookies" were not used. Technological approaches to deter someone gaining unauthorized access to the web server were used to prevent contamination and alteration of the data. As well, design methods were used to prevent abuse of the site. For example, at least 80% of the questions had to be answered or the survey program would not accept the data. Respondents were advised and given the opportunity to go back and answer more questions. The other choice was to exit the page, with the knowledge that the data had not been recorded. This latter option meant that when the "submit" button was activated, all previous answers were erased from the survey. Therefore, a respondent would have to invest considerable time to submit identical data repeatedly in order to compromise the research.

Thomas et al. (2000) note that this cost-effective approach results in cleaner data than those received on paper and pen surveys as data entry errors are bypassed. Responses are made by clicking a button on the computer screen, resulting in a forced choice and avoiding ambiguous responses. They suggest that Internet surveys are environmentally responsible as no paper is generated. As well, research costs such as postage are reduced. Using email, respondents can advise the researchers if they want to receive the study results, which in turn can also be sent to them by email. Computers may be accessed from home, work, Internet cafes or community organizations such as libraries or senior citizen centers. The relative anonymity between researcher and respondent is usually considered to be desirable.

As with all tools, there are benefits and limitations (see Chapter 1 in this volume). A frequent limitation of research is the homogeneity of the respondents. The Internet has the potential to reduce this problem considerably since respondents with disabilities, or those from different countries and time zones can participate. For example, Thomas, Stamler, Lafreniere, Out, and Delahunt (2002b) were able to compare American and Canadian respondents on several variables. American women reported receiving more nurse encouragement for all three breast health practices (breast self examination, clinical breast examination and mammogram) than did Canadian respondents. This gave rise to discussions about the role of nurses in both countries. Another national difference noted was the rate of breast cancer among the women responding. An unusually low percentage (4%) of Canadian respondents indicated that they had been diagnosed with breast cancer while a higher percentage (18%) of American respondents reported that they had received a breast cancer diagnosis. This difference may be due to more Canadian respondents hearing about the web site through the media, rather than specific web searches for information or support following a diagnosis. Other national differences could also be related to the variation and availability of resources for health education and support in the health care systems of the two countries. Interestingly, many women did not respond to the question, "country of residence" and only 2% of the sample reported residing in a country other than Canada. These women were not included in the further analyses and only those residing in Canada or the United States were considered when national differences were studied.

There were several unanticipated results from this research. As this project was completed several years ago when internet surveys were still quite novel, considerable media attention was garnered. Journalists and talk show hosts completed the survey and encouraged other women to do so. As well, Thomas and her colleagues (2000) found that some women participating in their study provided an unanticipated personal dimension by choosing to advise the researchers of their personal health situations. Sometimes their poignant health care experiences were about the wonderful treatment and support that they or their friends had received while at other times anger and frustration with the fallibility of women's bodies, treatment procedures and lack of support were expressed.

Initially, the survey site invited respondents to email the researchers with comments or questions. Many women did this after completing the survey and the volume of responses swamped the various inboxes of the researchers. To address this issue, these messages were directed to a separate account for this purpose and the researchers could answer them at regular intervals. A common theme from these messages was the desire for more information as well as requests for the "correct" answers to the questions on the survey.

From the great variety of women's stories, the researchers found that they had connected with a broad population of women. Since computer access was generally less available at the time the survey web site was set up and running, some respondents submitted printed surveys by regular mail. Information from these surveys indicated that a spouse or friend had usually printed off the survey and given it to the respondent for completion. Such surveys were not included in the data analysis as one of the purposes of this study was specifically to use the Internet as a research tool.

Lack of computer access and computer skills remains a major limitation of Internet research methodology. Literacy and language fluency are also required for responding to research surveys. As people representing a wider range of income and educational levels have more opportunity for on-line access, this tool will become increasingly effective for research. A guide to some practical issues in using the Internet as a research tool is provided in Table 3.

Table 3. Guide to Practical Issues in Using the Internet as a Research Tool (adapted from Thomas, Stamler, Lafreniere, Dumala, 2000)

- Utilize expertise in designing web site
- Obtain computer expertise to ensure anonymity of respondents and security of data
- Questionnaires should be reasonably brief
- Show approximate time to complete up front
- Include names and credentials of researchers
- Provide opportunity for feedback to be sent to researchers
- Be flexible so that modifications or updating can be made
- Recruit respondents to site by using varied marketing strategies
- Include graphics/visual images to reinforce respondents as they explore site

CONCLUSION

The Internet offers many possibilities as a research tool. As noted above, it has been used to study how and when people search for breast cancer information on the Internet, ways in which support groups assist breast cancer patients and their families, roles for art and aesthetics in breast cancer, ways that the Internet changes the experience of cancer for people and public monitoring of the quality of cancer care. A number of innovative research and educational uses have also been identified along with some practical issues, difficulties and personal experiences.

The Internet may not be the panacea for providing answers to the meaning of Life, the Universe and Everything (Dont Panic - 42 Hitchhikers Facts), but with some guidance, it does enable hitchhikers navigating through the virtual galaxy to obtain relevant breast cancer resources for their particular situations.

REFERENCES

[1] Adams, D., 1979, *The Hitchhiker's Guide to the Galaxy,* Pan Books, London.

[2] Blumenthal, D., 2000, 'Doctors in a Wired World: Can Professionalism Survive Connectivity?' *The Millbank Quarterly*, vol. 80, pp 525-46.

[3] Bruderle, E. and Valiga, T., 1994, 'Integrating the Arts and Humanities into Nursing Education', in P. Chinn and J. Watson, (eds.), *Art and Aesthetics in Nursing*, pp. 117-144, National League for Nursing Press, New York.

[4] Cancer Care Ontario, 2005, Retrieved April 28, 2005 from *<http://www.cancercare.on.ca/qualityindex/>*

[5] Dont Panic - 42 Hitchhikers Facts,, Retrieved April 28, 2005 from *<http://www.sci-find.co.uk/news/news-news91.html>*

[6] Eakin, E. and Strycker, M. 2001, 'Awareness and Use of Cancer Support and Information Resources by HMO Patients with Breast, Prostate, or Colon Cancer: Patient and Provider Perspectives,' *Psycho-Oncology*, vol. 10, pp. 103-13.

[7] Farber, J., Deschamps, M. and Cameron R., 2002, *Investigation and Assessment of the Navigator Role in Meeting the Information, Decisional and Educational Needs of Women with Breast Cancer in Canada*, Canadian Breast Cancer Initiative, Centre for Chronic Disease Prevention and Control, Health Canada. <*http:*//www.hc-sc.gc.ca/pphb-dgspsp/ ccdpc-cpcmc/cancer/publications/navigator_e.html>

[8] Fogel, J., et al, 2002, 'Internet Use and Social Support in Women with Breast Cancer', *Health Psychology*, vol. 21, no.4, pp. 398-404.

[9] Hoffman-Goetz, L. and Clarke, J., 2000, ' Quality of Breast Cancer Sites on the World Wide Web', *Canadian Journal of Public Health*, vol. 91, no.4, pp. 281-84.

[10] Hoshiko, B., 1985, 'Nursing Diagnosis at the Art Museum', *Nursing Outlook*, vol. 33, no.1, pp. 32-36.

[11] Lundin, M., Lundin, J., Helin, H. and Isola, J. 2004, 'A Digital Atlas of Breast Histopathology: An Application of Web Based Virtual Microscopy', *Journal of Clinical Pathology*, vol. 57, no.12, pp. 1288- 91.

[12] National Cancer Institute, 2003, Cancer Facts, Retrieved May 11, 2005, from *<http://cis.nci.nih.gov/fact/2_10.htm>*

[13] Mayer M. and Till, J., 1996, 'The Internet: A Modern Pandora's Box?' *Quality of Life Research*, vol. 5, no. 6, pp. 568- 71.

[14] Mohr, W., 1995, 'Integrating Esthetics into Nursing: Literature as a Suggested Modality', *Archives of Psychiatric Nursing*, vol. 9, no. 6, pp. 365-72.

[15] Robb, A. and Murray, R. 1992, 'Medical Humanities in Nursing: Thought Provoking', *Journal of Advanced Nursing*, vol. 17, pp. 1182-87.

[16] Rozmovits, L. and Ziebland, S., 2004, What do Patients with Prostate or Breast Cancer Want from an Internet Site? A Qualitative Study of Information Needs, *Patient Education and Counseling*, vol. 53, no.1, pp. 57-64.

[17] Roubidoux, M., Chapman, C. and Piontek, 2002, 'Development and Evaluation of an Interactive Web-based Breast Imaging Game for Medical Students', *Academic Radiology*, vol. 9, no. 10, pp. 1169-78.

[18] Santoro, E., 2003, 'Internet and Information on Breast Cancer: An Overview', Breast, vol. 12, no. 6, pp. 424-31.

[19] Satterlund,M., McCaul, K. and Sandgren, A., 2003, 'Information Gathering over Time by Breast Cancer Patients,' *Journal of Medical Internet Research*, vol.5, no. 3 *<http://www.jmir.org/2003/3/e15/>*

[20] Shon, J. and Musen, M., 1999, 'The Low Availability of Metadata Elements for Evaluationg the Quality of Medical Information on the World Wide Web', Proceedings of the American Medical Informatics Association Symposium, pp. 945-49.

[21] Teo, N., Paton,P. and Kettlewell, S., 2005, 'Use of an Interactive Web-based Questionnaire to Evaluate a Breast Cancer Website', *Breast*, vol.14, no.2, pp. 153-56.

[22] Thomas, B., Stamler, L., Lafreniere, K. Dumala, R., 2000, 'The Internet: An Effective Tool for Nursing Research with Women', *Computers in Nursing*, vol. 18, no.1, pp. 13-18.

[23] Thomas, B., Gold/Smith, S., Forrest, A. and Marshall, R., 2002a, 'Web Site Development: Applying Aesthetics to Promote Breast Health Education and awareness', *CIN: Computers, Informatics, Nursing*, vol. 20, no.5, pp. 184-90.

[24] Thomas, B., Stamler, L., Lafreniere, K., Out, J. and Delahunt, T., 2002b, 'Using the Internet: An Effective Tool for Nursing Research with Women', *Women and Health*, vol. 36, no.1, pp. 33-48.

[25] Thomas, B., Marshall, R., Gold/Smith, S. and Forrest, A., 2004, 'Visual Art and Breast Health Promotion: Artists' Perspectives', *Canadian Oncology Nursing Journal*, vol.14, no.4, pp. 233-43.

[26] Till, J., 2003, 'Evaluation of Support Groups for Women with Breast Cancer: Importance of the Navigator Role', *Health and Quality of Life Outcomes*, vol. 1. *<http://www.hqlo.com/content/1/1/16>*

[27] University of Windsor, 2001, Examining Our Breasts, Retrieved April 26, 2005, from *http://www.uwindsor.ca/eob*.

[28] Unruh, H., et al, 2004, Women's Approaches to the Use of New Technology for Cancer risk Information, *Women and Health*, vol. 40, no.1, pp. 59-78.

[29] Weissenberger, C., et al, 2004, Breast Cancer: Patient Information needs reflected in English and German Web Sites, *British Journal of Cancer*, vol. 91, no.8, pp. 1482-87.

[30] Winzelberg, et al, 2003, 'Evaluation of an Internet Support Group for Women with Primary Breast Cancer', *Cancer*, vol. 97, no. 5, pp. 1164-73.

[31] Ziebland, S., 2004, 'The Importance of Being Expert: The Quest for Cancer Information on the Internet', *Social Science and Medicine*, vol. 59, pp. 1783-93.

IN TRYING TO CONCLUDE......

Pranee Liamputtong

With the emergence of the Internet and the advancement of various online technologies, researchers are no longer limited to traditional means of information gathering and data collection.

(Johns et al., 2004: 105)

Engaging in online research is innovative and timely: in responding to the opportunities presented by the information age, electronic research methods will substantially enhance the development of methodologies that relate more closely to the needs of research participants.

(Seymour, 2001: 147-148)

The electronic communication continues to develop, expand and hence Internet communities will also continue to grow (Flicker et al., 2004). Thimbleby (1998: 1) contends, "we could be 'technological determinists'. The technology is amazing (and it certainly is). Therefore, it will do amazing things". In 2004 and 2005, at the time that we are writing our chapters, the advance of on-line communication has allowed such things as e-journals, e-books and virtual lectures, and hence there exists e-authors, e-readers, virtual lectures, and cyber presses. Selwyn and Robson (1998: 4) too suggests that the use of online methodologies in qualitative research (and quantitative research for that matter) is likely to increase in popularity in the near future. Numerous factors need to be brought under consideration if researchers wish to conduct online research. As Illingworth (2001) warns, researching online should not be seen as an easy option, as there are many issues to be carefully considered. And I have clearly laid some of these out through chapters in this book.

In the modern world, all things are in flux. As technology continues to expand and evolve, our research agenda and methodology will inevitably continue to be challenged. Brown (2002: 1), adopting Giddens's theory (1994), explicitly argues that, "as qualitative researchers, we are socially and historically situated agents. What we research, and how we choose to do it are inseparable from the period of reflexive modernity that we inhabit and that period happens to be one of rapid technological change. Technology developments directly impact on what we can achieve with qualitative research as a process". I, too, contend that, as a qualitative researcher, we need to embrace this new way of researching as a challenge. Having said this, I wish to articulate, as Strickland and colleagues (2003: 246) suggest, that "qualitative data collection over the internet needs to remain true to the philosophical stance of the qualitative approach". I will leave this book with what Brown (2002: 11) pleads in his technologically articulated paper that in what ever technological form we choose to conduct our research, "we should not lose sight of the interpretive researcher-led qualities of more traditional forms of qualitative research. Metaphorically, the computer desktop replaces the physical desktop, filing cabinet, and the floor of the researcher's office". Therefore, in conducting cyber research, we need to keep "the research process qualitative in the sense that it remains highly flexible, open-ended, and idiographic in practical application" (Brown 2002: 11).

The rapid advance of technology has great ramifications for us as online qualitative researchers. Online research not only challenges our assumptions of research methodology, but also ethical issues. What we have learnt from being the real world researcher may not be sufficient enough for us to continue our journey in the virtual world. As Flicker et al. (2004: 132) content, "the rapid pace of technological innovation challenges us to constantly reflect on our research practices". We need to continue our online research journeys and write about it; in the same way that all contributors have done in this volume. Only then, novice cyber researchers can learn from our mistakes and rewards. This will inevitably help future cyber researchers to continue a more ethical, practical and sensible research in cyberspace.

Dear All,
We have got to the time that we have to stop writing for this book.
I thank you all for such a wonderful job in writing your chapters.
Without you, it would have been impossible for me to bring this book to life.
But even though we stop for now, I would envisage that all of us will continue to do our research in cyberspace.
Perhaps.
I hope to be in touch with you again soon.
Perhaps.
Another collection!
Bye for now.
Pranee

REFERENCES

Brown, D., 2002, 'Going Digital and Staying Qualitative: Some Alternative Strategies for Digitizing the Qualitative Research Process', *Forum qualitative Social Research*, vol. 3, no. 2. <http://www.qualitative-research.net/fgs/fqs-eng.html>

Flicker, S., Haans, D. and Skinner, H., 2004, 'Ethical Dilemmas in Research on Internet Communities', *Qualitative Health Research*, vol. 14, no. 1, pp. 124-134.

Giddens, A., 1994, *Reflexive Modernisation*, Polity Press, Cambridge.

Illingworth, N., 2001, 'The Internet Matters: Exploring the Use of the Internet as a Research Tool', *Sociological Research Online*, vol. 6, no. 2. *<www.socresonline.org.uk/6/2/illingworth.html>*

Selwyn, N. and Robson, K., 1998, 'Using E-Mail as a Research Tool', Social Research Update 21. *<http://www.soc.surrey.ac.uk/sru/SRU21.html>*

Strickland, O.L., Moloney, M.F., Dietrich, A.S., Myerburg, S., Cotsonis, G.A. and Johnson, R.V., 2003, 'Measurement Issues Related to Data Collection on the World Wide Web', *Advances in Nursing Science*, vol. 26, no. 4, pp. 246-256.

Thimbleby, H., 1998, 'Personal Boundaries/Global Stage', *First Monday: Peer-Reviewed Journal On the Internet. <http://www.firstmonday.dk/issues/issue3_3/thimbleby/index.html>*

CONTRIBUTORS

Yeslem Al-Saggaf is a lecturer in Information Technology, an Associate Course Coordinator for the Master of Information Technology at Charles Sturt University, and a Research Fellow at the Centre for Applied Philosophy and Public Ethics (CAPPE). His PhD, which he received from Charles Sturt University in 2003, was in the area of online communities.

Melissa Altman is studying the process of producing subjectivity in the context of hegemonic discourse at Bowling Green State University. Her other research interests include postcolonial subjectivity, sexuality and desire, and rhetoric of technology and science.

Stephen Bradley is Senior Research Fellow CAMH, at the Department of Nursing, University of Central Lancashire, United Kingdom. Steve practised for over 20 years as a psychiatric nurse, including 8 years working with young people who challenge services. Steve's research is primarily qualitative, particularly taking a social constructionist approach to discourse/narrative inquiry. He teaches child and adolescent mental health issues on a number of courses at the university. He is a reviewer for the Journal of Child Health Care and the Journal of Psychiatric and Mental Health Nursing.

Janne Bromseth is a Ph.D student at Department for Interdisciplinary Studies of Culture, Norwegian University of Science and Technology. She has done research on the situated practises of creating community in mediated discussion groups within Nordic cultural contexts since 1997, and with ethical issues related to doing research online in particular. Her forthcoming dissertation focusses on social constructions of gender, sexuality and identity within Nordic queer online communities. The project is a part of the research-group 'When heterosexuality must explain itself', focussing on productions of heteronormativity through research and joint popular publications (see *http://www.hf.ntnu.no/hf/tverrfaglig/forskning/forskningsgrupper/kjonn/hetero-eng*).

Bernie Carter is Professor of Children's Nursing/Associate Head for Research and Development, Clinical Practice Research Unit, Department of Nursing, University of Central Lancashire, United Kingdom. Her clinical practice focused on children's surgery, and children's and neonatal intensive care prior to her moving into teaching and research. Bernie's current research is primarily qualitative and more specifically narrative in its approach. It covers three main areas (1) the impact of pain and chronicity on the lives of children/young people, (2) children's perspectives on the way that health care professionals interact with them, (3) multi-agency working practice with children with complex needs. She utilises a range of data generation techniques consonant with children's ways of expression including visual art based techniques, video and photography as well as interviews and focus groups. She is the Editor for the Journal of Child Health Care.

Wonshik Chee is Assistant professor of the University of Texas at San Antonio. He received his PhD in mechanical engineering from the University of California at Berkeley in 1997 and did his postdoctoral fellowship at the same institution. His expertise is control algorithm development including fuzzy logic control and Internet web programming, and his previous industrial and academic experiences were closely related to development of adaptive robust control systems for various mechatronic systems and Internet web programming in research projects. He has published widely in engineering journals and health-related journals.

Antoinette H. Cotton is a registered nurse and certified midwife currently employed as a lecturer at the School of Nursing, Family and Community Health, University of Western Sydney, Australia. Antoinette has research interests in critical thinking, critical reflective practice, global health, health care and education, as well as issues related to new technologies in health research. Antoinette's published works in refereed journals including: Clinical Nurse Specialist, Journal of Advanced Nursing, and Contemporary Nurse. Antoinette has also published articles relating to Internet and Web-based research in Contemporary Nurse, and Advances in Nursing Science.

Danielle Couch is a master student in the School of Public Health, La Trobe University, Australia. Danielle has worked broadly across the community, cultural, health and technology sectors in program development and communications. Her experiences working with an online community during the tech bubble fostered an ongoing interest in all things online, with a particular interest in why and how people choose to develop and maintain online relationships in their various forms.

Radhika Gajjala is Associate Professor in interpersonal communication/communication studies at Bowling Green State University, Ohio. She teaches courses on cyber culture, humanistic research methods, performing digitally mediated identities and feminist research methods in communication. Her research interests include new media technologies, critical theory, feminist theory, transnational communication, and postcolonial theory. She has been a member of the Spoon Collective for 10 years now and has founded and moderated several online lists related to gender and postcolonial theory. Since 1997 she has also been collaborating-both through Internet dialogue and through engagement in the field, with NGO fieldworkers examining alternative developmental models in order to benefit handloom weavers in South India. Her book "Cyberselves: Feminist Ethnographies of South Asian Women" was recently published by Altamira Press.

James Gillett is Assistant Professor jointly appointed in the Sociology Department and the Health Studies Programme at McMaster University in Hamilton, Ontario, Canada. His current research interests are in the cultural representations of health and illness and the approaches that people take toward their health and health care.

Michael Hardey is a Reader in Sociology at HYMS (Hull and York Medical School) and CASS (Department of Comparative and Applied Social Sciences, University of Hull). He has written extensively about the role of ICTS and mediated social relationships. This research has involved an engagement with ehealth, edating and eculture. In all these spheres, he has been concerned to develop theoretically innovative material that will help inform our understanding of life in the networked society. Readers can find his papers in journals including, Information, Communication and Society, Health, Sociology of Health and Illness, Sociales and Santé and Sociological Review.

Richard Hessler joined the University of Missouri faculty in 1971 and currently is Professor of Sociology there. His research includes several methodological studies, including an evaluation of consumer involvement in the research decision-making process. Most recently, he has conducted longitudinal studies on aging and longevity. Awards include The Distinguished Teaching Award, School of Medicine, Blue Chalk Award, College of Arts and Science, and a Fulbright Scholarship to Sweden.

Bibi Hølge-Hazelton is a senior researcher at the research unit of general practice in Copenhagen and Associate Professor at Learning Lab Denmark. She has an interest in gender, youth and health research and is currently occupied with developing transgressive qualitative methods including internet based and creative approaches.

Eun-Ok Im is Associate professor of the University of Texas at Austin. She received her PhD in nursing from the University of California, San Francisco in 1997, and had postdoctoral experience at the same institution. Her expertise is international cross-cultural women's health issues including menopause, cancer pain, and breast cancer. She has conducted nine studies on international cross-cultural women's health issues from a feminist perspective, and authored more than 40 articles published or accepted for publication in refereed journals. She is currently conducting three Internet studies that were funded by the National Institute of Health, the Oncology Nursing Foundation, and the Center for Health Promotion and Disease Prevention of The University of Texas at Austin.

Radwan Kharabsheh is a lecturer in International Business at the School of Commerce, Charles Sturt University. His research interests include organisational learning, international strategy and the South East Asia. His PhD, from Charles Sturt University, was on learning success in international joint ventures in Malaysia.

Pranee Liamputtong holds a position as Personal Chair in Public Health (a full professor) at the School of Public Health, La Trobe University, Melbourne, Australia. Pranee has previously taught in the School of Sociology and Anthropology and worked as a public health research fellow at the Centre for the Study of Mothers' and Children's Health, La Trobe University. Pranee has her particular interests on issues related to cultural and social influences on childbearing, childrearing and women's reproductive and sexual health. Pranee has published several books and a large number of papers in these areas. Her recent research method book is titled *Qualitative Research Methods, 2nd edition* (2005). She is now completing a book on *Researching the "Vulnerable"* for Sage in London. Pranee's new focus is on alternative methodology in research including the use of Internet and art-based methods in qualitative research.

Anthony P. Lombardo is a doctoral student in the Health and Behavioural Sciences program, Department of Public Health Sciences, Faculty of Medicine, University of Toronto, in Toronto, Ontario, Canada. He is the recipient of a Canada Graduate Scholarships Doctoral Scholarship, and his doctoral research will focus on aspects of health promotion and behaviour related to HIV/AIDS. His paper "(Web)Sites of Governmentality: Neo-Liberalism, the Internet and HIV/AIDS" was awarded best student paper in the 2003 Martin Levine Student Essay Competition of the Sociologists' AIDS Network. Anthony has also published in Symbolic Interaction.

Cindy Mendelson is Assistant Professor of Nursing at the University of New Mexico in the United States. She has baccalaureate degrees in both anthropology and nursing, a Master's degree in anthropology and her doctorate is in Nursing. She combines her interests in nursing and anthropology in her research of women's experiences in health and illness using an ethnographic approach. Her current work explores how women with lupus manage symptoms in the context of daily life experiences. As part of this program of research she has conducted studies of how women seek and provide support on internet communities, and is interested in the application of ethnographic forms of exploration of the formation of community on internet self-help sites.

Monika Merkes lives in Melbourne, Australia. Her research interests include social policy, online qualitative research, futures studies, e-democracy, and how new technologies affect our lives. She has published on these topics in peer reviewed journals and in online magazines and journals. In 2004, she completed a PhD at the School of Public Health, La Trobe University, Australia. Thesis topic: A longer working life for Australian women of the baby boom generation? - Women's voices and the social policy implications of an ageing female workforce. Monika works in local government in a social policy role.

Brian Mustanski has a doctorate in Clinical Psychology from Indiana University. He has conducted a number of Internet based studies focusing on various aspects of sexual health, including HIV/AIDS risk behaviors and sexual orientation. His study on how gay and lesbian college students define "having sex" was the first online study to receive IRB approval at Indiana University. His most recent study was an online daily diary investigation of the relationship between mood and sexual interest, behavior, and risk-taking. He has research interests in human sexuality, research and quantitative methodology, and behavior genetics.

Monique Solomon is a PhD student at the University of Calgary, Faculty of Communication and Culture. Her doctoral research is in e-health communication, specifically the impact of information communication technology on health care practices and applications. She received her Masters in Communication Studies from the University of Calgary and Bachelor of Arts in Psychology from the University of Victoria. As a Communications Consultant she has extensive professional experience in communications, media and marketing - particularly with health care organizations. As an Instructor at the University of Calgary she teaches professional and technical communication and is developing a course in e-health communication.

Barbara Thomas is Emerita Professor, in the Faculty of Nursing, University of Windsor, Windsor, Canada. She has taught undergraduate and graduate courses in health promotion and women's health issues. Her research interests are in the areas of health promotion and women's health, specifically breast health. She has used the Internet for both qualitative and quantitative research. Her publications can be found in a variety of national and international journals. Recently, she has done consulting in program evaluation and graduate education.

INDEX

A

F

G

J

K

L

M

Q

Y